D1258955

Pagliaros' COMPREHENSIVE GUIDE TO DRUGS AND SUBSTANCES OF ABUSE

Second Edition

Pagliaros' COMPREHENSIVE GUIDE TO DRUGS AND SUBSTANCES OF ABUSE

Second Edition

Louis A. Pagliaro, RPsych, MS, PharmD, PhD, FABMP, FPPR
Professor Emeritus and Former Professor of Pharmacopsychology
and Former Professor of Pharmacy and Pharmaceutical Sciences

and

Ann Marie Pagliaro, RN, BSN, MSN, PhD Candidate, FPPR
Professor Emeritus and Former Professor of Nursing and
Director, Substance Abusology and Clinical Pharmacology
Research Group

University of Alberta

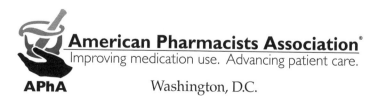
American Pharmacists Association®
Improving medication use. Advancing patient care.
APhA

Washington, D.C.

Editor: Nancy Tarleton Landis
Acquiring Editor: Sandra J. Cannon
Layout and Graphics: Michele A. Danoff, Graphics By Design
Cover Design: Mariam Safi, APhA Creative Services
Proofreading: Kathleen K. Wolter
Indexing: Louis A. Pagliaro

© 2009 by Louis A. Pagliaro and Ann Marie Pagliaro

Published by the American Pharmacists Association
2215 Constitution Avenue, N.W.
Washington, DC 20037-2985

APhA was founded in 1852 as the American Pharmaceutical Association.

To comment on this book via e-mail, send your message to the publisher at
aphabooks@aphanet.org.

Library of Congress Cataloging-in-Publication Data

Pagliaro, Louis A.
  Pagliaros' comprehensive guide to drugs and substances of abuse /
Louis A. Pagliaro and Ann Marie Pagliaro. -- 2nd ed.
    p. ; cm.
  Includes bibliographical references and index.
  ISBN 978-1-58212-131-4
  1. Drugs of abuse--Handbooks, manuals, etc. 2. Substance
abuse--Handbooks, manuals, etc. I. Pagliaro, Ann M. II. Title. III.
Title: Comprehensive guide to drugs and substances of abuse.
  [DNLM: 1. Substance-Related Disorders. 2. Psychotropic Drugs. WM
270 P1384p 2009]

  RM316.P34 2009
  615'.78--dc22
                                    2009010388

How to Order This Book

Online: www.pharmacist.com
By phone: 800-878-0729 (770-280-0085 from outside the United States)
VISA®, MasterCard®, and American Express® cards accepted

This text is dedicated to *all* who are suffering, or who have suffered,
as a result of the use of drugs and substances of abuse,
with the fervent hope that those who read this text will,
through understanding and applying the information presented,
help to alleviate their suffering.

Contents

List of Monographs

on Drugs and Substances of Abuse

Preface

to the Second Edition

Life, as we find it, is too hard for us; it brings us too many pains, disappointments, and impossible tasks. In order to bear it we cannot dispense with palliative measures.... There are perhaps three such measures: powerful deflections,[1] which cause us to make light of our misery; substitutive satisfactions,[2] which diminish it; and intoxicating substances,[3] which make us insensitive to it.

Sigmund Freud (1856–1939), Civilization and Its Discontents, *1931*

During the 5 years since the first edition of this text was published, the personal use of the drugs and substances of abuse has continued virtually unabated across North America, particularly among adolescents and young adults. In addition, new patterns of drug and substance use have been noted among several recent immigrant groups, particularly those who use the drugs and substances of abuse for ethno-medical or traditional healing (e.g., *Salvia divinorum*), for magico-religious ceremonies (e.g., *Ayahuasca*), or for socialization (e.g., *Catha edulis*). These drugs and substances of abuse also are being used in nontraditional ways by other North Americans, both adolescents and adults of both genders.

The adverse consequences of drug and substance use are myriad and are frequently noted by many segments of society. For example, parents at home and teachers in schools commonly observe behavioral problems related to drug and substance abuse among children and adolescents (e.g., methamphetamine-related aggression, cannabis-related learning disorders, fetal alcohol syndrome). Health care professionals in many settings are confronted on a daily basis with related disorders. Examples include methamphetamine-related dental caries and tooth loss, referred to as "meth mouth, in dental clinics; cocaine-induced psychosis in hospitals; heroin overdosages in emergency rooms; and the use of oxazepam for behavior management of residents in extended care facilities, especially at night, for the purpose of lowering staff ratios. Social care professionals increasingly observe the harmful effects of drug and substance use among the homeless, including mental and physical health problems (e.g., alcohol-induced Wernicke-Korsakoff syndrome and cirrhosis of the liver); in crisis centers (e.g., gamma-hydroxybutyrate-facilitated date rape); and in women's shelters (e.g., alcohol-related spousal abuse).

Law enforcement professionals see firsthand the results of drug and substance use on the streets, including violent drug-related crimes such as home invasions of marijuana "grow ops" and drive-by shootings and murders of rival gang members over "drug turf." Corrections officers also see the results (e.g., drug-related crime and commerce within jails and prisons). In courtrooms, judges, juries, and lawyers have front row seats for countless cases of drug-facilitated crimes of assault, vehicular manslaughter, and homicide associated with alcohol, amphetamine, cocaine, methamphetamine, and phencyclidine use.

In today's troubling and volatile context of drug and substance use, the basic purpose of this text has remained constant: to collect, analyze, and critique available published drug- and substance-use data and, through a process of careful and thorough reflective synthesis, to present a timely, authoritative, and scholarly reference on the individual drugs and substances of abuse and their pharmacology and patterns of use in North America. In addition, in response to requests by readers of the first edition of this text, we have made some significant changes to the second edition while preserving the first edition's well-received and useful features and format. To maintain a text of reasonable length and to facilitate readers' retrieval of desired information, we have eliminated the first edition's chapters on each of the three major classes of drugs and substances of abuse (the psychodepressants, the psychostimulants, and the psychodelics.[4,5] In this second edition, pertinent data have been updated and included in the respective drug monographs. Each monograph from the first edition has been thoroughly and extensively reviewed and revised as needed to ensure that the data are current and comprehensive. Finally, about a dozen new monographs have been added, reflecting new directions in North American drug and substance use.

Monographs

The text consists of monographs on more than 100 drugs and substances of abuse that are generally available in North America. The monographs are arranged in alphabetical order by generic or common name to facilitate rapid location and retrieval of data. Each monograph contains, when available, the following information: (1) name(s) of the drug or substance of abuse, including BAN and INN generic synonym(s) and brand or trade, chemical, and street name(s); (2) pharmacologic classification (see Appendix A); (3) a brief general overview of the drug or substance of abuse and its current availability; (4) dosage form(s) and route(s) of administration, including current patterns of use; (5) the purported mechanism of psychodepressant, psychostimulant, or psychodelic action; (6) pharmacodynamics (i.e., the time relationship between drug concentration and drug effect[s]) and pharmacokinetics (i.e., the mathematical modeling of the processes of drug absorption, distribution, metabolism, and excretion); (7) current approved indications for medical use and desired action or reason for personal use (i.e., why people choose to use or abuse a particular drug or substance of abuse, including ethno-medical use and magico-religious or ceremonial use); (8) basic toxicology, including associated acute and chronic adverse drug reactions, teratogenic and fetotoxic potential, and effects of maternal use on lactation and breast-fed neonates and infants; (9) physical and psychological abuse potentials[6]; (10) withdrawal syndrome; and (11) signs and symptoms of overdosage and its basic management (e.g., availability of specific antidotes). At the end of each monograph are notes providing further explanation of points discussed, as well as a list of current references that substantiate and support the data and offer additional information sources for interested readers.

Like the first edition, this text deliberately does not include dosages or prices for the drugs and substances of abuse.

Dosages. The omission of dosages and dosage ranges was not an oversight, nor was it related to any trepidation on our part—we have provided specific dosage guidelines and recommendations in the dozen clinical pharmacology texts that we have authored or co-edited for health care providers during the past 35 years. Our reason for not including dosages in this text is our respect for science and dosology. Sound dosage recommendations based on population data reflect a profound appreciation of individual variability and factors that contribute to it, such as maturation of body organs (e.g., in infants and children versus adults or elderly adults; gender; race, including genotype; and organ function, including hepatic and renal function).

In regard to drugs and substances of abuse, population data (or estimates thereof, generally obtained from large-scale clinical studies for the determination of safe and efficacious drug use) do not exist. All we have are case reports from the literature and from our own patient and research files. Further confounding this issue is the appreciation that drugs and substances of abuse that are illicitly produced and sold have no guarantee as to quality control in the manufacturing and labeling (i.e., packaging) processes. Thus, for example, the white tablet with a cartoon character embossed on it—even if it is the same drug or substance of abuse supplied by the same street drug dealer—may contain 50 mcg today, 55 mcg tomorrow, and 100 mcg 2 weeks from now. It also may contain various byproducts of chemical synthesis or a deliberate adulterant ("cut"). Thus, we have no established baseline from which to begin to generate valid and reliable dosage guidelines.[7]

In addition, even if dosage guidelines were available (e.g., for the licit and prescribed drugs of abuse and those that are illicitly obtained by diversion from hospitals, nursing homes, and pharmacies or purchased from easily accessed Internet sites, such as hydrocodone and oxymorphone), the endpoint is subjective and not easily measurable. Thus, how much of drug or substance X it will take to achieve the desired result of euphoria, or getting "high," will differ significantly among users.[8]

Prices. As with dosages, anecdotal data as well as DEA averages for various districts and regions are available on the street price of many of the drugs and substances of abuse. However, these data are not generalizable, nor are they consistent over time. Thus, they can be extremely misleading. Being subject to the controlling economic pressures of supply and demand in a totally unregulated and now global market, prices for the drugs and substances of abuse are subject to extreme variation.[9] In addition, as with other commodities, such as gasoline, the price can vary significantly on the same day and at the same time in different cities (e.g., Denver versus Honolulu). Furthermore, prices vary dramatically depending upon criminal connections and the quantity purchased. For example, the cost of BC Bud is significantly higher in Los Angeles and higher still in New York City than it is in Victoria or Vancouver, British Columbia. Also, cost often includes bartering for commodities in lieu of cash. For example, for BC Bud, transnational, large-scale trafficking deals commonly involve hand guns and other weapons or cocaine. Similarly, at the street level, sexual favors are often exchanged for a desired drug or substance of abuse (e.g., crack cocaine). In light of these confounding variables, we decided not to include reported street prices in the monographs on drugs and substances of abuse.

Appendices

Three appendices are included to facilitate the use of this text. Appendix A classifies the drugs and substances of abuse into three main categories: the psychodepressants, the psychostimulants, and the psychedelics. This taxonomy lists and places in a relational context, with subclassifications, all of the various drugs and substances of abuse included in the text. Appendix B lists and defines the FDA pregnancy categories, which are referred to in the monographs in regard to potential teratogenic effects when the drug or substance is used by adolescent girls or women who are pregnant or who may become pregnant. Appendix C defines the abbreviations used in this text.

Indices

This text contains two comprehensive indices. The subject index lists major topics and subtopics. The drug name index is an alphabetical list of generic names and virtually every brand/trade and street name commonly used for the drugs and substances of abuse in North America; it enables the reader who knows only a street name to identify and find information about the specific drug or substance of abuse.

We trust that readers will find this edition to be a user-friendly, practical, and comprehensive aid to quickly finding needed information concerning the drugs and substances of abuse. Furthermore, we trust that readers using the monographs will find them to be both informative (i.e., well supported by valid and reliable data) and, as shared with us by many readers of the first edition, "an interesting read."

LAP/AMP, 2009

Notes

1. Religion can be considered to be a "powerful deflection" in this context. For example, current suffering on earth is later rewarded in heaven.
2. Economic prosperity can be considered to be a "substitutive satisfaction" in this context. For example, the ability to purchase valued material possessions (e.g., luxury jewelry and automobiles; season tickets to the opera or professional sporting events) may assuage disappointment in a relationship or employment situation.
3. The drugs and substances of abuse are the "intoxicating substances" and, of all three palliative measures, are the most readily available to virtually everyone (i.e., people may not be religious and they may not be rich, but they can always avail themselves of a drug or substance of abuse).
4. Our use of the term "psychodelics" is explained in Appendix A.
5. Readers are referred to the first edition for additional background information on the following: general pharmacology of the drugs and substances of abuse; history of the drugs and substances of abuse; the Meta-Interactive Model of Drugs and Substances of Abuse; explanatory theories of drug and substance use; and general approaches to the treatment and management of substance use disorders.
6. That is, the potential of the drug or substance of abuse to produce physical or psychological dependence, or both. *Physical dependence* may occur when a drug or substance of abuse is regularly used over a prolonged period (i.e., weeks to months). This form of dependence is also referred to as *addiction*, which by definition requires the existence of two criteria: (1) tolerance—the need for an increasingly higher dosage in order to achieve the initial desired actions, and (2) the occurrence of a specific physically mediated (i.e., not mentally or psychologically mediated) withdrawal syndrome that occurs when the drug or substance of abuse is abruptly discontinued after regular long-term use and that is immediately alleviated by its resumed use. *Psychological dependence* may occur when a drug or substance of abuse is regularly used over a prolonged period (i.e., weeks to months). In this situation, users generally describe having a "craving" for the drug or substance of abuse and may come to feel "compelled" to use it (i.e., "loss of control"). By these definitions, cocaine, for example, is not physically addictive (i.e., use is not generally associated with physical dependence) because when

regular long-term use is abruptly discontinued, its associated withdrawal syndrome (i.e., "cocaine blues") cannot be alleviated by resumed use of cocaine. In this example, the user must wait until depleted dopamine levels are replenished in the brain (see Cocaine monograph). Obviously, not all drugs and substances of abuse are associated with physical dependence. However, all are associated with psychological dependence. Thus, although some of the drugs and substances of abuse may not cause physical dependence or *addiction*, they are included in this text because they may cause psychological dependence.

7. In this regard, we considered including dosage ranges, which could be provided for some of the pharmaceutically manufactured drugs and substances of abuse (e.g., alcohol, diazepam, morphine) for which pharmaceutical quality control issues are not significant. However, we decided against the inclusion of dosage ranges for this edition because illicit users generally do not follow published pharmaceutical guidelines in regard to dosage and method of administration. For example, a current pattern of use by adolescents and young adults is the combination use of crushed acetaminophen, diphenhydramine, and heroin, called "Cheese," which is sniffed intranasally (see the Diphenhydramine and Heroin monographs). Another pattern of use by adolescents and young adults is "pharming," in which combinations of drugs found in a family medicine cabinet are used without attention to dosage (see the Codeine and Diphenhydramine monographs).

8. This difference (i.e., intersubject variability) depends on the drug, the "set" (i.e., the highly individualized perception/definition of exactly what mental state defines being euphoric or "high," and past individual experiences with the particular drug or substance of abuse), and the setting (i.e., the environment of drug use). All three factors play a significant role.

9. These prices have significantly greater volatility than did the cost of a barrel of oil in 2008!

Preface

to the First Edition

If we could sniff or swallow something that would, for five or six hours each day, abolish our solitude as individuals, atone us with our fellows in a glowing exaltation of affection and make life in all its aspects seem not only worth living, but divinely beautiful and significant, and if this heavenly, world-transfiguring drug were of such a kind that we could wake up next morning with a clear head and an undamaged constitution—then, it seems to me, all our problems (and not merely the one small problem of discovering a novel pleasure) would be wholly solved and earth would become paradise.

Aldous Huxley (1894–1963), Brave New World, *1949*

We are in a time of significant economic, political, and social change. The attendant changes—including changes in family structures; reorientation of cultural, ethnic, and religious dominance and practices; globalization; and increasing adoption of pragmatic ethical and moral orientations—are all significantly affecting the professional and personal lives of each and every member of our society. Although health care professionals are acutely aware of these issues (often having to deal with them on a daily basis in their clinical practices), most seem oblivious to the fact that the use of drugs and substances of abuse has become ubiquitous in our society and presently is at an all time high. More than 50 years after Huxley's observation, new generations—of youth, in particular—seem to have vigorously renewed the quest to find an artificial paradise through the use of various drugs and substances of abuse. Basic core issues such as the ethics of drug and substance use and the decriminalization or legalization of drugs and substances of abuse have gained their own momentum for development, generally with little input from health care professionals. As the harmful effects of drug and substance use and its associated culture (e.g., family violence, fetal alcohol syndrome, gang violence, HIV infection, lung cancer, prostitution) draw heavily on health care dollars and take their daily toll on the overall personal and social well-being of our society, there is now an urgent need for these issues to be expediently and adequately addressed by health care professionals from all disciplines.

Naturally, some health care professionals, being content with the status quo or fearful of change, may wish that things just be left alone and remain as they are—or, perhaps more accurately, as they think they are. However, this wish cannot be granted—even if wish granting were possible—because, as noted by G. K. Chesterton, "If you leave a thing alone, you leave it to a torrent of change" (Orthodoxy, 1908). Thus, our only logical alternative is to become involved in the changes, to view change not as a threat but as an opportunity to broaden the positive impact that health care professionals have on the health and well-being of people who need their professional services—now more than ever.

Certainly, the optimal practice of virtually every health care professional—dentist, nurse, pharmacist, physician, psychologist, social worker—requires, if not detailed expertise in the area of drug and substance abuse, then, at a minimum, a substantial amount of specialized knowledge about the propensity of the drugs and substances of abuse to affect behavior, cognition, learning, memory, and thus virtually every other aspect of mental and physical health. This knowledge is essential in order for health professionals to be able to meet more competently and comprehensively the needs of their patients, many of whom will be using (or will have used) a drug or substance of abuse. For example, even the best nurse, physician, or psychologist in the world would more than likely be unsuccessful in the treatment of clinical depression if he or she did not know that the clinical depression was a direct result of the chronic use of a benzodiazepine (e.g., diazepam [Valium®], lorazepam [Ativan®], triazolam [Halcion®]) and did not recognize the adverse drug reaction (i.e., depression). The best psychologist or social worker in the world would more than likely be unsuccessful in helping a client to deal with financial difficulties or find and maintain gainful employment if the professional did not understand that the problem arose from the client's dependence on a particular drug or substance of abuse (e.g., alcohol, cocaine, heroin) and the amount of money needed to maintain this dependence.

To stem the increase in "double-doctoring" (i.e., obtaining prescriptions for the same complaint or disorder from more than one legitimate prescriber), physicians and other prescribers need to be aware of the abuse potential, signs and symptoms of intoxication, and current street (illicit) use patterns of the drugs they are prescribing. This same information is important for dispensing pharmacists to have. In order for drug information center and emergency department professionals to optimally triage reported cases of accidental ingestion (e.g., by children) and unintentional overdosage (i.e., by "users") of drugs and substances of abuse, information about the signs and symptoms of overdosages and related clinical sequelae is necessary.

In addition, to appropriately anticipate and respond to drug and substance abuse withdrawal syndromes, health care providers such as those working in addiction detoxification units, drug treatment settings, emergency departments, and intensive care units need to know the signs and symptoms and severity of the withdrawal syndromes. To suggest appropriate treatment options for patients, or the parents of pediatric patients, who are abusing drugs and substances of abuse, health care professionals need accurate information on physical dependence, psychological dependence, and withdrawal syndromes. For mental health care specialists (e.g., mental health nurses, psychiatrists, psychologists) to know whether the signs and symptoms they have observed in their patients (e.g., delusions, hallucinations) can be related to use of an abusable drug or substance, they need to have ready access to data on these drugs and substances (many of which are illicit and therefore not discussed in readily available standard pharmacopoeias or therapeutics texts). All health care providers need to know what specific drug or substance of abuse their patients are referring to when the user knows only the common "street name."

The purpose of this text is to present to the general health care professional a timely, authoritative, scholarly, referenced compilation and analysis of available data concerning the status, trends, and individual pharmacology of drug and substance abuse in North America. The text is designed to assist the health care provider in both learning more about the drugs and substances of abuse and retrieving required information quickly. It begins with an introduction to the issue of drug and substance abuse, followed by two major parts. Part I contains three chapters. Chapter 1, The Psychodepressants, provides an overview of the history and pharmacology of the opiates, sedative-hypnotics (including alcohol), and volatile solvents and inhalants. Chapter 2, The Psychostimulants, provides an overview of the history and pharmacology of the amphetamines and related drugs and substances, including caffeine, cocaine, and nicotine. Chapter 3, The Psychodelics, provides an overview of the history of cannabis in its various forms (e.g., marijuana, hashish, and hashish oil); the phenethylamines or "amphetamine-like psychodelics" (e.g., 3,4-methylenedioxyamphetamine [MDA]; 3,4-methylenedioxyethylamphetamine [MDE]; and 3,4-methylenedioxymethamphetamine [MDMA]); and the indoles, including lysergic acid amide (LSA), lysergic acid diethylamide (LSD), mescaline (peyote), and psilocin and psilocybin.

Part II contains individual monographs on more than 100 drugs and substances of abuse that are generally available in North America. The monographs are arranged in alphabetical order by generic or common name to facilitate rapid location and retrieval of necessary data. Each monograph contains, when available, the following information: name(s) of the drug or substance of abuse, including BAN and INN generic synonym(s), brand or trade name(s), and street name(s); pharmacologic classification; a brief overview of the drug or substance of abuse, including its availability and use patterns (current and historical); available dosage form(s) and route(s) of administration; the purported mechanism of psychodepressant, psychostimulant, or psychodelic action; pharmacodynamics and pharmacokinetics; current approved indications for medical use; desired action or reason for personal use (i.e., why people choose to use and abuse a particular drug or substance); basic toxicology, including associated acute and chronic adverse drug reactions, teratogenic and fetotoxic potential, and effects of maternal use on lactation and breast-fed neonates and infants; abuse potential; withdrawal syndrome; and overdosage, including signs and symptoms and its basic treatment. Each monograph concludes with a list of references that were of assistance in the preparation of the monograph and can be consulted by interested readers for additional information.

Years ago, in commenting on the ultimate consequences of drug and substance abuse for both the individual user and the society of which that individual is a member, we noted that "Drug and substance abuse kills the heart and murders the soul." Today, it is our fervent wish that, given the data regarding drug and substance abuse presented in this text, health care professionals will be better able to *heal* the heart and *enliven* the soul, making well those whose lives are adversely affected by drug and substance abuse.

LAP/AMP, 2004

Acknowledgments

The authors wish to acknowledge and thank Julian Graubart, APhA Senior Director, Books and Electronic Products, for his continuing faith in our ability to write and deliver high-quality manuscripts; Sandy Cannon, APhA acquisitions editor, for her assistance throughout this project; and Nancy Landis, copy editor, for her diligence and constructive feedback from start to finish.

In addition, we would like to express our sincere gratitude to our patients and students, both undergraduate and graduate, who, over the past 35 years, have helped us to learn more about and understand better the drugs and substances of abuse.

Monographs

ACETONE

Names

BAN or INN Generic Synonyms: Dimethyl ketone

Brand/Trade: Generally available by generic name

Chemical: 2-Propanone

Street: Nail Polish Remover; Sniff

Pharmacologic Classification

Psychodepressant, volatile solvents & inhalants: volatile solvent (ketone)

Brief General Overview

Acetone is a colorless, flammable, volatile liquid that is commercially produced and is usually used as a solvent for the removal of nail polish. The use of acetone as an *inhalant* is primarily observed in children and is most often limited to one-time experimental use at the encouragement of a friend (i.e., playmate, schoolmate) or older sibling. A noted exception to this usual pattern of use involves the widespread chronic use of acetone as an inhalant, and other volatile solvents (see Volatile Solvents & Inhalants monograph), by Canadian Aboriginal and Native American children and adolescents, particularly those who reside on Indian reserves and reservations where there are high levels of poverty.[1]

Dosage Forms and Routes of Administration

Acetone is chemically synthesized and made commercially available to the public in a variety of liquid products that contain acetone alone or as one of several ingredients (e.g., fingernail polish remover such as Cutex®). Acetone is generally self-administered either by directly inhaling the acetone fumes from the product container or by pouring the acetone onto a rag and inhaling the fumes while the rag is held over the nose and mouth.[2] The liquid product is often heated (e.g., over a car radiator, furnace radiator, or stovetop) to increase volatility and thus enhance pulmonary availability and absorption. This method of use has often resulted in combustion of the flammable liquid product and burns to the face, head, and hands of the user.

Mechanism of CNS Action

Acetone causes a dose-related depression of the brain and spinal cord similar to that observed with various other psychodepressants. However, the exact mechanism of action has not been determined. See the Volatile Solvents & Inhalants monograph.

Pharmacodynamics/Pharmacokinetics

In cases of acetone poisoning, the elimination half-life for acetone has been reported to be ~24 hours. Additional valid and reliable data are not available.

Current Approved Indications for Medical Use

None[3]

Desired Action/Reason for Personal Use

Alcohol-like disinhibitory euphoria or "high"; sensory distortions

Toxicity

Acute: Cognitive impairment; dizziness; drowsiness; eye irritation (chemical burns); headache; impaired judgment; muscle weakness; nausea; psychomotor impairment; pulmonary irritation; vomiting

Chronic: Cough; mental depression; memory impairment; respiratory impairment[4]; thirst (persistent)

Pregnancy & Lactation: Data on the effects of acetone inhalation by adolescent girls and women who are pregnant or breast-feeding are not generally available. Studies of female laboratory personnel exposed during pregnancy to various organic solvents, including acetone, have indicated a significant reduction in their ability to produce offspring (i.e., fecundability ratios). On the basis of these studies, and to err on the side of safety, adolescent girls and women who are pregnant or breast-feeding should avoid inhaling acetone. Additional valid and reliable data are needed.

Abuse Potential

Physical dependence: None (USDEA: not a scheduled drug)
Psychological dependence: Low to moderate

Withdrawal Syndrome

An acetone withdrawal syndrome associated with regular, long-term use has not been substantiated. If it does exist, it probably is relatively mild.

Overdosage

Published data on the medical management of overdosage related to acetone abuse are unavailable. After users who have overdosed have been removed from the source of acetone, including acetone on clothing, and provided with adequate ventilation, they should be carefully monitored and symptomatically managed for at least 2 days.

Notes

1. Gasoline is by far the most commonly abused volatile solvent among Native American children and adolescents (see Gasoline monograph for additional information).
2. A variation of this method of use involves placing the acetone-soaked rag in a plastic sandwich bag and then inhaling the acetone fumes while the bag is held tightly over the nose and mouth.
3. Acetone occasionally has been used as a topical preparation for cleansing skin sites before application of adhesive leads for electrocardiography.
4. The inhalation of acetone fumes has been specifically linked to damage of the mucous membranes that line the respiratory tract. This pulmonary damage is a direct consequence of its irritant effects.

References

Arts, J.H., Mojet, J., van Gemert, L.J., et al. (2002). An analysis of human response to the irritancy of acetone vapors. Critical Reviews in Toxicology, 32(1), 43-66.

Jones, W. (2000). Elimination half-life of acetone in humans: Case reports and review of the literature. Journal of Analytical Toxicology, 24(1), 8-10.

Noraberg, J., & Arlien-Soborg, P. (2000). Neurotoxic interactions of industrially used ketones. Neurotoxicology, 21(3), 409-418.

Wennborg, H., Bodin, L., Vainio, H., et al. (2001). Solvent use and time to pregnancy among female personnel in biomedical laboratories in Sweden. *Occupational and Environmental Medicine, 58*(4), 225-231.

ALCOHOL

Names

BAN or INN Generic Synonyms: Ethanol

Brand/Trade: Available in various concentrations as beer, wine, and distilled spirits or as a component of office and household products (e.g., cleaning products [Lysol® spray]; and personal hygiene products [Listerine® mouthwash; Mennen® aftershave])

Chemical: Ethyl alcohol

Street: Ale; Amber Brew; Angel's Food; Aperitif; Barley Broth; Beggar Boy's Ass; Beverage; Bevvie; Bitch Piss; Booze; Bottle; Brew; Brewskeez; Brewskis; Cold One; Cordials; Courage in a Bottle; Daddy's Juice; Daddy's Soda; Daily Mail; Diddle; Drink; Fire Water; Grandpa's Cough Syrup; Grog; Hard Stuff; Hooch; Juice; Knock-me-down; Likker; Liquid Courage; Liquor; Malt; Moonshine; Night-cap; Old Boy; Pimp Juice; Piss; Plonk; Porter; Road Soda; Rocket Fuel; Sauce; Shooters; Shrub; Spirits; Suds; Thirst-aid; *Vino*

Pharmacologic Classification

Psychodepressant, sedative-hypnotic: miscellaneous

Brief General Overview

Alcohol abuse is endemic in North American society (and almost every other society in the world), with an overall lifetime prevalence of between 10% and 20%.[1] Alcohol abuse can occur at any time during the life span between early childhood and old age.

Problematic patterns of alcohol use, including binge drinking (i.e., consumption of five or more alcoholic drinks on one occasion) are a significant problem, particularly among Canadian Aboriginal and Native American adolescents and adults. The rate of binge drinking, both in terms of numbers of binge drinkers and numbers of episodes, is increasing among men. Currently, men account for more than 80% of the binge drinkers in North America.

Although problematic patterns of alcohol use are traditionally regarded as being, and reported to be, significantly higher in men, more recent findings suggest equal rates in women. Problematic patterns of alcohol use are observed in people of all races, ethnic and socioeconomic backgrounds, and sexual orientations. They also may be observed in members of some religious groups, including those that specifically proscribe the use of alcohol (e.g., fundamentalist Muslims, Seventh Day Adventists), although rates in these groups are reportedly significantly lower than those observed in the general population.

Dosage Forms and Routes of Administration

Alcoholic beverages (e.g., beer, distilled spirits, wine) produced by legal brewers and distillers are legally available to adults in bars, grocery stores, liquor stores, pharmacies, and restaurants. Alcoholic beverages also are directly prepared by some users (e.g., "home brew," homemade wines) for their own personal use. Although these beverages are generally used socially without serious harmful consequences, there are several problematic patterns of use. For example, a significant number of homeless or "street" people, particularly those who have a variety of significant economic, health, and social problems, are regular, long-term users of alcohol. Physically and psychologically dependent on alcohol, these men and women, who usually are unable to purchase or otherwise obtain alcoholic beverages, may obtain and drink commercially prepared alcohol-containing food products (e.g., Chinese cooking wine, vanilla extract) or nonfood products (i.e., those that are not intended for human consumption, such as aftershave lotions, Lysol® spray disinfectant, and shoe polish) in an effort to get "high," as well as to prevent or minimize the occurrence of the alcohol withdrawal syndrome.

New patterns of problematic use also continue to develop. For example, the concomitant consumption of alcoholic beverages and caffeine-containing "energy drinks" (see Caffeine monograph) has increased significantly over the past 5 years. The typical person who displays this pattern of use is a European-American man in his 20s who attends college or university. These men usually participate in intramural athletics, generally are involved in fraternity social activities, and commonly believe that drinking energy drinks allows them to maintain their sobriety while consuming more alcohol than usual during a drinking episode (i.e., to prevent drunkenness). Unfortunately, these young men have been found to be significantly more likely to drink to intoxication (i.e., become drunk) more frequently than matched controls and to engage in alcohol-related high-risk behaviors, including driving a motor vehicle when drunk and engaging in unprotected sex with multiple partners.

Mechanism of CNS Action

The exact molecular mechanism by which alcohol exerts its psychodepressant action has not been determined. Alcohol appears to modify the membrane environment of the gamma-aminobutyric acid (GABA)-receptor complex. Thus, the affinity for both endogenous GABA and other exogenous sedative-hypnotics, such as barbiturates or benzodiazepines, is significantly increased (i.e., GABAergic inhibition is enhanced). Acute alcohol consumption significantly decreases overall brain glucose metabolism, which may also result in psychodepressant effects.

Pharmacodynamics/Pharmacokinetics

The pharmacokinetics of alcohol vary depending on genetic and other factors. For example, alcohol absorption from the gastrointestinal (GI) tract, although usually fairly complete, is influenced by atrophic gastritis, carbonation of the alcoholic beverage or any other beverage consumed concomitantly (e.g., "rum and coke" mixed drink, shot of whiskey followed with a beer chaser), concentration of the alcoholic beverage consumed, drinking pattern, presence and type of meal consumed in relation to ingesting alcohol, time of day, and other factors.

Alcohol is highly metabolized to acetaldehyde (i.e., 95% to 98%) with the remainder excreted in unchanged form in the breath, perspiration, and urine. Metabolism occurs primarily in the liver and is mediated by the enzyme alcohol dehydrogenase, which has a relatively low Michaelis-Menten constant (km) of 0.05 to 0.1 gram/L and displays genetic polymorphism. In addition, the hepatic microsomal enzyme CYP2E1, which has a higher km (0.5 to 0.8 gram/L) and also is inducible,[2] plays a minor but significant role in the hepatic metabolism of alcohol.

As a rule of thumb for the average person, the consumption of one alcoholic beverage (e.g., one shot of distilled liquor or one can of beer or one glass of wine) increases the blood alcohol concentration by 0.02 gram% (i.e., 20 mg/100 mL). Conversely, each hour elapsed since the termination of alcohol consumption will result in a decrease in the blood alcohol concentration by 0.02 gram%.[3]

Current Approved Indications for Medical Use[4]

Antidote for methanol poisoning[5]

Desired Action/Reason for Personal Use

Anxiety/stress reduction; disinhibition (decrease sexual or social inhibitions); euphoria or "high"; mood elevation; prevention/self-management of the alcohol withdrawal syndrome; relaxation; sense of well-being; also, purposely administered to others, with or without their knowledge, in the context of perpetration of a drug-facilitated crime (e.g., robbery; sexual assault, including date rape)[6]

Toxicity (also see Table 1 on pages 8–9)

Acute: Accidental injuries or fatalities (e.g., related to drownings, falls, or motor vehicle crashes[7]); cognitive impairment; coma; disinhibition; drowsiness; hallucinations; memory impairment, including alcoholic blackouts; psychomotor impairment; respiratory depression; slurred speech

Chronic: Accidental injuries (e.g., falls, motor vehicle crashes), increased risk and frequency; ascites; cancer, particularly breast cancer in women,[8] and cancer of the esophagus, rectum, and throat in both men and women; cardiac disease, including cardiac dysrhythmias, cardiomyopathy, coronary artery disease, and sudden death[9]; cirrhosis of the liver; dementia[10]; folic acid deficiency; gastritis; hepatitis; mental depression; neurotoxicity[11]; peripheral neuropathy; physical dependence; premature death[12]; psychological dependence; psychosis; sexual assault, risk for[13]; sexual impairment, males; self-neglect; suicide, risk for[14]; violent injuries, risk for[15]; Wernicke-Korsakoff syndrome

Pregnancy & Lactation: Alcohol is a known human teratogen with the potential to adversely affect the pregnancies of almost all girls and women who drink during pregnancy. The observed effects, noted throughout history and formally documented since the 1960s, have been collectively known as the fetal alcohol syndrome (FAS). More recently, FAS has been further conceptualized as the fetal alcohol spectrum disorder (FASD) in an effort to better identify the wide range of effects that alcohol use during pregnancy may have on embryonic and fetal growth and development and, later, growth and development during childhood and adolescence.

FAS, which was originally linked to heavy drinking during pregnancy, has now been associated with regular maternal consumption of two or more alcoholic drinks per day during pregnancy or isolated periods of binge drinking during pregnancy.[16] In a large sample of women with pregnancies that resulted in a live birth, 14% engaged in preconception binge drinking. These women tended to be single and of European American descent. They were likewise found to be more likely to continue to both drink alcohol and smoke tobacco during their pregnancies. In North America, Canadian Aboriginal peoples and Native Americans have the highest rates of FAS.

The malformations and adverse effects associated with FAS can be classified into four categories: CNS dysfunction, growth retardation, characteristic facies (shown in Figure 1), and associated physical anomalies. Intrauterine growth retardation is common, as is mental retardation. An increased rate of learning disorders, including attention disorders (e.g., attention-deficit/hyperactivity disorder, or ADHD) is seen in older children with FAS, even when their IQ scores are within normal range.

Alcohol is excreted in significant amounts in breast milk. The related taste and odor appear to decrease milk consumption by breast-fed neonates and infants. Adolescent girls and women who are breast-feeding should avoid drinking alcoholic beverages.

Abuse Potential

Physical dependence: High (USDEA: not a scheduled drug)
Psychological dependence: High

Withdrawal Syndrome

A classic alcohol withdrawal syndrome has been long noted in people who are physically dependent on alcohol and abruptly discontinue its use. The alcohol withdrawal syndrome may begin within a few hours after the last drink of alcohol was consumed and may last for up to 7 days (as long as alcohol is not consumed). Signs and symptoms of alcohol withdrawal generally include agitation, anhedonia, anxiety, hallucinations, hypertension, illusions, insomnia, irritability, nausea, sweating, tachycardia, tremors, and vomiting. In severe cases, sometimes referred to in the literature as "resistant alcohol withdrawal," tonic–clonic (grand mal) seizures can occur, usually within the

FIGURE 1

Common Craniofacial Characteristics Associated with Fetal Alcohol Syndrome

Reprinted from Pagliaro, L.A., & Pagliaro, A.M. (2004). *Pagliaros' comprehensive guide to drugs and substances of abuse.* Washington, D.C.: American Pharmacists Association.

Eyes
1. Ptosis (drooping lid)
2. Strabismus (squint)
3. Shortened palpebral fissure (opening between eyelids)
4. Epicanthal fold

Ears
5. Smaller or larger than normal, malformed, or low set

Nose
6. Low nasal bridge
7. Short with high or upturned nasal tip

Mouth
8. Philtrum (groove in upper lip): underdeveloped or absent
9. Micrognathia (small jaw) or retrognathia (posteriorly displaced jaw)
10. Teeth: absent enamel, malformed, or maloccluded
11. Wide mouth
12. Thin vermilion border of upper lip

Head
13. Microcephaly (small head size)
14. Abnormally shaped cranium
15. Mid-face hypoplasia (broad, flat face)
16. Narrow, receding forehead

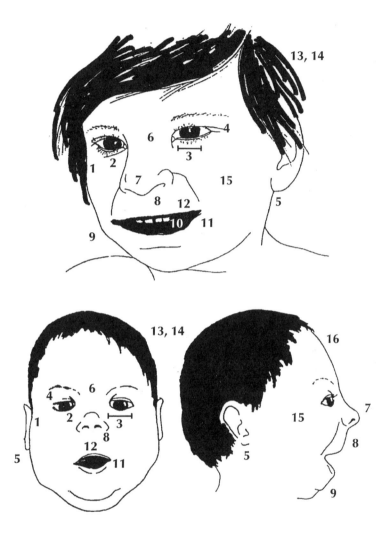

first 12 to 24 hours following the discontinuation of alcohol use. If untreated, a late complication is delirium tremens (DTs), which may generally occur 6 or more days after the last drink of alcohol was consumed. Signs and symptoms of DTs include agitation (severe), confusion, delirium, diarrhea, disorientation, fever, hallucinations (often bizarre and extremely frightening), hypertension, hyperthermia, mydriasis, nausea, sweating (profuse), and tachycardia. Cardiovascular collapse may occur if DTs is left untreated, and may be fatal. Medical management of DTs generally involves hospitalization, the cautious administration of long-acting benzodiazepine pharmacotherapy, and careful monitoring of body systems.

TABLE 1
Acute (A) and Chronic (C) Adverse Effects Associated with Alcohol Use in Adults

Absenteeism from work (A) (C)
Accidents, general (e.g., drownings, falls) (A) (C)
Abusive and aggressive behavior, physical and psychological (A) (C)
Alcoholic blackouts (A) (C)
Alcoholic ketoacidosis (A) (C)
Anemia (C)
Angina pectoris (A) (C)
Arteriosclerosis (C)
Ascites (C)
Ataxia (A)
Breast cancer (C)
Cardiac dysrhythmias (C)
Cardiovascular heart disease (C)
Cardiovascular morbidity and mortality (C)
Child abuse, physical and psychological (A) (C)
Cirrhosis of the liver (C)
Cognitive dysfunction/impairment (A) (C)
Coma (A) (C)
Criminal behavior (A) (C)
Decreased immune response (C)
Diabetes mellitus (C)
Dilated cardiomyopathies (C)
Dysfunctional parenting (A) (C)
Dysmenorrhea (C)
Elder abuse, physical and psychological (A) (C)
Esophageal varices (C)
Fetal alcohol syndrome (A) (C)
Formication (A) (C)
Gastritis (A) (C)
Gastrointestinal bleeding (C)
Guilt (A) (C)
Hallucinations (A)
Hangover (A)
Heart disease (C)
Hepatic failure (C)
Hepatitis (C)
Hypertension (C)
Hypertriglyceridemia (C)
Hypoglycemia (A) (C)
Korsakoff's psychosis (C)
Malnutrition (e.g., thiamine deficiency) (C)
Memory dysfunction (A) (C)
Mental depression (A) (C)
Motor vehicle crashes (A)
Neuropathy (C)
Neurotoxicity (A) (C)
Nystagmus (A)
Osteoporosis (C)
Pancreatitis (A) (C)
Peripheral neuropathy (C)
Physical dependence (C)
Psychological dependence (C)
Psychomotor impairment (A)
Psychosis (A)

(continued)

TABLE 1 (continued)
Acute (A) and Chronic (C) Adverse Effects Associated with Alcohol Use in Adults

Reflexes, impaired (A)
Respiratory depression (A)
Self-neglect (A) (C)
Sexual dysfunction (males) (A)
Sexual inhibitions, decreased (A)
Slurred speech (A)
Social problems (e.g., absence from work, arguments with family members, divorce) (A) (C)
Spousal abuse, physical and psychological (A) (C)
Suicide (A) (C)
Victimization (e.g., physical assault, sexual assault) (A) (C)
Violent behavior, including homicide, physical assault, and rape (A)
Wernicke-Korsakoff syndrome (C)
Work productivity, decreased (A) (C)

Source: Adapted from Pagliaro, L.A., & Pagliaro, A.M. (2004). *Pagliaros' comprehensive guide to drugs and substances of abuse.* Washington, DC: American Pharmacists Association.

Overdosage

Alcohol overdosage is generally self-limited by the occurrence of sleep related to the psychodepressant action of alcohol. However, if blood alcohol concentrations become high enough, centrally mediated respiratory depression can occur and may be fatal. The blood alcohol concentration and respiratory status should be carefully monitored. Appropriate medical support of body systems is required, with attention to maintaining respiratory function. There is no known antidote.

Notes

1. The range of percentages is due to differences in the many definitions that are used in regard to what constitutes alcohol abuse. For example, if abuse were synonymous with the *DSM-IV-TR* definition, then 10% would be the more accurate percentage.
2. This type of metabolism may help to explain the higher clearance rates for alcohol sometimes observed in heavy drinkers who have relatively normal liver function and who do not display the usual hepatic dysfunction often associated with long-term, heavy drinking.
3. These estimates should be considered to be initial, rough, or "ballpark" estimates only.
4. Alcoholic beverages (e.g., whiskey, brandy) have been medically used in the past as tonics or stimulants and to aid sleep (i.e., as a nightcap). Although these uses are generally considered obsolete, alcohol continues to be used as a vehicle for many oral liquid drug formulations (e.g., cough and cold products).
5. Fomepizole (Antizol®) generally is the antidote of choice for this indication. It also is currently the drug of first choice for emergency medical management of ethylene glycol (i.e., antifreeze) poisoning. Generally, fomepizole is used with appropriate medical support of body systems, including the restoration and maintenance of fluid and electrolyte balance.
6. Alcohol is the oldest and, currently, the most commonly used drug or substance of abuse for the facilitation of sexual assault.
7. Motor vehicle crashes are the leading cause of death in North American adolescent boys and young men 16 to 24 years of age, and alcohol use contributes significantly to these crashes.
8. Breast cancer in women appears to be mediated by alcohol dehydrogenase II gene polymorphism. In addition, it is believed that the congeners of alcohol that are formed during the brewing process may be the major contributory factor to the increased risk of rectal cancer associated with the ingestion of beer in men. This latter hypothesis is substantiated by the observation of significantly less risk when alcohol is consumed in the form of wine or distilled spirits.

9. Alcohol is a known myocardial depressant (i.e., left ventricular cardiac [systolic] function displays progressive decline in a dose-dependent manner with alcohol). However, several studies have suggested a cardioprotectant effect associated with low alcohol consumption patterns (i.e., one to seven typical alcoholic drinks per week). Conversely, chronic heavy alcohol consumption has been directly related to elevated blood pressure and the development of congestive heart failure.

10. Occurring at the highest rate in elderly chronic heavy drinkers (with the exception of senile dementia [i.e., Alzheimer's dementia]).

11. The neurotoxicity may be a direct toxic effect of regular long-term alcohol exposure on serotonin receptors.

12. Increased risk for men in all adult age groups, particularly men 35 to 44 years of age.

13. Not a direct pharmacologic effect of alcohol use, but alcohol use has consistently been highly correlated with being a victim of sexual assault.

14. Suicide is significantly correlated with alcohol use disorders. Suicide also is related to the mental depression directly caused by the ingestion of alcohol.

15. Like sexual assault, violent injuries are not a direct pharmacologic effect of alcohol use. However, alcohol use has consistently been highly correlated with being a victim of violent injuries. Therefore, the more one drinks and the more frequently one becomes intoxicated, the greater the risk for violent injury.

16. Some research has suggested that maternal use of as little as 15 mL (0.5 ounce) of absolute alcohol per day (i.e., the equivalent of one average alcoholic drink per day) significantly increases the risk for negative neurobehavioral outcomes for the neonates and infants (e.g., lower cognitive performance, slower infant reaction times). We consistently recommend that pregnant women completely avoid drinking alcohol.

References

Banks, S.M., Pandiani, J.A., Schacht, L.M., et al. (2000). Age and mortality among white male problem drinkers. *Addiction, 95*(8), 1249-1254.

Barceloux, D.G., Bond, G.R., Krenzelok, E.P., et al. (2002). American Academy of Clinical Toxicology practice guidelines on the treatment of methanol poisoning. *Journal of Clinical Toxicology, 40*(4), 415-446.

Berggren, U., Eriksson, M., Fahlke, C., et al. (2002). Is long-term heavy alcohol consumption toxic for brain serotonergic neurons? Relationship between years of excessive alcohol consumption and serotonergic neurotransmission. *Drug and Alcohol Dependence, 65*(2), 159-165.

Deng, X.S., & Deitrich, R.A. (2007). Ethanol metabolism and effects: Nitric oxide and its interaction. *Currents in Clinical Pharmacology, 2*(2), 145-153.

Fetal alcohol syndrome—Alaska, Arizona, Colorado, and New York, 1995-1997. (2002). *MMWR. Morbidity and Mortality Weekly Reports, 51*(20), 433-435.

Hack, J.B., Hoffmann, R.S., & Nelson, L.S. (2006). Resistant alcohol withdrawal: Does an unexpectedly large sedative requirement identify these patients early? *The Journal of Medical Toxicology, 2*(2), 55-60.

Hall, J.A., & Moore, C.B. (2008). Drug facilitated sexual assault—A review. *Journal of Forensic and Legal Medicine, 15*(5), 291-297.

Halsted, C.H., Villanueva, J.A., Devlin, A.M., et al. (2002). Metabolic interactions of alcohol and folate. *The Journal of Nutrition, 132*(8 Suppl), 2367S-2372S.

Harris, R.A., Trudell, J.R., & Mihic, S.J. (2008). Ethanol's molecular targets. *Science Signals, 1*(28), re7.

Involvement by young drivers in fatal alcohol-related motor-vehicle crashes—United States, 1982-2001. (2002). *MMWR. Morbidity and Mortality Weekly Reports, 51*(48), 1089-1091.

Jacobson, S.W., Chiodo, L.M., Sokol, R.L., et al. (2002). Validity of maternal report of prenatal alcohol, cocaine, and smoking in relation to neurobehavioral outcome. *Pediatrics, 109*(5), 815-825.

Kelly, T.M., Cornelius, J.R., & Lynch, K.G. (2002). Psychiatric and substance use disorders as risk factors for attempted suicide among adolescents: A case control study. *Suicide and Life-Threatening Behavior, 32*(3), 301-312.

Lee, W.K., & Regan, T.J. (2002). Alcoholic cardiomyopathy: Is it dose-dependent? *Congestive Heart Failure, 8*(6), 303-306.

Liskow, B.I., Powell, B.J., Penick, E.C., et al. (2000). Mortality in male alcoholics after ten to fourteen years. *Journal of Studies on Alcohol, 61*(6), 853-861.

Martinotti, G., Nicola, M.D., Reina, D., et al. (2008). Alcohol protracted withdrawal syndrome: The role of anhedonia. *Substance Use & Misuse, 43*(3-4), 271-284.

Matsumoto, H., & Fukui, Y. (2002). Pharmacokinetics of ethanol: A review of the methodology. *Addiction Biology, 7*(1), 5-14.

Mennella, J.A. (2001). Regulation of milk intake after exposure to alcohol in mothers' milk. *Alcoholism, Clinical and Experimental Research, 25*(4), 590-593.

Mennella, J.A., & Garcia-Gomez, P.L. (2001). Sleep disturbances after acute exposure to alcohol in mothers' milk. *Alcohol, 25*(3), 153-158.

Mitic, W., & Greschner, J. (2002). Alcohol's role in the deaths of BC children and youth. *Canadian Journal of Public Health, 93*(3), 173-175.

Naimi, T.S., Brewer, R.D., Mokdad, A., et al. (2003). Binge drinking in the United States. *JAMA: The Journal of the American Medical Association, 289*(1), 70-75.

Norberg, A., Jones, W.A., Hahn, R.G., et al. (2003). Role of variability in explaining ethanol pharmacokinetics: Research and forensic applications. *Clinical Pharmacokinetics, 42*(1), 1-31.

O'Brien, M.C., McCoy, T.P., Rhodes, S.D., et al. (2008). Caffeinated cocktails: Energy drink consumption, high-risk drinking, and alcohol-related consequences among college students. *Academic Emergency Medicine, 15*(5), 453-460.

Oneta, C.M., Pedrosa, M., Ruttimann, S., et al. (2001). Age and bioavailability of alcohol. *Zeitschrift fur Gastroenterology, 39*(9), 783-788.

Ramchandani, V.A., Bosron, W.F., & Li, T.K. (2001). Research advances in ethanol metabolism. *Pathologie-Biologie (Paris), 49*(9), 676-682.

Ramchandani, V.A., Kwo, P.Y., & Li, T.K. (2001). Effect of food and food composition on alcohol elimination rates in healthy men and women. *Journal of Clinical Pharmacology, 41*(12), 1345-1350.

Scott-Ham, M., & Burton, F.C. (2005). Toxicology findings in cases of alleged drug-facilitated sexual assault in the United Kingdom over a 3-year period. *Journal of Clinical Forensic Medicine, 12*(4), 175-186.

Spies, C.D., Sander, M., Stangl, K., et al. (2001). Effects of alcohol on the heart. *Current Opinions in Critical Care, 7*(5), 337-343.

Sturmer, T., Wang-Gohrke, S., Arndt, V., et al. (2002). Interaction between alcohol dehydrogenase II gene, alcohol consumption, and risk for breast cancer. *British Journal of Cancer, 87*(5), 519-523.

Thomas, V.S., & Rockwood, K.J. (2001). Alcohol abuse, cognitive impairment, and mortality among older people. *Journal of the American Geriatrics Society, 49*(4), 415-420.

Volkow, N.D., Ma, Y., Zhu, W., et al. (2008). Moderate doses of alcohol disrupt the functional organization of the human brain. *Psychiatry Research, 162*(3), 205-213.

ALFENTANIL

Names

BAN or INN Generic Synonyms: None

Brand/Trade: Alfenta®

Chemical: N-(1-(2-(4-Ethyl-4,5-dihydro-5-oxo-1h-tetrazol-1-yl)ethyl)-4-(methoxymethyl)-4-piperidinyl)-n-phenylpropanamide

Street: None

Pharmacologic Classification

Psychodepressant, opiate analgesic: pure agonist (synthetic)

Brief General Overview[1]

Alfentanil is a potent synthetic opiate analgesic.

Dosage Forms and Routes of Administration

Alfentanil is commercially available from licit pharmaceutical manufacturers as an aqueous solution for intravenous injection. People who abuse alfentanil are primarily hospital employees (e.g., nurses, nursing assistants, pharmacists, pharmacy technicians, physicians) who self-inject alfentanil intravenously. These users are rare because of the potency of alfentanil (i.e., its great potential for fatal overdosage errors) and its propensity to cause chest wall rigidity in up to one-third of users. Alfentanil, for these same reasons, is very seldom found "on the street." In addition, its short elimination half-life and relatively short duration of action (i.e., 30 minutes) would require almost continuously repeated injection to achieve and maintain the desired effects or to prevent the onset of the opiate analgesic withdrawal syndrome in users who are physically dependent.

Mechanism of CNS Action

See the Opiate Analgesics monograph.

Pharmacodynamics/Pharmacokinetics

The onset of alfentanil's action is virtually immediate following intravenous injection. It is moderately protein bound (i.e., 92%) and has an apparent volume of distribution of ~1 L/kg. Alfentanil is metabolized primarily by dealkylation and oxidation by the hepatic microsomal CYP3A4 enzyme system to noralfentanil and N-phenylpropionamide. Cytochrome CYP3A5, which is polymorphically expressed, also plays a role in the metabolism of alfentanil and may be responsible for observed interindividual variability in its pharmacodynamics and pharmacokinetics. Less than 1% of an injected dose of alfentanil is excreted in unchanged form in the urine. The drug's mean total body clearance is ~6 mL/kg/minute and clearance is reduced in the presence of hepatic dysfunction (e.g., hepatic cirrhosis). The elimination half-life of alfentanil is ~90 minutes.

Current Approved Indications for Medical Use

Analgesia as adjunct to anesthesia and mechanical ventilation[2]; pain, moderate to severe

Desired Action/Reason for Personal Use

Euphoria

Toxicity

Acute: Apnea; bradycardia; dizziness; hypotension; nausea; skeletal muscle rigidity, particularly of the chest wall and truncal muscles; somnolence; respiratory depression; vomiting

Chronic: Valid and reliable data are not available. See the Opiate Analgesics monograph for general related information.

Pregnancy & Lactation: Valid and reliable data are not available. See the Opiate Analgesics monograph for general related information.

Abuse Potential

Physical dependence: High (USDEA Schedule II; high abuse potential)
Psychological dependence: High

Withdrawal Syndrome

Valid and reliable data are not available. See the Opiate Analgesics monograph for general related information.

Overdosage

Valid and reliable data are not available. See the Opiate Analgesics monograph for general related information.

Notes

1. Alfentanil should not be confused with *alphamethylfentanyl* (AMF). AMF, chemical name N-phenyl-N-[1-(1-phenylpropan-2-yl)-4-piperidyl] propanamide, was synthesized in 1979 in an early effort to create a new form of opiate analgesic drug that could avoid legal control by either the FDA or USDEA laws and regulations. Thus, it became the first generally recognized "designer drug" (i.e., a drug designed to get around the law).

   AMF was extremely potent and soon became known "on the street" as the mythical *China White*—the "perfect" opiate analgesic. However, its potency quickly led to the demise of its use. Following numerous overdosage deaths related to its use, AMF was placed on USDEA Schedule I (use is prohibited) in 1981—only 2 years after its original synthesis. Since that time, over one dozen related analogues of fentanyl have been synthesized and used "on the street." The extreme potency of these opiate analgesic analogues and their corresponding increased risk for fatal overdosage have minimized their current use.

2. Alfentanil is used as an adjunct to general anesthesia in combination with barbiturates or nitrous oxide. It also is used to facilitate compliance and tolerance in mechanically ventilated patients.

References

Hagelberg, N., Kajander, J.K., Nagren, K., et al. (2002). Mu-receptor agonism with alfentanil increases striatal dopamine D2 receptor binding in man. *Synapse, 45*(1), 25-30.

Mariero Klees, T., Sheffels, P., Thummel, K.E., et al. (2005). Pharmacogenetic determinants of human liver microsomal alfentanil metabolism and the role of cytochrome P450 3A5. *Anesthesiology, 102*, 550-556.

McMunnigall, F., & Welsh, J. (2008). Opioid withdrawal syndrome on switching from hydromorphone to alfentanil. *Palliative Medicine, 22*(2), 191-192.

ALPHA-METHYLTRYPTAMINE

Names

BAN or INN Generic Synonyms: 3-(2-Aminopropyl) indole

Brand/Trade: None

Chemical: alpha-Methyltryptamine

Street: 3-IT; AMT; IT-290; Spirals

Pharmacologic Classification

Psychodelic, LSD-like psychodelic: indole/tryptamine

Brief General Overview

Alpha-methyltryptamine (AMT) is a long-acting tryptamine (i.e., indoethylamine) psychodelic. It reportedly has activity as a monoamine oxidase inhibitor A (MAOI-A) and was medically used as an antidepressant in the former Soviet Union during the 1960s. Although AMT was never clinically used as an antidepressant in North America, its homologue, alpha-ethyltryptamine (AET), was used during the 1960s for this indication.[1] On the east and west coasts of the United States (e.g., in California, Florida, and New York), it has been a popular "designer drug" used mainly by college-age men and women at dance clubs and raves. During the past 5 years, AMT use has increased among both high school students and U.S. military personnel.

Dosage Forms and Routes of Administration

AMT is generally available in powder or crystal form, often packed into capsules. Both forms are orally ingested, inhaled (i.e., smoked), or intranasally snorted.[2] Several detailed recipes for the chemical synthesis of AMT are available on the Internet, where AMT also can be illicitly obtained from several U.S. and foreign chemical companies.

Mechanism of CNS Action

The exact mechanism of AMT's CNS action has not been determined, but it appears to be related, in large part, to AMT's affinity for serotonin (5-hydroxytryptamine, or 5-HT) receptors, particularly 5-HT2.[3] Dopamine D2-receptor agonism also appears to mediate the CNS actions of AMT. In addition, AMT has demonstrated inhibition of serotonin reuptake.

Pharmacodynamics/Pharmacokinetics

AMT's onset of action is ~30 minutes after inhalation (i.e., smoking) or intranasal snorting and 1 to 2 hours after oral ingestion. Effects generally persist for 12 to 24 hours. Additional valid and reliable data are not available.

Current Approved Indications for Medical Use

None

Desired Action/Reason for Personal Use

Auditory distortions; empathy; euphoria; feelings of "love"; hallucinations; increased energy; visual distortions

Toxicity

Acute: Anxiety; bruxism; diarrhea; elevated blood pressure; feelings of depersonalization; headache; insomnia; irritability; jaw clenching; mydriasis; nausea; nervousness; psychomotor impairment (mild); restlessness; tachycardia; unpleasant smell and taste; vomiting

Chronic: Valid and reliable data are not available.

Pregnancy & Lactation: Valid and reliable data are not available.

Abuse Potential

Physical dependence: None to low (USDEA Schedule I; use is prohibited)
Psychological dependence: Low

Withdrawal Syndrome

An AMT withdrawal syndrome has not been reported.

Overdosage

Several deaths have been related to AMT use. There is no known antidote. Additional valid and reliable data are needed.

Notes

1. AET has not been in clinical use in North America for several decades and is currently a USDEA Schedule I drug (use is prohibited).
2. Intranasal snorting of AMT has been associated with an intense intranasal burning sensation.
3. This proposed mechanism of action is very similar to that of lysergic acid diethylamide (LSD; see monograph), with which AMT shares most of its CNS actions.

References

Boland, D.M., Andollo, W., Hime, G.W., et al. (2005). Fatality due to acute α-methyltryptamine intoxication. *Journal of Analytical Toxicology, 29*(5), 394-397.

Drug Enforcement Administration (DEA), Department of Justice. (2004, September 29). Schedules of controlled substances: Placement of α-methyltryptamine and 5-methoxy-N,N-diisopropyltryptamine into schedule I of the Controlled Substances Act. Final rule. *Federal Register, 69*(188), 58950-3.

Leinwand, D. (2002, July 22). Dangerous club-drug knockoffs surge. *USA Today.* Available: http://www.usatoday.com/news/nation/2002-07-22-drug-fakes_x.htm.

ALPRAZOLAM

Names

BAN or INN Generic Synonyms: None

Brand/Trade: Alprazolam Intensol®; Apo-Alpraz®; Novo-Alprazol®; Nu-Alpraz®; Xanax®; Xanax TS®

Chemical: 8-Chloro-1-methyl-6-phenyl-4H-s-triazolo[4,3-α][1,4]benzodiazepine

Street: Coffins; Dog Bones; Footballs; Forgetful Pills; Fo's; Four Bars; French Fries; Gold Bars; Green Bars; Handlebars; Jellybeans; Nutragrain Bars; School Buses; Sticks; Totem Poles; White Bars; Xan-Bars; Xannies; X-Boxes; Z-Bars; Zan Bars; Zannies; Zanny Bars

Pharmacologic Classification

Psychodepressant, sedative-hypnotic: benzodiazepine

Brief General Overview

Alprazolam was first synthesized in 1973. Currently, it is among the top three abused benzodiazepines in North America. Among adults, a high rate of alprazolam abuse is found in women 30 to 50 years of age who are generally university educated, working in a professional capacity (e.g., schoolteacher or principal), and taking prescription alprazolam under their physician's guidance for the management of an anxiety or mood disorder.[1] Among youth, abusers are most likely to be adolescent boys of African or Hispanic descent.

Dosage Forms and Routes of Administration

Alprazolam is produced by licit pharmaceutical manufacturers and is available in various oral and sublingual tablet formulations. It is usually orally ingested or used sublingually.

Mechanism of CNS Action

Alprazolam and other benzodiazepines cause dose-related CNS depression varying from mild depression of cognitive and psychomotor performance to hypnosis. The exact mechanism of action for the anxiolytic and antipanic actions of alprazolam has not been determined, but it appears to involve an interaction with benzodiazepine receptors (types 1 and 2 [BZD-1 and BZD-2]) at several sites within the CNS, particularly in the cerebral cortex and limbic system. This action also may be mediated by, or work in concert with, gamma-aminobutyric acid, an inhibitory neurotransmitter. See also the Benzodiazepines monograph.

Pharmacodynamics/Pharmacokinetics

Alprazolam is rapidly and well absorbed following oral ingestion ($F = 0.9$), and the extent of absorption is not affected by co-ingestion of food. Blood concentrations are proportional to the dose ingested, and peak blood concentrations are achieved within 1 to 2 hours. Alprazolam is ~80% bound to plasma proteins and has an apparent volume of distribution of ~1 L/kg. Alprazolam is extensively metabolized in the liver to an active metabolite, alpha-hydroxyalprazolam, and is excreted primarily in the urine (~20% in unchanged form). It has a mean elimination half-life of ~12 hours (range, 7 to 16 hours) and a mean total body clearance of 50 mL/minute.

Current Approved Indications for Medical Use

Symptomatic management of anxiety disorders (e.g., acute anxiety, generalized anxiety disorder, panic attacks)

Desired Action/Reason for Personal Use

Anxiety/stress reduction; euphoria or "high"; also, purposely administered to others without their knowledge in the context of perpetration of a drug-facilitated crime (e.g., robbery; sexual assault, including date rape)

Toxicity

Acute: Ataxia; blurred vision; cognitive impairment; confusion; constipation; decreased sex drive; disinhibition; dizziness; drowsiness; dysarthria; fatigue; headache; incoordination; increased appetite; irritability; lightheadedness; memory impairment; mental depression; weight change (loss or gain)

Chronic: Physical dependence; psychological dependence

Pregnancy & Lactation: FDA Pregnancy Category D (see Appendix B). Safety of alprazolam use by adolescent girls and women who are pregnant has not been established. Alprazolam use during pregnancy has not been directly implicated in fetal harm. Additional valid and reliable data are needed. (Also see the Benzodiazepines monograph.)

Safety of alprazolam use by adolescent girls and women who are breast-feeding has not been established. Additional valid and reliable data are needed.

Abuse Potential

Physical dependence: Moderate (USDEA Schedule IV; low potential for abuse)
Psychological dependence: Moderate to high

Withdrawal Syndrome

Signs and symptoms of the alprazolam withdrawal syndrome may occur when long-term alprazolam pharmacotherapy, or regular personal use, is abruptly discontinued for any reason (e.g., unavailability, prescribed reduction of dosage, doses missed because of forgetfulness or hospitalization). Thus, alprazolam pharmacotherapy, or regular personal use, should be gradually discontinued.

Overdosage

Signs and symptoms of alprazolam overdosage include coma, confusion, diminished reflexes, incoordination, and somnolence. Death has been associated with alprazolam overdosage alone or in combination with alcohol use. Alprazolam overdosage requires emergency medical support of body systems, with attention to increasing alprazolam elimination. The benzodiazepine receptor antagonist flumazenil (Anexate®, Romazicon®) may be required.[2]

Notes

1. Women who have a confirmed paternal history of alcoholism reportedly are at greatest risk for the development of problematic patterns of alprazolam use.
2. Caution is required because flumazenil antagonism may precipitate the alprazolam withdrawal syndrome in people who are physically dependent on alprazolam.

References

Erdman, K., Stypinski, D., Combs, M., et al. (2007). Absence of food effect on the extent of alprazolam absorption from an orally disintegrating tablet. *Pharmacotherapy, 27*(8), 1120-1124.

Evans, S.M., Levin F.R., & Fischman, M.W. (2000). Increased sensitivity to alprazolam in females with a paternal history of alcoholism. *Psychopharmacology, 150*(2), 150-162.

Forrester, M.B. (2006). Alprazolam abuse in Texas, 1998-2004. *Journal of Toxicology and Environmental Health, Part A: Current Issues, 69*(3-4), 237-243.

Kintz, P., Villain, M., Chèze, M., et al. (2005). Identification of alprazolam in hair in two cases of drug-facilitated incidents. *Forensic Science International, 153*(2-3), 222-226.

Peters, R.J. Jr., Meshack, A.F., Kelder, S.H., et al. (2007). Alprazolam (Xanax) use among southern youth: Beliefs and social norms concerning dangerous rides on "handlebars." *Journal of Drug Education, 37*(4), 417-428.

AMANITA MUSCARIA

Names

BAN or INN Generic Synonyms: None

Brand/Trade: None

Chemical: See "Mechanism of CNS Action"

Street: Flesh of the Gods; Fly Agaric[1]; Soma

Pharmacologic Classification

Psychodelic, LSD-like psychodelic: indole

Brief General Overview

Amanita muscaria is a wild mushroom that grows in much of Asia, Europe, and North America, particularly near birch, fir, larch, oak, and pine trees. The Amanita mushrooms were widely used by native Siberian tribes[2] and most likely are the "soma" praised in over 100 verses of the *Rig Veda*.[3] Currently, North American users are typically high school and college or university students of both genders, predominantly of European descent.

Dosage Forms and Routes of Administration

The *Amanita muscaria* mushroom typically is harvested, dried, and then orally ingested to achieve the desired psychodelic action.[4,5]

Mechanism of CNS Action

The psychodelic action of *Amanita muscaria* mushrooms is due to several naturally occurring alkaloids, including ibotenic acid, muscarine, and muscimol. Chemical decarboxylation of ibotenic acid to muscimol, which occurs during the process of drying the mushrooms, produces the most potent and stable form of the psychodelic. However, the exact molecular mechanism of action has not been determined.

Pharmacodynamics/Pharmacokinetics

Valid and reliable data are not available.

Current Approved Indications for Medical Use

None

Desired Action/Reason for Personal Use

Euphoria; peaceful sleep; sensory distortion (e.g., hallucinations, illusions)

Toxicity[6]

Acute: Diarrhea; dizziness; hallucinations, primarily auditory and macropsia; incoordination; muscle jerking or twitching; nausea; numbness of the limbs; psychosis; sleep (deep); vomiting

Chronic: Paranoia; violent behavior, including self-mutilation

Pregnancy & Lactation: Data are not available. On the basis of the reported pharmacologic effects of *Amanita muscaria* and related psychodelics, it is expected that teratogenic potential is low. However, active psychodelic chemicals are likely excreted in human breast milk, and adolescent girls and women are therefore advised to refrain from breast-feeding if they are using *Amanita muscaria*. Additional valid and reliable data are needed.

Abuse Potential

Physical dependence: None (USDEA: not a scheduled drug)
Psychological dependence: Low

Withdrawal Syndrome

A specific *Amanita muscaria* withdrawal syndrome has not been reported.

Overdosage

Signs and symptoms of *Amanita muscaria* overdosage are intensified expected pharmacologic actions, including anticholinergic effects, hallucinations, and muscle jerking or twitching. Death is generally from cardiac arrest and may be preceded by delirium, convulsions, or deep coma. The prognosis of *Amanita muscaria* overdosage is usually good with symptomatic medical management. However, death due solely to overdosage of *Amanita muscaria* has been noted infrequently.[7] Although not an antidote, physostigmine has been used to counter the anticholinergic effects associated with *Amanita muscaria* overdosage.

Notes

1. Called Fly Agaric because it is commonly used to kill household flies. However, it appears that Fly Agaric does not actually kill flies, but rather renders them unconscious.
2. Written confirmation of use by various indigenous Siberian tribes dates back to the mid-1600s; this use has been largely supplanted by alcohol use (e.g., vodka).
3. The *Rig Veda* is a collection of poems and hymns written by Aryans as they migrated from the North into what today is India. These verses, written almost 4000 years ago, are considered by many scholars to be the foundation of modern-day Hinduism.
4. Several reports, primarily historical, have noted that drinking the urine of those intoxicated with *Amanita muscaria* produces a similar state of intoxication in the urine drinker. No related scientific data are available, but it is quite conceivable that the principal psychoactive chemicals found in *Amanita muscaria* are excreted significantly in unchanged form in the urine and hence are capable of eliciting their expected pharmacologic action in urine drinkers.
5. Non-psychodelic mushrooms are often deliberately contaminated with psychodelic tryptamines in order to produce a psychodelic action. They are then sold as "psychodelic mushrooms" to unknowing buyers.
6. The ingestion of *Amanita muscaria* mushrooms generally produces distinct characteristic effects with auditory and visual hallucinations and alternating phases of drowsiness and agitation. The agitation phase also can produce seizures.
7. Deaths have been frequently reported with the unintentional or accidental ingestion of related *Amanita* mushrooms, particularly *Amanita phalloides* (i.e., the "Death Cap").

References

Brvar, M., Mozina, M., & Bunc, M. (2006). Prolonged psychosis after Amanita muscaria ingestion. *Wiener Klinische Wochenschrift, 118*(9-10), 294-297.

Michelot, D., & Melendez-Howell, L.M. (2003). Amanita muscaria: Chemistry, biology, toxicology, and ethnomycology. *Mycological Research, 107*(Part 2), 131-146.

Oda, T., Tanaka, C., & Tsuda, M. (2004). Molecular phylogeny and biogeography of the widely distributed Amanita species, A. muscaria and A. pantherina. *Mycological Research, 108*(Part 8), 885-896.

Satora, L., Pach, D., Butryn, B., et al. (2005). Fly agaric (Amanita muscaria) poisoning, case report and review. *Toxicon, 45*(7), 941-943.

Tsujikawa, K., Mohri, H., Kuwayama, K., et al. (2006). Analysis of hallucinogenic constituents in Amanita mushrooms circulated in Japan. *Forensic Science International, 164*(2-3), 172-178.

AMOBARBITAL (See Barbiturates)

AMPHETAMINE (See Amphetamines)

AMPHETAMINES

Names

BAN or INN Generic Synonyms: Amfetamines

Brand/Trade: See the individual amphetamine monographs: Dextroamphetamine, Methamphetamine, and Mixed Amphetamines

Chemical: (±)-alpha-Methylphenethylamine[1] (see also the Dextroamphetamine, Methamphetamine, and Mixed Amphetamines monographs)

Street: A; Ace; Accelerant; Affe; Aimies; Amf; AMP; Amp; Amphets; Amps; Amy; A-Plus; A-Train; Back Dex; Bass; B-Bomb; Beaners; Beans; Bennie; Bennies; Bens; Benz; Benzedrine; Benzidrine; Billy; Billy Whiz; Biphetamine; Bippies; Black and White; Black Beauties; Black Birds; Black Bombers; Black Cadillacs; Black Dex; Black Mollies; Blacks; Blueberries; Blue Boy; Blue Mollies; Bomber Pilots; Brain Pills; Brain Ticklers; Brownies; Browns; Bumblebees; Cartwheels; Chalk; Chicken Powder; Christina; Christmas Tree; Coast to Coast; Co-Pilot; Crank; Crisscross; Cross Tops; Crossroads; Crystal; Dex; Dexie; Dexies; Dexy; Diet Coke; Diet Pills; Dolls; Dominoes; Double Cross; Drex; Drivers; Eye Opener; Eye Openers; Fives; Fly Boy; Footballs; Forwards; French Blue; Gas; GBs; Go; Go-ee; Greenies; Head Drugs; Head Fruit; Hearts; Horse Heads; Jam; Jam Cecil; Jelly Baby; Jelly Bean; Jolly Bean; Jugs; L.A.; L.A. Turnaround; Leeper; Lid-Popper; Lid Proppers; Lightning; Little Guys; Louie; Marathons; Marching Powder; Meth; Mini Beans; Minibennie; Mollies; Morning Shot; Nineteen; Nugget; Oranges; Peaches; Pep Pills; Pink Hearts; Pixies; Purple Hearts; Rhythm; Rippers; Road Dope; *Rosa*; Roses; Smurfs; Snap; Sparkle Plenty; Sparklers; Speed; Splash; Splivins; Sprinkles; Stars; Strawberry Shortcake; Sulph; Sweeties; Sweets; Tens; Thrusters; Tic-Tacs; TR-6s; Truck Drivers; Turnabouts; Uppers; Uppies; U.S.P.; Wake-a-Mines; Wake-Up Pills; Wake Ups; West-Coast; West Coast Turnarounds; White Cross; Whities; Whiz; Zoom (Also see the Dextroamphetamine, Methamphetamine, and Mixed Amphetamines monographs.)

Pharmacologic Classification

Psychostimulant, amphetamines

Brief General Overview

The amphetamines,[1] as sympathomimetics, are chemically related to ephedrine (see monograph), the active ingredient of the ancient herb ephedra.[2] Ephedra was first medically used more than 5000 years ago in China.[3] Although ephedrine was chemically isolated from the plant form in the late 1800s, its sympathomimetic actions were not generally recognized until the early 1920s when its use as an alternative to epinephrine for the treatment of nasal congestion and bronchoconstriction was explored. Ephedrine was soon touted as superior to epinephrine because it could be orally ingested or inhaled, had a longer duration of action, and displayed predictable actions with fewer adverse and toxic effects. However, researchers and medical practitioners became concerned that natural supplies of ephedrine would soon be depleted, stimulating researchers in Europe, Japan, and the United States to search for a synthetic substitute. The divergent research directions taken by these scientists led to the synthesis of the amphetamines: amphetamine sulfate, dextroamphetamine, and methamphetamine.

The psychostimulant action of amphetamine was discovered in Los Angeles in 1927 by Gordon Alles, a young research chemist. Having reviewed ephedrine research, he concluded that phenylisopropylamine (i.e., amphetamine), a volatile base synthesized during the late 1800s, was the best candidate for further research. Performing animal experiments and also experimenting on himself, he discovered that Benzedrine® (racemic or dextro-levo-amphetamine) and Dexedrine® (the "right-handed" isomer of Benzedrine®) had powerful central stimulant actions in addition to the peripheral alpha-adrenergic and beta-adrenergic actions characteristic of the indirectly acting sympathomimetics. They also could be orally ingested or inhaled, with Dexedrine® surpassing Benzedrine® in alleviating fatigue, increasing alertness, and creating "euphoric confidence." Methamphetamine, the N-methyl analogue of dextrorotatory amphetamine, was synthesized by Japanese scientists in 1919. This form of amphetamine has remained the most potent member of this class of psychostimulants (see Methamphetamine monograph).

Since their introduction into clinical practice in the 1930s as a nasal decongestant, the amphetamines have been used to treat, with limited therapeutic success, both mental depression and obesity. During this time, the various amphetamines (e.g., dextroamphetamine, methamphetamine) also have been widely used in North America for their psychostimulant actions—to "get high," "have fun," or "freak out." Up to the late 1980s, most amphetamine use involved the illicit use of prescription diet pills (i.e., Dexedrine®).[4] During the past two decades, illicitly produced methamphetamine has been the most heavily used form of amphetamine, although other forms, including prescription mixed amphetamines (Adderall®, Adderall XR®) also are used, particularly by parents and siblings of children who are being medically managed for ADHD with the mixed amphetamines (see monograph). Current research indicates that approximately 5% of North Americans have used amphetamines at some time in their lives and that the highest rate of use is found among adolescent boys and men, 20 to 40 years of age, of European descent. A timeline of the history and use of the amphetamines is presented in Table 2.

Dosage Forms and Routes of Administration

The amphetamines are produced for medical use through chemical synthesis by licit pharmaceutical manufacturers. However, an overwhelming majority of amphetamine production across North America is by clandestine illicit laboratories (i.e., Meth labs) that can be found in numerous locations ranging from basement suites to warehouses oper-

TABLE 2

Historical Timeline of the Amphetamines

1887	Amphetamine synthesized in Germany by L. Edeleano.[a]
1910	Amphetamines tested in laboratory animals.
1919	Methamphetamine synthesized in Japan.
1927	Intrigued by the work of Edeleano, research chemist Gordon Alles self-administers amphetamine and notes its psychostimulant effects, including euphoria. Sympathomimetic actions of amphetamine (e.g., bronchodilation, increased blood pressure) discovered. Amphetamine used to treat bronchial asthma.[b]
1930s	Research at the University of Minnesota on the psychological effects of the amphetamines results in student participants spreading the word that these "new drugs" enable them to remain awake all night for studying or having fun. Many former users of illegal cocaine switch to legally available amphetamines.
1932	Benzedrine® (amphetamine) nasal inhaler marketed as a nonprescription product to treat nasal congestion.
1935	Amphetamine medically used to treat narcolepsy.
1936	Adverse effects associated with amphetamine use (e.g., insomnia, physical collapse) are recognized at an alarming rate among university students, and national media warn the public about the dangers of amphetamine use. Media references to "brain," "pep," and "superman" lead to increased public curiosity rather than discouraging use.
1937	Amphetamine medically used to treat minimal brain dysfunction.[c]
WW II	Amphetamines widely distributed to both Allied and Axis soldiers and pilots to diminish fatigue and thus promote combat performance.
1940s	Intravenous methamphetamine use becomes epidemic in Japan after WW II. Professional football players begin to use amphetamines to enhance performance.
1950s	At least seven different nasal inhalers containing large amounts of amphetamine are available for purchase at drug or grocery stores without prescription. Amphetamine is obtained from the easily opened inhalers by various techniques limited only by users' ingenuity (e.g., dissolving the amphetamine from the amphetamine-impregnated cotton fillers of the inhalers in alcohol or coffee and then orally ingesting the beverage, chewing the cotton filters or swallowing them whole). Because of their availability, inhaler products and other amphetamine formulations (e.g., injectables, oral tablets) are used by tens of thousands of North Americans, including athletes (e.g., to run farther or faster), college students (e.g., to "cram" for exams), and trailer truck drivers (e.g., to stay awake during long hauls).
1960s	Amphetamines widely prescribed to treat mental depression and exogenous obesity. Potential for amphetamines to cause physical and psychological dependence becomes widely recognized. However, they continue to be medically used and abused by "delinquent," "derelict," "addict subculture," or "socially marginalized" populations. Although it is not widely known, President John F. Kennedy is regularly prescribed amphetamines by one of his attending physicians, Max Jacobson (known as "Dr. Feelgood"), and becomes addicted.
1970	Over 30 different amphetamine products legally produced by North American pharmaceutical companies. Legal prescriptions exceed 40 million annually. Federal Controlled Substances Act of 1970 significantly reduces legal production and use of amphetamines in the United States.
1980	Most amphetamine use replaced by cocaine. However, by the mid 1990s interest in amphetamines is renewed among adolescents and adults as an economic alternative. Renewed interest also stimulated by increased availability of injectable and smokable forms of methamphetamine (e.g., Crystal Meth, Ice) initially supplied to the continental United States from the Pacific Rim.
1995	Mexican criminal gangs begin to dominate methamphetamine production and commerce in the continental United States. Most methamphetamine is produced in "superlabs" capable of producing 10 pounds or more of methamphetamine per day (see Methamphetamine monograph). The purer form of illicit methamphetamine (i.e., Crystal Meth) becomes widely available across North America and is smoked in much the same way as Crack Cocaine (see Cocaine monograph).

(continued)

TABLE 2 (continued)
Historical Timeline of the Amphetamines

1996	Comprehensive Methamphetamine Control Act of 1996 broadens controls on chemical precursors of methamphetamine, including ephedrine, phenylpropanolamine, and pseudoephedrine.
2000	*Yaba*, an oral methamphetamine formulation, becomes popular in California, particularly among Asian youth. It is produced in microtablet form, usually in combination with caffeine, primarily in Burma, and is imported from Burma and Thailand, where use is widespread. In North America, 4% of adults report having tried methamphetamine at least once. High school seniors report significantly greater lifetime use (i.e., 7.9%). Use is highest in western, southwestern, and midwestern sections of the country. Methamphetamine Anti-Proliferation Act passed by U.S. Congress to strengthen sentencing guidelines.
2005	Amphetamine laboratories range from well-organized, highly efficient operations capable of producing 50 kg (110 pounds) of amphetamine per week to university laboratories to kitchens or bathrooms in small apartments that produce less than 30 grams (1 ounce) per week. A substantial percentage of the illicit amphetamine production and sale in North America is handled by well-organized criminal gangs (e.g., Asian criminal youth gangs; Hells Angels outlaw motorcycle gangs; Mexican Mafia).
2009	Amphetamines, including methamphetamine, continue to be a major commodity for international organized crime syndicates (e.g., Asian crime syndicates) and outlaw motorcycle gangs (e.g., Hells Angels) operating in North America. An estimated 5% of North Americans have used amphetamines at some time in their lives. The highest rate of abuse is found among adolescent boys and men (20 to 40 years of age) of European descent.

[a]Amphetamine was originally known as phenylisopropylamine.
[b]A related psychostimulant and sympathomimetic, ephedrine (see monograph) was used for the same indication. However, because it is a natural plant product, its availability was limited.
[c]Minimal brain dysfunction is the name previously used for attention-deficit/hyperactivity disorder (ADHD).
Source: Adapted from Pagliaro, L.A., & Pagliaro, A.M. (2004). *Pagliaros' comprehensive guide to drugs and substances of abuse*. Washington, DC: American Pharmacists Association.

ated by Hells Angels and other biker gangs to university chemistry laboratories. When used illicitly, the amphetamines are orally ingested, intravenously injected (i.e., "mainlined"), intranasally sniffed (snorted), and inhaled (i.e., smoked). (For additional details, see the Dextroamphetamine, Methamphetamine, and Mixed Amphetamines monographs.)

Mechanism of CNS Action

Amphetamines are members of the phenylisopropylamine chemical family. They are noncatechol, sympathomimetic amines. The amphetamines have potent actions on both the central and peripheral nervous systems. Centrally, their action is similar to that of the endogenous catecholamine neurotransmitters: the biogenic amines dopamine, epinephrine, norepinephrine, and serotonin. Compared with ephedrine and other catecholamines, the amphetamines produce greater CNS stimulation (e.g., enhanced alertness, increased psychomotor activity, and suppressed feelings of drowsiness or fatigue). Thus, since the initial synthesis of amphetamines, these actions have made them attractive as performance enhancers to a variety of people, including aircraft pilots, athletes, college and university students, entertainers, long-distance truck drivers, soldiers, and surgeons.

The amphetamines are indirect-acting psychostimulants. As such, they stimulate the release of biogenic amines (e.g., dopamine, norepinephrine, serotonin) from presynaptic nerve terminal storage vesicles in the midbrain and inhibit their reuptake, primarily by blocking the plasmalemmal dopamine transporter and the vesicular monoamine transporter-2. These actions result in CNS stimulation and other expected pharmacologic effects, including abnormal dilation of the pupils (mydriasis), bronchodilation, contraction of the urinary bladder sphincter, increased blood pressure, and loss of appetite (anorexia). The amphetamines also inhibit, to varying degrees, monoamine oxidase. The clinical significance of this action has not been clearly established. A simplified, stylized representation of the principal sites and mechanisms of the psychostimulant action of the amphetamines is shown in Figure 2.

FIGURE 2
Psychostimulant Action of the Amphetamines

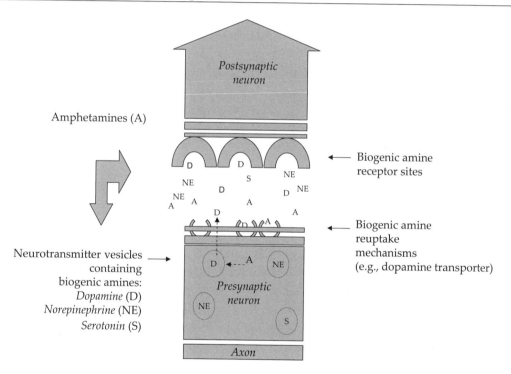

Pharmacodynamics/Pharmacokinetics

The amphetamines are readily absorbed after oral ingestion and are widely distributed in body tissues. They are lipid soluble and thus readily cross the blood–brain barrier after oral ingestion, inhalation (smoking), intravenous injection, or intranasal sniffing (snorting). Urinary excretion is pH dependent; amphetamine elimination is increased in acidic urine and decreased in alkaline urine. Thus, regular, long-term amphetamine users commonly consume oral antacids (e.g., Tums® [calcium carbonate]), which alkalinize their urine, to both enhance and prolong the pharmacologic actions of the amphetamines. (See the Dextroamphetamine, Methamphetamine, and Mixed Amphetamines monographs for additional information.)

Current Approved Indications for Medical Use[5]

Attention-deficit/hyperactivity disorder; exogenous obesity; narcolepsy

Desired Action/Reason for Personal Use

Alertness, vigilance or wakefulness; appetite or hunger suppression; decreased fatigue; euphoria; exhilaration (intense); heightened feeling of well-being; physical endurance[6]; rapid flow of ideas; weight maintenance or loss

Toxicity

Acute: Abdominal cramps; agitation; anorexia; anxiety; blurred vision; cardiac dysrhythmias; chills; CNS stimulation; constipation; death, secondary to amphetamine-related accident or homicide; dizziness; dry mouth; flushing; headache; hypertension; increased sex drive; insomnia; mydriasis; myocardial infarction; nausea; nervousness; restlessness; seizures; stroke; sudden death[7]; sweating; tachycardia; talkativeness; tics; tremor; urinary retention; violent behavior

Chronic: Agitation; cardiomyopathy; compulsive, stereotyped grooming behavior; dermatoses, severe; dopamine transporter reduction (and associated cognitive and motor impairment); hallucinations; hepatitis secondary to the use of contaminated needles and syringes, unsafe sex, and activities involving the fecal–oral route; hyperactivity; insomnia, marked; irritability; neurological impairment (e.g., working memory impairment); paranoia; physical dependence; preoccupation with how things work; psychological dependence; psychosis[8]; punding (e.g., taking mechanical things, such as an automobile engine or clock, apart and attempting to put them back together again); stereotypic behavior (persistent repetition of senseless movements, phrases, or words); weight loss

Pregnancy & Lactation: FDA Pregnancy Category C (see Appendix B). Safety of amphetamine use by adolescent girls and women who are pregnant has not been established. Additional valid and reliable data are needed.

Safety of amphetamine use by adolescent girls and women who are breast-feeding has not been established. Amphetamines are excreted in breast milk. Neonates and infants may display expected pharmacologic actions (e.g., irritability, weight loss). Adolescent girls and women who are breast-feeding should not use amphetamines.

Abuse Potential

Physical dependence: High (USDEA Schedule II; high potential for abuse)
Psychological dependence: High

Withdrawal Syndrome

Although an amphetamine withdrawal syndrome has not been specifically identified, available data suggest that abrupt discontinuation after long-term, high-dosage pharmacotherapy, or regular personal use, may result in extreme fatigue, mental depression, and sleep pattern changes on EEG.

Overdosage

Signs and symptoms of acute amphetamine overdosage include agitation, constipation, hallucinations, panic, paranoia, overstimulation, restlessness, rapid respirations (tachypnea), seizures, and tremor. Depression and fatigue usually follow the CNS stimulation. Other signs and symptoms include abdominal cramps, circulatory collapse, diarrhea, dysrhythmias, hypertension or hypotension, nausea, and vomiting. Hyperpyrexia (i.e., elevated body temperature) and rhabdomyolysis (i.e., an acute, sometimes fatal reaction caused by the destruction of skeletal muscle) can also occur. Fatal amphetamine overdosage usually is preceded by convulsions and coma. Acute amphetamine overdosage requires emergency medical support, with attention to increasing amphetamine elimination.[9] There is no known antidote.

Notes

1. The name *amphetamine* was derived by using selected letters of the name of the original chemical structure, *alphamethylphenethylamine*.
2. There are more than 50 species of ephedra, and ephedrine is found in many, including *Ephedra equisetina*, *Ephedra sinica*, and *Ephedra vulgaris*.
3. Ephedrine, a constituent of the medicinal herb *Ma Huang*, was brewed and orally ingested as a tea in ancient China and continues to be widely used today in traditional Chinese medicine.
4. During that period, as today, a significant number, but a minority, of amphetamine users intravenously injected amphetamine. This method of use was known as "shooting crank," or "shooting-up speed." Most users injected the amphetamine into the veins in the antecubital fossa of the anterior forearm. Intravenous sites on the hand, foot, leg, neck, and groin also were commonly used by regular long-term amphetamine users, particularly when their usual injection sites became infected or when their veins became damaged from overuse.
5. Also widely prescribed and used by military personnel in many countries, including the United States, in virtually every war since WW II (1939–1945), when it was first formally used to decrease battle fatigue and increase alertness and vigilance.
6. Amphetamines prolong tolerance to anaerobic metabolism and thus can be of benefit to athletes whose sports require intense anaerobic metabolism (e.g., basketball, cycling, football, and ice-hockey). Use among semiprofessional and professional athletes engaged in these sports, although banned and not recommended because of associated well-known adverse effects, is quite common.
7. Sudden death can occur in children, adolescents, and adults who are using amphetamines. Users with heart defects or other serious heart conditions are at particular risk.
8. Amphetamine-induced psychosis is often clinically indistinguishable from schizophrenia, being differentiated in most cases by a history of amphetamine use. It is frequently characterized by aggressive or violent behavior, hallucinations, and paranoid delusions.
9. Induction of vomiting is generally not recommended because of the risk for precipitating the onset of seizures and resultant aspiration of vomitus or other injury.

References

Anglin, M.D., Burke, C., Perrochet, B., et al. (2000). History of the methamphetamine problem. *Journal of Psychoactive Drugs, 32*(2), 137-141.

Brecht, M.L., von Mayrhauser, C., & Anglin, M.D. (2000). Predictors of relapse after treatment for methamphetamine use. *Journal of Psychoactive Drugs, 32*(2), 211-220.

Caldwell, J.A., & Caldwell, J.L. (2005). Fatigue in military aviation: An overview of US military-approved pharmacological countermeasures. *Aviation, Space, and Environmental Medicine, 76*(7 Supplement), C39-C51.

Chang, L., Ernst, T., Speck, O., et al. (2002). Perfusion MRI and computerized cognitive test abnormalities in abstinent methamphetamine users. *Psychiatry Research, 114*(2), 65-79.

Cho, A.K., & Melega, W.P. (2002). Patterns of methamphetamine abuse and their consequences. *Journal of Addictive Diseases, 21*(1), 21-34.

Darke, S., Ross, J., & Kaye, S. (2001). Physical injecting sites among injecting drug users in Sydney, Australia. *Drug and Alcohol Dependence, 62*(1), 77-82.

Davidson, C., Gow, A.J., Lee, T.H., et al. (2001). Methamphetamine neurotoxicity: Necrotic and apoptotic mechanisms and relevance to human abuse and treatment. *Brain Research. Brain Research Reviews, 36*(1), 1-22.

Fleckenstein, A.E., Volz, T.J., Riddle, E.L., et al. (2007). New insights into the mechanism of action of amphetamines. *Annual Review of Pharmacology and Toxicology, 47*, 681-698.

Forrester, M.B. (2007). Adderall abuse in Texas, 1998-2004. *Journal of Toxicology and Environmental Health, Part A: Current Issues, 70*(7), 658-664.

George, A.J. (2000). Central nervous system stimulants. *Baillière's Best Practice & Research Clinical Endocrinology & Metabolism, 14*(1), 79-88.

Harris, D., & Batki, S.L. (2000). Stimulant psychosis: Symptom profile and acute clinical course. *The American Journal on Addictions, 9*(1), 28-37.

Hutin, Y.J., Sabin, K.M., Hutwagner, L.C., et al. (2000). Multiple modes of hepatitis A virus transmission among methamphetamine users. *American Journal of Epidemiology, 152*(2), 186-192.

Shearer, J., Wodak, A., Mattick, R.P., et al., (2001). Pilot randomized controlled study of dexamphetamine substitution for amphetamine dependence. *Addiction, 96*(9), 1289-1296.

Srisurapanont, M., Jarusuraisin, N., & Kittirattanapaiboon, P. (2001). Treatment for amphetamine withdrawal. *Cochrane Database of Systematic Reviews* (4), CD003021.

Volkow, N.D., Chang, L., Wang, G.J., et al. (2001). Association of dopamine transporter reduction with psychomotor impairment in methamphetamine abusers. *American Journal of Psychiatry, 158*(3), 377-382.

White, R. (2000). Dexamphetamine substitution in the treatment of amphetamine abuse: An initial investigation. *Addiction, 95*(2), 229-238.

Zhu, B.L., Oritani, S., Shimotouge, K., et al. (2000). Methamphetamine-related fatalities in forensic autopsy during 5 years in the southern half of Osaka city and surrounding areas. *Forensic Science International, 113*(1-3), 443-447.

ARECA NUT (See *Betel cutch*)

ARECOLINE (See *Betel cutch*)

ARMODAFINIL

Names

BAN or INN Generic Synonyms: R-Modafinil

Brand/Trade: Nuvigil®

Chemical: z-[(R)-(Diphenylmethyl)sulfinyl]acetamide

Street: None

Pharmacologic Classification

Psychostimulant: miscellaneous

Brief General Overview

Armodafinil is the "r" isomer of modafinil (see Modafinil monograph). In 2007, it was introduced into clinical practice in the United States for the medical management of various sleep disorders, including hypersomnia and narcolepsy (see "Current Approved Indications for Medical Use").

Dosage Forms and Routes of Administration

Armodafinil is produced in North America by licit pharmaceutical manufacturers and is available as an oral tablet. At this time, abuse appears to be primarily restricted to people for whom armodafinil was legitimately prescribed.

Mechanism of CNS Action

Armodafinil's mechanism of action appears to be distinct from those of other psychostimulants, such as cocaine and methamphetamine. The exact mechanism of its CNS action has not been determined, but it appears to primarily involve (1) stimulation of α_1-adrenergic receptors and (2) binding to dopamine transporter (DAT) and consequently inhibiting dopamine reuptake.

Pharmacodynamics/Pharmacokinetics

Armodafinil is readily absorbed following oral ingestion, with peak blood concentration achieved within 2 hours in the fasting state. The ingestion of food delays peak blood concentration by 2 to 4 hours. Armodafinil is moderately bound to plasma proteins (i.e., ~60%) and has a mean apparent volume of distribution of 42 L. It is extensively metabolized in the liver, with less than 10% excreted in unchanged form in the urine. Amide hydrolysis is the major metabolic pathway, with metabolism by CYP3A4/5 being the next major metabolic pathway. The two major resulting metabolites are R-modafinil acid and modafinil sulfone. The half-life of elimination is ~15 hours, and armodafinil's total body clearance is ~33 mL/minute.

Current Approved Indications for Medical Use

Narcolepsy; obstructive sleep apnea/hypopnea syndrome (adjunctive pharmacotherapy)[1]; shift-work sleep disorder

Desired Action/Reason for Personal Use

CNS stimulation (i.e., enhanced alertness, vigilance, and wakefulness); euphoria; feelings of confidence

Toxicity

Acute: Abdominal pain; agitation; anorexia; anxiety; dizziness; dry mouth; headache; insomnia; mental depression; nausea; nervousness; rashes, severe[2]; suicidal ideation; sweating; thirst

Chronic: Psychological dependence

Pregnancy & Lactation: FDA Pregnancy Category C (see Appendix B). Safety of armodafinil use by adolescent girls and women who are pregnant has not been established. Valid and reliable data are needed.

Safety of armodafinil use by adolescent girls and women who are breast-feeding has not been established. It is not known if armodafinil is excreted in breast milk. Valid and reliable data are needed.

Abuse Potential

Physical dependence: Low (USDEA Schedule IV; low potential for abuse)
Psychological dependence: Low

Withdrawal Syndrome

An armodafinil withdrawal syndrome has not been reported.

Overdosage

Signs and symptoms of acute armodafinil overdosage are associated with its CNS stimulant and sympathomimetic actions. These signs and symptoms may include agitation, anxiety, confusion, dizziness, disorientation, excitation, headache, hypertension, insomnia, irritability, nausea, nervousness, palpitations, tachycardia, and tremor. Acute armodafinil overdosage requires emergency medical support with attention to increasing armodafinil elimination. There is no known antidote.

Notes

1. Armodafinil helps alleviate daytime sleepiness but has no effect on sleep apnea.
2. Rashes may be life threatening (rare, < 1%) and include Stevens-Johnson syndrome, or toxic epidermal necrolysis.

References

Dinges, D.F., Arora, S., Darwish, M., et al. (2006). Pharmacodynamic effects on alertness of single doses of armodafinil in healthy subjects during a nocturnal period of acute sleep loss. *Current Medical Research and Opinion, 22*(1), 159-167.

Harsh, J.R., Hayduk, R., Rosenberg, R., et al. (2006). The efficacy and safety of armodafinil as treatment for adults with excessive sleepiness associated with narcolepsy. *Current Medical Research and Opinion, 22*(4), 761-774.

Hirshkowitz, M., Black, J.E., Wesnes, K., et al. (2007). Adjunct armodafinil improves wakefulness and memory in obstructive sleep apnea/hypopnea syndrome. *Respiratory Medicine, 101*(3), 616-627.

Lankford, D.A. (2008). Armodafinil: A new treatment for excessive sleepiness. *Expert Opinion on Investigational Drugs, 17*(4), 565-573.

Nishino, S., & Okuro, M. (2008). Armodafinil for excessive sleepiness. *Drugs Today, 44*(6), 395-414.

Roth, T., White, D., Schmidt-Nowara, W., et al. (2006). Effects of armodafinil in the treatment of residual excessive sleepiness associated with obstructive sleep apnea/hypopnea syndrome: A 12-week, multicenter, double-blind, randomized, placebo-controlled study in nCPAP-adherent adults. *Clinical Therapeutics, 28*(5), 689-706.

ATOMOXETINE

Names

BAN or INN Generic Synonyms: Tomoxetine

Brand/Trade: Strattera®

Chemical: (-)-N-Methyl-3-phenyl-3-(o-tolyloxy)-propylamine

Street: None

Pharmacologic Classification

Psychostimulant, miscellaneous

Brief General Overview

Atomoxetine is a phenylpropanolamine derivative that was approved for use in the United States by FDA in 2002. It is generally considered to be a non-psychostimulant. However, on the basis of its chemical structure and mechanisms of action, we include it in the special category of miscellaneous psychostimulants.[1]

Dosage Forms and Routes of Administration

Atomoxetine is legally produced by pharmaceutical manufacturers in North America. It is generally available in oral capsule form. At this time, abuse appears to be primarily restricted to family members and acquaintances of people for whom atomoxetine has been prescribed.

Mechanism of CNS Action

The exact mechanism of atomoxetine's CNS action has not been determined. However, both atomoxetine and its primary metabolite are active presynaptic selective norepinephrine reuptake inhibitors (i.e., inhibitors of norepinephrine transporter). In addition, they appear to increase dopamine levels in the prefrontal cortex by an as yet unknown mechanism.

Pharmacodynamics/Pharmacokinetics

Atomoxetine is rapidly and moderately absorbed following oral ingestion ($F = 0.63$). Food has minimal effect on its absorption. Atomoxetine is extensively metabolized in the liver by CYP2D6 to its primary active metabolite, 4-hydroxyatomoxetine. It is highly bound to plasma proteins (~98%) and has a volume of distribution of ~0.85 L/kg. Greater than 80% of the atomoxetine dose is excreted in the urine as 4-hydroxyatomoxetine-O-glucuronide. Of the remainder, <17% is excreted in the feces as 4-hydroxyatomoxetine-O-glucuronide and <3% is excreted as unchanged atomoxetine in the urine. The mean elimination half-life of atomoxetine is 5 hours.

   Poor metabolizers of CYP2D6 (i.e., people with reduced activity in the CYP2D6 pathway), who account for <10% of the North American population, have higher plasma concentrations of atomoxetine and a prolonged mean elimination half-life of ~21 hours. The primary metabolite remains 4-hydroxyatomoxetine, which is rapidly glucuronidated.

Current Approved Indications for Medical Use

Attention-deficit/hyperactivity disorder

Desired Action/Reason for Personal Use

Alertness, vigilance or wakefulness; appetite or hunger suppression; decreased fatigue; euphoria (mild)

Toxicity

Acute: Anorexia; blood pressure increase (small); constipation; dizziness; dry mouth; dyspepsia; headache; heart rate, increase (small); insomnia; irritability; motor tic; nausea; seizures (rare); sweating; urinary retention; vomiting

Chronic: Liver damage (hepatitis), severe (rare); suicide-related events (i.e., attempts and/or ideation)

Pregnancy & Lactation: FDA Pregnancy Category "not established." Safety of atomoxetine use by adolescent girls and women who are pregnant has not been established. It is not known if atomoxetine crosses the human placenta. Additional valid and reliable data are needed.

Safety of atomoxetine use by adolescent girls and women who are breast-feeding has not been established. Atomoxetine appears to be excreted in human breast milk. Adolescent girls and women who are breast-feeding should not use atomoxetine.

Abuse Potential

Physical dependence: None to low (USDEA Schedule: not a scheduled drug; low potential for abuse)
Psychological dependence: Low to moderate

Withdrawal Syndrome

An atomoxetine withdrawal syndrome has not been reported.

Overdosage

Signs and symptoms of atomoxetine overdosage include abnormal behavior, agitation, dry mouth, hyperactivity, mydriasis, seizures, and tachycardia. No deaths have been directly attributed to atomoxetine overdosage. Atomoxetine overdosage requires emergency medical support, with attention to increasing atomoxetine elimination. There is no known antidote.

Note

1. Atomoxetine was originally developed as an antidepressant, similar to fluoxetine (Prozac®). However, initial clinical trials failed to demonstrate significant antidepressant efficacy.

References

Eiland, L.S., & Guest, A.L. (2004). Atomoxetine treatment of attention-deficit/hyperactivity disorder. *The Annals of Pharmacotherapy, 38*(1), 86-90.

Heil, S.H., Holmes, H.W., Bickel, W.K., et al. (2002). Comparison of the subjective, physiological, and psychomotor effects of atomoxetine and methylphenidate in light drug users. *Drug and Alcohol Dependence, 67*(2), 149-156.

Jasinski, D.R., Faries, D.E., Moore, R.J., et al. (2008). Abuse liability assessment of atomoxetine in a drug-abusing population. *Drug and Alcohol Dependence, 95*(1-2), 140-146.

Ledbetter, M. (2005). Atomoxetine use associated with onset of a motor tic. *Journal of Child and Adolescent Psychopharmacology, 15*(2), 331-333.

Morrison, H. (2008). Atomoxetine and suicidal behaviour: Update. *Canadian Adverse Reaction Newsletter, 18*(3), 7.

Párraga, H.C., Párraga, M.I., & Harris, D.K. (2007). Tic exacerbation and precipitation during atomoxetine treatment in two children with attention-deficit/hyperactivity disorder. *International Journal of Psychiatry in Medicine, 37*(4), 415-424.

Purper-Ouakil, D., Fourneret, P., Wohl, M., et al. (2005). Atomoxetine: A new treatment for Attention Deficit/Hyperactivity Disorder (ADHD) in children and adolescents. *Encephale, 31*(3), 337-348.

Sears, J., & Patel, N.C. (2008). Development of tics in a thirteen-year-old male following atomoxetine use. *CNS Spectrums, 13*(4), 301-303.

Simpson, D., & Plosker, G.L. (2004). Atomoxetine: A review of its use in adults with attention deficit hyperactivity disorder. *Drugs, 64*(2), 205-222.

Wilens, T.E., Adler, L.A., Weiss, M.D., et al. (2008). Atomoxetine treatment of adults with ADHD and comorbid alcohol use disorders. *Drug and Alcohol Dependence, 96*(1-2), 145-154.

AYAHUASCA (See Harmala alkaloids)

BARBITURATES

Names

BAN or INN Generic Synonyms: None

Brand/Trade: See the individual monographs: Pentobarbital, Phenobarbital, and Secobarbital

Chemical: See the individual monographs: Pentobarbital, Phenobarbital, and Secobarbital

Street: Abbots; Backwards; Barbs; Barbies; Blue Angels; Blue Devils; Blues; Blue Velvet; Chill Pills; Christmas Trees; Dolls; Downers; F-66s; Goofballs; Gorilla Pills; Mexican Yellows; Nembies; Peanuts; Phennies; Pinks; Pink Ladies; Purple Hearts; Rainbows; Red Bullets; Red Devils; Red Jackets; Reds; Secs; Seggy; Sex; Sleepers; Stoppers; Stumble-Bumbles; Tooies; Twos; Whites; Yellow Jackets; Yellows

Pharmacologic Classification

Psychodepressant, sedative-hypnotic: barbiturate

Brief General Overview

Chemically, the barbiturates are members of the family of substituted pyrimidines. They are structurally derived from barbituric acid, which has no intrinsic CNS activity of its own. The barbiturates are generally grouped into four categories according to the duration of their psychodepressant actions: (1) ultrashort-acting, 15 minutes to 3 hours (e.g., thiopental [Pentothal®]); (2) short-acting, 3 to 6 hours (e.g., amobarbital [Amytal®], pentobarbital [Nembutal®], secobarbital [Seconal®]); (3) intermediate-acting, 6 to 12 hours (e.g., butabarbital); and (4) long-acting, 12 to 24 hours (e.g., phenobarbital).

During the 1950s, 1960s, and 1970s, people who abused the barbiturates commonly "overused" their prescribed barbiturate capsules and tablets, maintaining their supplies by frequently obtaining early refills. During the same period, "street use" of the barbiturates was primarily by users who intravenously injected illicitly diverted barbiturate capsules. The intravenous injection of the highly alkaline barbiturates placed users at significant risk for gangrene and loss of the injected limb if the injection was inadvertently made into an artery instead of a vein.[1] During the 1970s, the commercial introduction of the benzodiazepines increased and, by the end of the 20th century, the medical use of the barbiturates largely disappeared along with their illicit use.

Dosage Forms and Routes of Administration

The barbiturates are produced by licit pharmaceutical manufacturers and are available in a wide variety of dosage formulations, including injectables (for intramuscular and intravenous use); oral capsules, elixirs, and tablets; and rectal suppositories. Users divert legitimate supplies of the barbiturates by a variety of means (e.g., "double-doctoring," burglary of pharmacies).

Mechanism of CNS Action

The barbiturates depress the sensory cortex, decrease motor activity, and alter cerebellar function. In addition, they can produce, through their dose-related psychodepressant action, all levels of CNS depression, ranging from mild sedation and hypnosis to anesthesia, deep coma, and death. However, the exact mechanisms by which barbiturates achieve their psychodepressant actions have not been determined.

A current theory that is helpful in explaining the mechanisms of action of the barbiturates is that they bind to receptor sites adjacent to the gamma-aminobutyric acid (GABA) receptor. This binding results in the retention of GABA at its receptor and an increased influx of chloride ions through the associated chloride ion channels, which produces neuronal inhibition. This proposed mechanism of action is similar to that proposed for the action of the benzodiazepines (see monograph), with the exception that each of the two classes of sedative-hypnotics acts at distinct receptor sites that probably are adjacent to the GABA receptor site and surround the chloride ion channel. A simplified, stylized representation of the principal sites and mechanisms of the psychodepressant action of the barbiturates is shown in Figure 3.

Of clinical significance, the barbiturates induce the production of drug-metabolizing enzymes in the liver and are thus referred to as hepatic enzyme inducers. These enzymes (i.e., the cytochrome P450 hepatic microsomal isoenzymes) are responsible for the metabolism of several other classes of drugs, including the barbiturates themselves (i.e.,

FIGURE 3
Psychodepressant Action of the Barbiturates

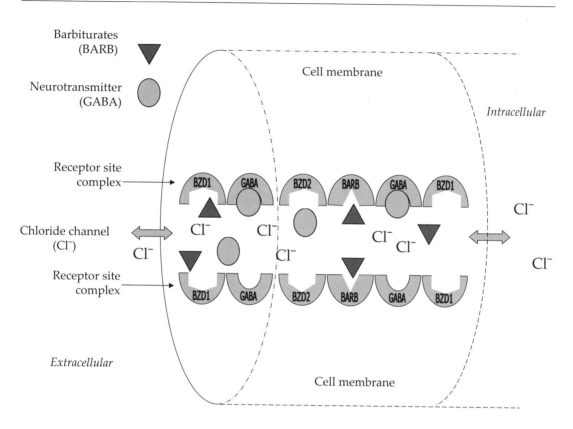

the barbiturates stimulate [auto-induce] their own metabolism). Because the barbiturates are hepatic enzyme inducers, their concomitant use can affect the dosing requirements of other drugs or substances that are metabolized by the liver. For example, concomitant use of a barbiturate can necessitate an increase in the dosage of another drug (e.g., warfarin [Coumadin®]) to obtain its desired action (appropriate degree of anticoagulation). Similarly, when use of the barbiturate is discontinued, a decrease in the dosage of the other drug is usually required in order to avoid toxicity (e.g., hemorrhage in the example of concomitant warfarin use). Because of hepatic enzyme autoinduction, the barbiturates, when used chronically, have a shorter duration of action, so a larger dosage is needed to obtain the desired effects (i.e., tolerance develops).

Pharmacodynamics/Pharmacokinetics

Barbiturates display wide variability in regard to absorption after oral ingestion. The onset of action generally occurs within 10 to 60 minutes. They are rapidly distributed to all body fluids and tissues, and, because they are weak acids, they achieve high concentrations in the brain, kidney, and liver. Their lipid solubility is the main factor in their wide distribution. Barbiturates are bound to plasma and tissue proteins. The degree of binding associated with the various barbiturates also is a direct function of their lipid solubility. Thiopental, which is used as a general anesthetic, is the most lipid-soluble barbiturate and is ~65% plasma protein bound. Duration of action, which is related to the rate of distribution throughout the body, varies among patients and in the same patient from time to time. Barbiturates are metabolized primarily by the hepatic microsomal enzyme system. The inactive metabolites are excreted as conjugates of glucuronic acid. These metabolites are excreted in the urine and, to a lesser extent, in the feces. See the individual barbiturate monographs (Pentobarbital, Phenobarbital, and Secobarbital) for additional information.

Current Approved Indications for Medical Use

Anxiety disorders; seizure disorders (partial and tonic–clonic seizures); sleep disorders (insomnia)

Desired Action/Reason for Personal Use

Alcohol-like disinhibitory euphoria or "high"; anxiety/stress reduction; prevention/self-management of the barbiturate withdrawal syndrome

Toxicity[2]

Acute: Angioedema; apnea; arthralgia; bradycardia; cognitive impairment; coughing; exfoliative dermatitis; fever; headache; hyperkinesia; hypotension; laryngospasm; memory impairment; myalgia; nystagmus, sustained; psychomotor impairment; slurred speech; somnolence; syncope; unsteady gait

Chronic: Confusion; chronic fatigue; hepatic damage; impaired judgment; irritability; insomnia; mental depression; physical dependence; psychological dependence; psychomotor impairment; reduced sex drive; suppression of REM sleep

Pregnancy & Lactation: FDA Pregnancy Category D (see Appendix B). Barbiturate use during pregnancy has been associated with congenital malformations (i.e., birth defects). After ingestion, barbiturates readily cross the placental barrier and are distributed throughout the placenta and embryonic and fetal tissues. The highest concentration is found in the brain and the liver. The use of barbiturates during pregnancy also has been associated with a significantly increased rate of hemorrhagic disease of the newborn. Generally, this disorder is readily correctable with appropriate vitamin K_1 (phytonadione) pharmacotherapy for the neonate. Neonates born to mothers who used barbiturates throughout the last trimester of pregnancy also may display signs and symptoms of the barbiturate withdrawal syndrome, such as irritability and seizures. Delayed onset of these signs and symptoms of withdrawal may occur up to 14 days after delivery. Adolescent girls and women who are pregnant should not use barbiturates.

Safety of barbiturate use by adolescent girls and women who are breast-feeding has not been established. Small amounts of barbiturates are excreted in breast milk. However, the breast milk concentrations may be sufficient to cause expected pharmacologic actions in breast-fed neonates and infants, including drowsiness and lethargy. Concentrations also may be sufficient both to cause physical dependence in breast-fed neonates and infants and to stimulate hepatic microsomal enzyme metabolism. Adolescent girls and women who are breast-feeding should not use barbiturates.

Abuse Potential

Physical dependence: High (USDEA Schedule II or III; high or moderate, respectively, potential for abuse)
Psychological dependence: High

Withdrawal Syndrome

Abrupt discontinuation of regular long-term barbiturate use may result in the barbiturate withdrawal syndrome, signs and symptoms of which may be fatal and include convulsions and delirium. The signs and symptoms of barbiturate withdrawal may begin as early as 12 to 24 hours after the barbiturate was last used and usually peak in 1 to 7 days. The barbiturate withdrawal syndrome tends to be more severe when higher dosages are used and when short- or intermediate-acting barbiturates are used. Regular long-term barbiturate use should be discontinued gradually.

Phenobarbital substitution is often used to medically manage short- or intermediate-acting barbiturate withdrawal, in much the same way as diazepam substitution is used to medically manage alcohol or short-acting benzodiazepine withdrawal. Phenobarbital is beneficial for this use because, as a long-acting barbiturate, it causes less fluctuation in blood concentration during withdrawal, has a higher therapeutic index, produces signs and symptoms of toxicity (e.g., ataxia, slurred speech, nystagmus) that are more easily recognized and treated, and is not usually associated with disinhibition euphoria, which makes it much less likely to be abused.

Overdosage[3]

The ingestion of 1 gram (1000 mg) of most barbiturates produces serious overdosage in adults. The signs and symptoms of barbiturate overdosage may be confused with alcohol intoxication or various neurological disorders. Generally, the ingestion of 2 to 10 grams of barbiturates is fatal. The signs and symptoms of acute barbiturate overdosage include CNS and respiratory depression, which may progress to Cheyne-Stokes respirations, areflexia, slightly constricted pupils (in severe overdosage, pupils may show paralytic dilation), decreased urine production (oliguria), tachycardia, hypotension, lowered body temperature, and coma. A typical shock syndrome (i.e., apnea, circulatory collapse, respiratory arrest, and death) may occur. In addition to other complications (e.g., pneumonia), extreme barbiturate overdosage may result in cessation of all electrical activity in the brain. This effect is reportedly fully reversible unless hypoxia-induced damage has occurred. Barbiturate overdosage requires emergency medical support, with attention to increasing barbiturate elimination. There is no known antidote.

Notes

1. The alkaline pH of the dissolved barbiturate capsules is such that injection into an artery can cause severe arterial spasms. These spasms, in turn, can result in loss of adequate blood supply to the associated limb or digit distal to the site of injection and, consequently, gangrene.
2. Users are at particular risk for accidental injuries, including falls, motor vehicle crashes, and power tool injuries, because of the actions of the barbiturates on the CNS that result in both cognitive and psychomotor impairment.
3. The use of a barbiturate, as well as barbiturate overdosage, may occur unknowingly to the user—for example, when street heroin is adulterated ("cut") with barbiturates or when barbiturate-containing

analgesic combination products, such as Fiorinal® (which contains aspirin, butalbital, and caffeine), are used without careful attention to the contents of the combination product.

References

Adlaf, E.M., Paglia, A., Ivis, F.J., et al. (2000). Nonmedical drug use among adolescent students: Highlights from the 1999 Ontario Student Drug Survey. *CMAJ: Canadian Medical Association Journal, 162*(12), 1677-1680.

Holbrook, I., Sinclair, M., Turley, P., et al. (2001). Positive screening tests for barbiturates in urine samples in the York area over a 1-year period. *Annals of Clinical Biochemistry, 38*(Part 5), 559-560.

Loder, E., & Biondi, D. (2003). Oral phenobarbital loading: A safe and effective method of withdrawing patients with headache from butalbital compounds. *Headache, 43*(8), 904-909.

McLean, W., Boucher, E.A., Brennan, M., et al. (2000). Is there an indication for the use of barbiturate-containing analgesic agents in the treatment of pain? Guidelines for their safe use and withdrawal management. Canadian Pharmacists Association. *Canadian Journal of Clinical Pharmacology, 7*(4), 191-197.

Romero, C.E., Baron, J.D., Knox, A.P., et al. (2004). Barbiturate withdrawal following Internet purchase of Fioricet. *Archives of Neurology, 61*(7), 1111-1112.

Tobias, J.D. (2000). Tolerance, withdrawal, and physical dependence after long-term sedation and analgesia of children in the pediatric intensive care unit. *Critical Care Medicine, 28*(6), 2122-2132.

Vetulani, J. (2001). Drug addiction. Part I. Psychoactive substances in the past and present. *Polish Journal of Pharmacology, 53*(3), 201-214.

BENZENE (See Volatile solvents & inhalants)

BENZODIAZEPINES

Names

BAN or INN Generic Synonyms: None

Brand/Trade: See the individual benzodiazepine monographs: Alprazolam, Bromazepam, Chlordiazepoxide, Clonazepam, Diazepam, Estazolam, Flunitrazepam, Flurazepam, Lorazepam, Nitrazepam, Oxazepam, Temazepam, and Triazolam

Chemical: See the individual benzodiazepine monographs

Street: Benzoids; Benzos; Candy Downers; Chill Pills; Downers; Gone Time; Goofers; Jellies; *La Rocha*; Tranks; Tranqs; Tranx[1]

Pharmacologic Classification

Psychodepressant, sedative-hypnotic: benzodiazepine

Brief General Overview

The benzodiazepines are the most widely prescribed class of psychoactive drugs in the world. Because of their therapeutic efficacy, high therapeutic index, and lower abuse potential, they are clinically preferred over other sedative-hypnotics—including the barbiturates, which they have virtually replaced over the past 50 years. Unfortunately, many benzodiazepine users develop problematic patterns of use.

Most people begin to use benzodiazepines when they are prescribed for the symptomatic management of a benzodiazepine-responsive medical disorder (e.g., anxiety disorder; sleep disorder). However, when regular, short-term use exceeds 30 days, the potential for both physical and psychological dependence increases. These users generally find that they need their prescribed benzodiazepine more often and sometimes at a higher dosage, for a longer period of time. They also may use their benzodiazepine in combination with other drugs and substances of abuse, including alcohol, cannabis (marijuana), and opiate analgesics. For example, a common combination, referred to "on the street" as "Tem-Tems," is temazepam and buprenorphine (see monograph).

Reportedly, alprazolam (Xanax®), clonazepam (Rivotril®), and diazepam (Valium®) are the most frequently abused benzodiazepines in North America. Women and the elderly account for the majority of people who display problematic patterns of use. People who have alcoholism and problematic patterns of polydrug use are also at particularly high risk. These users can be characterized by two distinct patterns of use: (1) regular, long-term relatively low dosage oral use; and (2) short-term high dosage intravenous use.

Dosage Forms and Routes of Administration

The benzodiazepines are widely available from several licit pharmaceutical manufacturers in a number of injectable, oral, rectal, and sublingual dosage forms. All of the dosage forms are associated with the development of problematic patterns of benzodiazepine use. However, in North America, the oral dosage form is most often used, followed by the injectable dosage form, and the drugs are usually obtained by medical prescription or over the Internet. In addition to oral ingestion, some users may grind the oral dosage form to a fine powder for intranasal sniffing (i.e., snorting).

Mechanism of CNS Action

The benzodiazepines cause dose-related CNS depression ranging from mild impairment of cognitive and psychomotor functions to hypnosis. They appear to act at the benzodiazepine receptors (types 1 and 2 [BZD-1 and BZD-2]). These receptors are found at several sites in the CNS, particularly in the cerebral cortex and the limbic system. The benzodiazepine receptors are found primarily in conjunction with the GABA-receptor complex and predominantly in association with the $GABA_A$ receptor.[2] Thus, it appears that the benzodiazepines elicit their pharmacologic actions by potentiating the actions of GABA, a major inhibitory neurotransmitter, within the CNS.[3] A simplified, stylized representation of the principal sites and mechanisms of action of the benzodiazepines is shown in Figure 4.

Pharmacodynamics/Pharmacokinetics

The benzodiazepines are generally well absorbed after oral ingestion. Food can sometimes delay the rate, but generally not the extent, of absorption. Some benzodiazepines (e.g., flurazepam) undergo extensive first-pass hepatic metabolism. The benzodiazepines

FIGURE 4
Psychodepressant Action of the Benzodiazepines

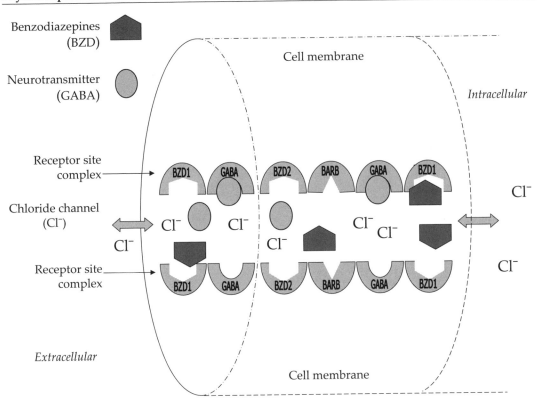

are highly bound to plasma proteins and are widely distributed throughout body tissues. The benzodiazepines and their metabolites readily cross the blood–brain and placental barriers, and they are excreted in breast milk.

Most benzodiazepines are metabolized mainly by the hepatic microsomal enzyme system. Therefore, liver dysfunction can significantly affect metabolism and predispose patients to toxicity. Exceptions include lorazepam, oxazepam, and temazepam, which are metabolized primarily by urinary conjugation to more water-soluble (i.e., polar) glucuronide derivatives that are subsequently excreted in the urine.

On the basis of their duration of action, the benzodiazepines are commonly classified as short-acting (i.e., triazolam), intermediate-acting (i.e., alprazolam, bromazepam, lorazepam, oxazepam, and temazepam), and long-acting (i.e., chlordiazepoxide, clorazepate, diazepam, and flurazepam). The duration of action is generally well correlated with the volume of distribution of the various benzodiazepines, which in turn is correlated with their degree of lipid solubility. See the individual benzodiazepine monographs for additional information.

Current Approved Indications for Medical Use

Anxiety disorders, short-term symptomatic management generally less than 30 days; seizure disorders; sleep disorders: insomnia, short-term systematic management generally fewer than 10 consecutive nights; substance-related disorders: alcohol withdrawal,[4] prevention/management of the alcohol withdrawal syndrome[5]

Desired Action/Reason for Personal Use

Alcohol-like disinhibitory euphoria or "high"; anxiety/stress reduction; also, purposely administered to others without their knowledge in the context of perpetration of a drug-facilitated crime (e.g., robbery; sexual assault, including date rape)

Toxicity[6,7]

Acute: Amnesia, particularly anterograde; ataxia; inattentiveness; blurred vision; cognitive impairment; confusion; diplopia; dizziness; drowsiness; dysarthria; memory impairment, particularly episodic, or explicit, and short-term; muscle weakness; psychomotor impairment; slurred speech; somnolence; vertigo

Chronic: Apathy; emotional instability; lethargy; memory impairment; mental depression; physical dependence; psychological dependence; rebound anxiety; rebound insomnia

Pregnancy & Lactation: FDA Pregnancy Category D (see Appendix B). The benzodiazepines readily cross the placental barrier and often achieve fetal blood concentrations that are equal to or higher than maternal blood concentrations. Regular, long-term maternal use of benzodiazepines during pregnancy or use near term may result in the neonatal benzodiazepine withdrawal syndrome characterized by hypotonia ("floppy baby syndrome"), poor sucking behavior, reduced Apgar scores, respiratory depression, and tremor. Maternal use during labor may be associated with expected psychodepressant pharmacologic actions including neonatal sedation and respiratory depression. Adolescent girls and women who are pregnant should not use benzodiazepines.

Benzodiazepines are excreted in breast milk, generally in concentrations sufficient to cause sedation and potential physical dependence in breast-fed neonates and infants. The benzodiazepine withdrawal syndrome may occur in breast-fed infants if their mothers discontinue regular, long-term benzodiazepine pharmacotherapy, or regular personal use, or if they discontinue breast-feeding. Adolescent girls and women who are breast-feeding should not use benzodiazepines.

Abuse Potential

Physical dependence: Low to moderate (USDEA Schedule IV; low potential for abuse)
Psychological dependence: Moderate to high

Withdrawal Syndrome

A withdrawal syndrome has been associated with abrupt discontinuation of regular long-term benzodiazepine pharmacotherapy or regular personal use. Signs and symptoms range from mild dysphoria and rebound anxiety and insomnia to more severe signs and symptoms such as abdominal and muscle cramps, delirium, hallucinations, nightmares, paranoid ideation, sweating, toxic psychosis, and tremors. Signs and symptoms of the benzodiazepine withdrawal syndrome have included life-threatening seizures at dosages within the recommended range for some benzodiazepines (e.g., alprazolam [Xanax®]). People who have histories of seizure disorders are at particular risk for seizures. The severity and duration of the withdrawal syndrome appear to be related to the dosage and duration of benzodiazepine pharmacotherapy or regular personal use.

Signs and symptoms of the benzodiazepine withdrawal syndrome have been associated with rapid reductions in dosage and abrupt discontinuation of use. Therefore, rapid reductions in dosage and abrupt discontinuation of use should be avoided when possible. The signs and symptoms of benzodiazepine withdrawal involving short- or intermediate-acting benzodiazepines may be managed by resumption of benzodiazepine use or a medically planned withdrawal program. Withdrawal programs usually involve replacing the shorter-acting benzodiazepine (e.g., alprazolam [Xanax®], midazolam [Versed®], or triazolam [Halcion®]) with a long-acting benzodiazepine (e.g., diazepam [Valium®]). The dosage is then gradually reduced over a specified period of time to minimize or prevent signs and symptoms of withdrawal until the benzodiazepine is no longer needed.[8]

Minor signs and symptoms of benzodiazepine withdrawal generally peak within 3 to 7 days following discontinuation of use and dissipate within 2 to 4 weeks. These signs and symptoms usually can be managed without medical intervention. However, the onset of the withdrawal syndrome and its duration depend on the particular benzodiazepine used, its pattern of use (i.e., dosage used, length of time used, and regularity of use), and its half-life of elimination. For example, signs and symptoms of withdrawal may not begin until up to 3 weeks after discontinuing the use of a long-acting benzodiazepine, such as diazepam (see monograph; also see related discussion in "Pregnancy & Lactation").

Overdosage

Signs and symptoms of benzodiazepine overdosage include coma, confusion, diminished reflexes, incoordination, and somnolence. Respiratory arrest is more common with short-acting benzodiazepines (e.g., alprazolam [Xanax®], midazolam [Versed®], and triazolam [Halcion®]). Benzodiazepine overdosage is usually not fatal, because the benzodiazepines possess a high LD_{50}. However, fatalities commonly occur when overdosages involve the use of benzodiazepines in combination with alcohol or opiate analgesics. Benzodiazepine overdosage requires emergency medical support of body systems, with attention to increasing benzodiazepine elimination. The benzodiazepine receptor antagonist flumazenil (Anexate®, Romazicon®) may be required.[9]

Notes

1. During the 1950s, pharmaceutical advertisers coined the term "tranquilizer" for the benzodiazepines specifically to promote their use as the "new wonder drugs." Strong advertising campaigns were developed to convince both patients and their physicians that these drugs were indicated to provide relief from the everyday stresses of modern life (i.e., to make hectic lives more tranquil) and, as a result, the drugs became commonly known as "tranquilizers" by patients and health care professionals alike. The advertising campaigns were so successful that the benzodiazepines became the top selling drugs across North America for three decades.

   However, pharmacologically, the benzodiazepines should be referred to only as sedative-hypnotics. The only "tranquilizers" that have ever been available for clinical use are the "antipsychotic tranquilizers" (e.g., chlorpromazine [Thorazine®], clozapine [Clozaril®], haloperidol [Haldol®]), which we prefer to call antipsychotics for pharmacologic reasons.

2. The α-1 subunit of the $GABA_A$ receptor has a preponderance of BZD-1 receptors, while the α-2, α-3, and α-5 subunits have a preponderance of BZD-2 receptors.

3. They purportedly do so by binding to the benzodiazepine receptors within the GABA receptor complex. Thus, allosterically, they appear to change the conformation of the complex and increase the affinity for GABA, which is the major inhibitory neurotransmitter in the CNS.

4. Benzodiazepine pharmacotherapy should be initiated only after alcohol use has been discontinued. People who have alcohol use disorders are at particular risk for the development of benzodiazepine dependence (both physical and psychological).
5. It is estimated that up to 40% of North Americans who have an alcohol abuse disoder have abused benzodiazepines at some point, often to ameliorate the alcohol withdrawal syndrome.
6. Intravenous use of benzodiazepines carries the risk of significant morbidity directly associated with injection of the drugs, including abscesses and infections at injection sites; deep vein thrombosis; gangrene, which may require partial or complete amputation of the involved extremity; hepatitis B and C; HIV infection; thrombophlebitis; and tissue necrosis.
7. Users are at particular risk for accidental injuries, including falls, motor vehicle crashes, and power tool injuries because of the psychodepressant actions of the benzodiazepines that result in both cognitive and psychomotor impairment.
8. An equivalent daily dosage of diazepam is often therapeutically substituted for the benzodiazepine being discontinued. This dosage is gradually reduced every 2 weeks, as tolerated, until completely discontinued.
9. Caution is required because flumazenil antagonism may precipitate the benzodiazepine withdrawal syndrome in people who are physically dependent on benzodiazepines.

References

Barbanoj, M.J., Urbano, G., Antonijoan, R., et al. (2007). Different acute tolerance development to EEG, psychomotor performance and subjective assessment effects after two intermittent oral doses of alprazolam in healthy volunteers. *Neuropsychobiology, 55*(3-4), 203-212.

Bateson, A.N. (2002). Basic pharmacologic mechanisms involved in benzodiazepine tolerance and withdrawal. *Current Pharmaceutical Design, 8*(1), 5-21.

Lane, S.D., Cherek, D.R., & Nouvion, S.O. (2008). Modulation of human risky decision making by flunitrazepam. *Psychopharmacology, 196*(2), 177-188.

Licata, S.C., & Rowlett, J.K. (2008). Abuse and dependence liability of benzodiazepine-type drugs: GABA$_A$ receptor modulation and beyond. *Pharmacology Biochemistry and Behavior, 90*(1), 74-89.

Longo, L.P., & Johnson, B. (2000). Addiction: Part I. Benzodiazepines—side effects, abuse risk and alternatives. *American Family Physician, 61*, 2121-2128.

Malcolm, R.J. (2003). GABA systems, benzodiazepines, and substance dependence. *The Journal of Clinical Psychiatry, 64*(Suppl 3), 36-40.

Mintzer, M.Z., & Griffiths, R.R. (2007). A triazolam/amphetamine dose-effect interaction study: Dissociation of effects on memory versus arousal. *Psychopharmacology, 192*(3), 425-440.

Neutal, C.I. (2005). The epidemiology of long-term benzodiazepine use. *International Review of Psychiatry, 17*(3), 189-197.

Puustinen, J., Nurminen, J., Kukola, M., et al. (2007). Associations between use of benzodiazepines or related drugs and health, physical abilities and cognitive function: A non-randomized clinical study in the elderly. *Drugs & Aging, 24*(12), 1045-1059.

Rowlett, J.K., Duke, A.N., & Platt, D.M. (2007). Abuse and dependence liability of GABA$_A$-receptor modulators. In S.J. Enna & H. Möhler (Eds.), *The GABA Receptors* (3rd ed., (pp. 143-168). Totowa, NJ: Humana.

Smith, T.H. (2001). Type A gamma-aminobutyric acid (GABAA) receptor subunits and benzodiazepine binding: Significance to clinical syndromes and their treatment. *British Journal of Biomedical Science, 58*(2), 111-121.

Stewart, S.H., & Westra, H.A. (2002). Benzodiazepine side-effects: From the bench to the clinic. *Current Pharmaceutical Design, 8*(1), 1-3.

BETEL CUTCH

Names

BAN or INN Generic Synonyms: None

Brand/Trade: None in North America

Chemical: See "Mechanism of Action"

Street: *Amaska*; *Areca* Nut; *Areca Quid*; *Arequier*; *Betal*; *Betal Quid*; *Betel* Nut; *Betel Quid*; *Catechu*; *Cutch*; *Gutkha*; *Hmarg*; *Maag*; Marg; *Mawa*; *Paan*; Pan; *Pan Masala*; *Pinang*; *Pinlang*; *Pugua*; *Quid*; *Supai*; *Ugam*

Pharmacologic Classification

Psychostimulant, miscellaneous: pyridine alkaloids (natural)

Brief General Overview

Betel cutch (*betel quid*, *betel* nut, *paan*, or *quid*) is composed of the nut of the acacia palm (*Areca catechu*), the leaf of the *betel* pepper (*Piper betel*), and calcium hydroxide (lime).[1] It is chewed on a regular basis by over 600 million people worldwide (i.e., one-tenth of the world's population), particularly in Cambodia, Fiji, Guam, India, Malaysia, New Guinea, Pakistan, the Philippines, and Taiwan. Copious amounts of bright red saliva are produced when it is chewed. *Betel cutch* is the fourth most used psychoactive substance in the world after alcohol, caffeine, and nicotine (i.e., tobacco).

Dosage Forms and Routes of Administration

Betel cutch is either freshly prepared directly by the user or, quite commonly, purchased, much like fast food, from a *betel cutch* stand where it is prepared for ready use.[2] It is generally prepared in one of two ways: The fresh *betel* nut[3] is simply wrapped in a *betel* leaf (*Piper chavica betel*), or a *betel* leaf and some lime paste (slaked lime)[4] are sandwiched between the two halves of a cut *betel* nut. Chewing *betel cutch*, a practice common among adolescents and young adults, mostly males, usually begins as a cultural or ethnic social norm.[5] However, the practice is often accompanied by the development of physical and psychological dependence. The unnecessary morbidity and mortality related to the use of *betel cutch*, and the associated excessive ingestion of tannin, is staggering in many developing countries.[6]

Mechanism of CNS Action

The exact mechanism of the psychostimulant action of *betel cutch* has not been determined. However, its action is believed to be primarily due to the pyridine alkaloids found in *betel* nut, particularly arecoline. Arecoline, which is a ganglionic stimulant and a parasympathomimetic, binds as an agonist to both muscarinic and nicotinic acetylcholine receptors.

Pharmacodynamics/Pharmacokinetics

Valid and reliable data are not available.

Current Approved Indications for Medical Use[7]

None

Desired Action/Reason for Personal Use

Alertness; arousal of sexual desire; euphoria; generalized sensation of warmth; psychostimulation (mild)

Toxicity

Acute: Asthma, exacerbation; blurred vision; cardiac dysrhythmias; cholinergic actions (e.g., salivation, sweating, urinary incontinence); diarrhea; dizziness; dyspnea; flushing; hypotension; increased appetite[8]; mydriasis; myocardial infarction (rare); nausea; psychosis, acute; tachycardia; vomiting

Chronic: Cholinergic crisis; diabetes mellitus; gum recession; hepatic cancer; hypertension; kidney disease; leukoplakia; metabolic syndrome; milk-alkali syndrome; oral cancers; oral lichenoid lesion; oral submucosa fibrosis; pharyngeal cancers; physical dependence; psychological dependence; squamous cell carcinoma; staining of oral mucosa; tooth staining, red-brown to black

Pregnancy & Lactation: Available data suggest slightly reduced birth weight, as with other mild psychostimulants, including caffeine (see monograph). Additional valid and reliable data are needed.

Abuse Potential

Physical dependence: Moderate (USDEA: not a scheduled drug)
Psychological dependence: Moderate

Withdrawal Syndrome

Valid and reliable data are not available.

Overdosage

Betel cutch overdosage can be fatal as a result of significant cholinergic and related cardiovascular effects.[9] Severe cases of overdosage require emergency medical support. There is no known antidote. Additional valid and reliable data are needed.

Notes

1. Other common ingredients, which are dependent on local custom and individual user taste and preference, include smokeless (chewing) tobacco and spices (e.g., anise seed, cardamom, cinnamon, clove, fennel, and nutmeg).
2. In most countries where *betel cutch* is commonly used, its production, purchase or sale, and use are legal. For example, in Taiwan, curbside dealers legally prepare and sell fresh *betel cutch* to passing motorists in a way similar to the sale of newspapers or hot dogs from the curbside in most major North American cities.
3. In many countries, the *betel* nut is dried, cured, and flavored prior to use.

4. The lime (calcium hydroxide) is often obtained by burning coral or seashells.
5. Use in North America is uncommon, except by recent immigrants, because (1) *betel nuts* are not native to North America and thus the supply is limited; (2) users prefer freshly prepared *betel cutch*; and (3) North Americans generally find the copious blood-red saliva produced by *betel cutch* chewing to be unaesthetic.
6. *Betel* nut is very high in tannins. Immature nuts may contain up to 50% tannins; levels tend to decrease as the nut matures. Processed mature *betel* nuts typically contain ~10% tannins. Tannins are believed to be the primary carcinogen in *betel cutch*.
7. Traditionally, *betel cutch* has been used as folk medicine to treat a wide range of diseases and conditions, including alcoholism, cough, dysmenorrhea, dyspepsia, impotence, intestinal worms, joint pain, leprosy, and toothache.
8. The increased appetite has been clearly associated with obesity among users, which in turn has been associated with diabetes mellitus, hypertension, and the metabolic syndrome.
9. Probably most likely to occur in users who have preexisting cardiovascular disease or dysfunction.

References

Avon, S.L. (2004). Oral mucosal lesions associated with use of quid. *Journal of the Canadian Dental Association, 70*(4), 244-248.

Chang, M.C., Ho, Y.S., Lee, P.H., et al. (2001). Areca nut extract and arecoline induced the cell cycle arrest but not apoptosis of cultured oral KB epithelial cells: Association of glutathione, reactive oxygen species and mitochondrial membrane potential. *Carcinogenesis, 22*(9), 1527-1535.

Chang, W.C., Hsiao, C.F., Chang, H.Y., et al. (2006). Betel nut chewing and other risk factors associated with obesity among Taiwanese male adults. *International Journal of Obesity, 30*(2), 359-363.

Chou, C.Y., Cheng, S.Y., Liu, J.H., et al. (2008, July 23). Association between betel-nut chewing and chronic kidney disease in men. *Public Health Nutrition*, 1-5.

Deng, J.F., Ger, J., Tsai, W.J., et al. (2001). Acute toxicities of betel nut: Rare but probably overlooked events. *Journal of Toxicology. Clinical Toxicology, 39*(4), 355-360.

Guh, J.Y., Chuang, L.Y., & Chen, H.C. (2006). Betel-quid use is associated with the risk of the metabolic syndrome in adults. *The American Journal of Clinical Nutrition, 83*(6), 1313-1320.

Guy, J.Y., Chen, H.C., Tsai, J.F., et al. (2007). Betel-quid use is associated with heart disease in women. *The American Journal of Clinical Nutrition, 85*(5), 1229-1235.

Kang, I.M., Chou, C.Y., Tseng, Y.H., et al. (2007). Association between betelnut chewing and chronic kidney disease in adults. *Journal of Occupational and Environmental Medicine, 49*(7), 776-779.

Lin, W.Y., Chiu, T.Y., Lee, L.T., et al. (2008). Betel nut chewing is associated with increased risk of cardiovascular disease and all-cause mortality in Taiwanese men. *The American Journal of Clinical Nutrition, 87*(5), 1204-1211.

Núñez-de la Mora, A., Jesmin, F., & Bentley, G.R. (2007). Betel nut use among first and second generation Bangladeshi women in London, UK. *Journal of Immigrant and Minority Health, 9*(4), 299-306.

Parmar, G., Sangman, P., Vashi, P., et al. (2008). Effect of chewing a mixture of areca nut and tobacco on periodontal tissues and oral hygiene status. *Journal of Oral Science, 50*(1), 57-62.

Thomas, S.J., Harris, R., Ness, A.R., et al. (2008). Betel quid not containing tobacco and oral leukoplakia: A report on a cross-sectional study in Papua New Guinea and a meta-analysis of current evidence. *International Journal of Cancer, 123*(8), 1871-1876.

Tsai, Y.S., Lee, K.W., Huang, J.L., et al. (2008). Arecoline, a major alkaloid of areca nut, inhibits p53, represses DNA repair, and triggers DNA damage response in human epithelial cells. *Toxicology, 249*(2-3), 230-237.

Tseng, C.H. (2008). Betel nut chewing is associated with hypertension in Taiwanese type 2 diabetic patients. *Hypertension Research, 31*(3), 417-423.

Yang, M.J., Chung, T.C., Yang, M.J., et al. (2001). Betel quid chewing and risk of adverse birth outcomes among aborigines in eastern Taiwan. *Journal of Toxicology and Environmental Health, Part A: Current Issues, 64*(6), 465-472.

Yang, M.S., Lee, C.H., Chang, S.J., et al. (2008). The effect of maternal betel quid exposure during pregnancy on adverse birth outcomes among aborigines in Taiwan. *Drug and Alcohol Dependence, 95*(1-2), 134-139.

Yap, S.F., Ho, P.S., Kuo, H.C., et al. (2008). Comparing factors affecting commencement and cessation of betel quid chewing behaviour in Taiwanese adults. *BMC Public Health, 8*, 199.

Yen, A.M., Chiu, Y.H., Chen, L.S., et al. (2006). A population-based study of the association between betel-quid chewing and the metabolic syndrome in men. *The American Journal of Clinical Nutrition, 83*(5), 1153-1160.

BROMAZEPAM

Names

BAN or INN Generic Synonyms: None

Brand/Trade: Lectopam®; Lexotan®

Chemical: 7-Bromo-1,3-dihydro-5-(2-pyridyl)-2H-1,4-benzodiazepin-2-one

Street: None

Pharmacologic Classification

Psychodepressant, sedative-hypnotic: benzodiazepine

Brief General Overview

First synthesized in 1969, bromazepam is a "general use" benzodiazepine.

Dosage Forms and Routes of Administration

Bromazepam is available in oral tablet form from licit pharmaceutical manufacturers.[1] People who illicitly use bromazepam generally ingest the tablets orally.

Mechanism of CNS Action

Bromazepam is a benzodiazepine with anxiolytic and sedative actions. It has been demonstrated to impair the initial stage of visual information processing and to significantly increase electrophysiological measures of cortical interhemispheric coherence. Its exact mechanism of psychodepressant action has not been determined, but it appears to work in concert with the inhibitory neurotransmitter GABA. See also the Benzodiazepines monograph.

Pharmacodynamics/Pharmacokinetics

Bromazepam is well and rapidly absorbed from the GI tract after oral ingestion. Peak blood concentrations are achieved within 1 to 4 hours. Its mean elimination half-life is ~12 hours (range, 8 to 19 hours). Bromazepam is metabolized in the liver and is excreted in the urine in the form of conjugated metabolites. It has no active metabolites.

Current Approved Indications for Medical Use

Anxiety disorders

Desired Action/Reason for Personal Use

Alcohol-like disinhibitory euphoria or "high" (relatively mild); anxiety/stress reduction; also, purposely administered to others without their knowledge in the context of the perpetration of a drug-facilitated crime (e.g., robbery; sexual assault, including date rape)

Toxicity

Acute: Ataxia; blurred vision; cognitive impairment; confusion; dizziness; drowsiness; dry mouth; hypotension; hypothermia; mental depression; muscle weakness; pruritus; slurred speech; tachycardia

Chronic: Physical dependence; psychological dependence

Pregnancy & Lactation: FDA Pregnancy Category "not established." Safety of bromazepam use by adolescent girls and women who are pregnant has not been established. See the Benzodiazepines monograph. Additional valid and reliable data are needed.

Safety of bromazepam use by women who are breast-feeding has not been established. Additional valid and reliable data are needed.

Abuse Potential

Physical dependence: Low to moderate (USDEA: not a scheduled drug)
Psychological dependence: Moderate

Withdrawal Syndrome

A bromazepam withdrawal syndrome similar to the withdrawal syndrome associated with alcohol and other benzodiazepines has been observed upon abrupt discontinuation of regular long-term bromazepam pharmacotherapy or regular personal use. This syndrome is characterized by abdominal cramps, irritability, memory impairment, nervousness, rebound anxiety, and vomiting. Regular long-term use should be discontinued gradually in order to avoid this syndrome.

Overdosage

Signs and symptoms of bromazepam overdosage include drowsiness (excessive), incoordination (ataxia), impaired vision, depressed reflexes, and coma. Hypotension and respiratory depression may occur with overdosages involving large amounts of bromazepam. Bromazepam overdosage requires emergency medical support, with attention to increasing bromazepam elimination. The benzodiazepine antagonist flumazenil (Anexate®, Romazicon®) may be required.[2]

Notes

1. Bromazepam (Lectopam®) is manufactured and used for legitimate medical indications in Canada, but not in the United States.
2. Caution is required because flumazenil antagonism may precipitate the bromazepam withdrawal syndrome in people who are physically dependent on bromazepam.

References

Busto, U.E., Kaplan, H.L., Wright, C.E., et al. (2000). A comparative pharmacokinetic and dynamic evaluation of alprazolam sustained-release, bromazepam, and lorazepam. *Journal of Clinical Psychopharmacology, 20*(6), 628-635.

Michaud, K., Romain, N., Giroud, C., et al. (2001). Hypothermia and undressing associated with non-fatal bromazepam intoxication. *Forensic Science International, 124*(2-3), 112-114.

Puga, F., Sampaio, I., Veiga, H., et al. (2007). The effects of bromazepam on the early stage of visual information processing (P100). *Arquivos de Neuro-psiquiatria, 65*(4A), 955-959.

Sampaio, I., Puga, F., Veiga, H., et al. (2007). Influence of bromazepam on cortical interhemispheric coherence. *Arquivos de Neuro-psiquiatria, 65*(1), 77-81.

Villain, M., Chèze, M., Dumestre, V., et al. (2004). Hair to document drug-facilitated crimes: Four cases involving bromazepam. *Journal of Analytical Toxicology, 28*(6), 516-519.

4-BROMO-2,5-DIMETHOXYPHENETHYLAMINE

Names

BAN or INN Generic Synonyms: 2-Bromo-2,5-diphenoxyphenethylamine

Brand/Trade: None[1]

Chemical: 4-Bromo-2,5-dimethoxyphenethylamine

Street: 2's; 2-CB; 2-CBs; 2C-B; 2C-Bs; A2C-B; A2CBs; BDMPEA; BDMPEAs; Bees; Bromo; Bromos; Erox; MFTs; Nexus; Nexus Jr; Spectrums; Toonies; Two's; Venus

Pharmacologic Classification

Psychodelic, amphetamine-like psychodelic: phenethylamine

Brief General Overview

4-Bromo-2,5-dimethoxyphenethylamine (2C-B) is a psychodelic that was first synthesized in 1974 by Alexander Shulgin as an "entactogen." After a brief period of use, it fell out of vogue and was not commonly used again until approximately 20 years later when Nexus® tablets began to be imported from South Africa. The effects of 2C-B are similar to those produced by other psychodelics but are dependent in large measure on the user's mindset and the setting in which it is used. In addition, the margin of safety of 2C-B (i.e., the difference between a dose that results in a "pleasurable trip" and one that results in a "bad trip") is quite narrow. 2C-B is often misrepresented and sold as 3,4-methylenedioxymethamphetamine (MDMA, Ecstasy; see monograph) because of its relatively narrow therapeutic index. It also is produced in Germany and sold as Erox® tablets that list the active ingredient as a "brominated phenethylamine."

Dosage Forms and Routes of Administration

2C-B is produced by illicit clandestine laboratories across North America.[2] It is generally available in oral gelatin capsules (gel-caps) or oral tablets and is orally ingested.[3] Most users in the United States are adolescents or young adults of European descent, 15 to 30 years of age (i.e., high school and college or university students). 2C-B is considered to be a "club" drug and is most often available in related venues (e.g., raves, "techno parties," and urban nightclubs). It also is commonly available at "circuit parties."[4] Within these contexts, 2C-B is rarely used alone; it is often used with lysergic acid diethylamide (LSD) and MDMA. When used with LSD, the combination is known as a "banana split" and when used with MDMA it is known as a "party pack."

Mechanism of CNS Action

The exact mechanism of 2C-B's psychodelic action has not been determined. However, 2C-B has a high affinity for serotonin receptors in the CNS, and this receptor affinity appears to be central to its mechanism of action.

Pharmacodynamics/Pharmacokinetics

The psychodelic action of 2C-B has its onset 20 to 30 minutes after oral ingestion and generally peaks within 1 to 2 hours. The duration of action is 3 to 8 hours. Additional valid and reliable data are not available.

Current Approved Indications for Medical Use

None

Desired Action/Reason for Personal Use

Diminish impotence or frigidity; empathy; erotic sensual sensations (at lower dosages); euphoria; hallucinations, LSD-like (at higher dosages); perceptual enhancement (i.e., increased receptivity to sensory input); sexual arousal or desire; state of passive relaxation (at lower dosages); synesthesia (e.g., seeing a sound)

Toxicity

Acute: chills; delusions (morbid, with higher dosages); hallucinations (generally terrifying, with higher dosages); hypertension; hyperthermia; nausea; nervousness; tachycardia; trembling

Chronic: Tolerance (associated with 2C-B use more frequently than once per week)

Pregnancy & Lactation: Valid and reliable data are not available.

Abuse Potential

Physical dependence: None to low (USDEA Schedule I; use is prohibited)
Psychological dependence: Low

Withdrawal Syndrome

A 2C-B withdrawal syndrome has not been reported.

Overdosage

No fatalities specifically associated with 2C-B have been reported. There is no known antidote. Additional valid and reliable data are needed.

Notes

1. Although never legally manufactured in North America, 2C-B was produced during the 1990s in South Africa under the brand/trade name Nexus®. Misrepresented as a "natural product," it was imported and distributed legally across North America until it became a controlled substance.
2. It has also been illicitly synthesized and smuggled into the United States from South Africa.
3. It also has been sold in "blotter" or "stamp" transmucosal delivery systems and in powder form for intranasal sniffing (snorting).
4. "Circuit party" is the term used for social gatherings of gay and bisexual men for the purposes of dancing, social interaction, and sex. These "parties" generally take place on weekends and may occur in neighborhood homes (i.e., "local circuit parties") or homes, hotels, and other venues a geographic distance from a participant's own home (i.e., "distant circuit parties").

References

Bell, S.E., Burns, D.T., Dennis, A.C., et al. (2000). Rapid analysis of ecstasy and related phenethylamines in seized tablets by Raman spectroscopy. *Analyst, 125*(3), 541-544.

Carmo, H., Hengstler, J.G, de Boer, D., et al. (2005). Metabolic pathways of 4-bromo-2,5-dimethoxyphenethylamine (2C-B): Analysis of phase I metabolism with hepatocytes of six species including human. *Toxicology, 206*(1), 75-89.

World Health Organization. (2001). WHO expert committee on drug dependence. Thirty-second report. *World Health Organization Technical Report, 903*(1-5), 1-26.

BUPRENORPHINE

Names

BAN or INN Generic Synonyms: None

Brand/Trade: Buprenex®; Subutex®

Chemical: 21-Cyclopropyl-7-α-[(s)-1-hydroxy-1,2,2-trimethylpropyl]-6,14-endo-ethano-6,7,8,14-tetrahydrooripavine

Street: Tems

Pharmacologic Classification

Psychodepressant, opiate analgesic: mixed agonist/antagonist (synthetic)

Brief General Overview

Buprenorphine is a synthetic opiate analgesic that was first synthesized in 1976. It has a mixed agonist/antagonist action. Like methadone (see monograph), it produces cross-tolerance to other opiate analgesics and has thus been used as substitution or replacement therapy for the treatment of illicit heroin use. Its highest abuse liability appears to occur in heroin users who are not opiate dependent (e.g., "chippers").

Dosage Forms and Routes of Administration

Buprenorphine is available in North America from licit pharmaceutical manufacturers in injectable formulations for intramuscular or intravenous use, primarily for pain relief, and as sublingual tablets, primarily for the management of opiate analgesic dependence. A buprenorphine transdermal delivery system also has been developed. Users almost always self-inject buprenorphine intravenously (often in combination with a benzodiazepine). Virtually all of these users are enrolled in, or are associated with, long-term buprenorphine programs for the treatment of their opiate analgesic dependence. Studies indicate that these users reflect the following sociodemographic characteristics: 80% men; 50% European Americans; 25% African Americans; 25% Hispanic Americans; 60% welfare recipients or other social assistance recipients; and 80% with dual diagnoses.[1]

Mechanism of CNS Action

Buprenorphine's exact mechanism of psychodepressant action has not been determined, but it probably exerts its analgesic action by binding to mu-opiate receptors, for which it has high affinity. Although it may be classified as a partial agonist, under conditions for recommended use it acts much like a classic mu agonist such as morphine. However, unlike other opiate analgesic agonists or agonist/antagonists, buprenorphine appears to dissociate from its receptor sites. This unusual dissociation from receptor sites may account for its longer duration of action compared with morphine, unpredictable reversal by opiate analgesic antagonists, and apparently lower potential for the development of physical dependence.

Pharmacodynamics/Pharmacokinetics

Buprenorphine is rapidly, but variably (i.e., 40% to 90%), absorbed after intramuscular injection. Pharmacologic actions after intramuscular injection occur within ~15 minutes. Peak effects are achieved within 1 hour, with analgesic action persisting for 6 hours or longer. Onset and time to peak actions are shortened (i.e., within 30 minutes) with intravenous injection. It is highly (96%) plasma protein bound, primarily to α and β globulins, with little binding to plasma albumin. Its apparent volume of distribution is ~100 L. Buprenorphine is virtually completely metabolized in the liver. It has a mean elimination half-life of ~2 hours (range, 1 to 7 hours) and a total body clearance of 1.3 L/minute.

Current Approved Indications for Medical Use

Pain, moderate to severe; opiate analgesic dependence (substitutive maintenance pharmacotherapy)[2]

Desired Action/Reason for Personal Use

Euphoria; generalized sensation of warmth ("rush"); prevention/self-management of the opiate analgesic withdrawal syndrome[3]

Toxicity

Acute: Bradycardia; cognitive impairment; constipation; dizziness; drowsiness; headache; hypotension; hypoventilation; miosis; nausea; sedation; sweating (excessive); and vomiting. Use of the buprenorphine transdermal delivery system also has been associated with dermatitis, erythema, and pruritus at the application site.

Chronic: Hepatitis (associated with intravenous use); HIV infection (associated with intravenous use); physical dependence; psychological dependence

Pregnancy & Lactation: FDA Pregnancy Category C (see Appendix B). Safety of buprenorphine use by adolescent girls and women who are pregnant has not been established. A mild neonatal buprenorphine abstinence (withdrawal) syndrome characterized by enhanced Moro reflex, shortened periods of sleep after feeding, and tremors commonly occurs within 12 hours of birth and lasts for up to 5 days. Adolescent girls and women who are pregnant, and who are not physically dependent on opiate analgesics, should avoid buprenorphine use.[4]

Safety of buprenorphine use by women who are breast-feeding has not been established. The amount of buprenorphine that is excreted in breast milk is unknown. However, extradural administration of buprenorphine to the mother during cesarean section reportedly suppresses neonatal breast-feeding. As a precaution, adolescent girls and women who are breast-feeding should not use buprenorphine. Additional valid and reliable data are needed.

Abuse Potential

Physical dependence: Moderate (USDEA Schedule III; limited abuse potential)
Psychological dependence: Moderate

Withdrawal Syndrome

A buprenorphine withdrawal syndrome has not been reported. This is most likely because of the mixed opiate analgesic agonist/antagonist action of buprenorphine.[5]

Overdosage[6]

Clinical experience with buprenorphine overdosage is limited in North America. Buprenorphine's antagonist action may be observed at dosages somewhat above the usual recommended dosage. Dosages within the therapeutic range may produce clinically significant respiratory depression in certain patients (e.g., patients who are elderly, frail, or debilitated; those who have respiratory disorders; and young children). Buprenorphine overdosage requires emergency medical support, with attention to maintaining respiratory and cardiovascular function. Mechanical ventilation may be required because the respiratory depression produced by buprenorphine, a partial opiate analgesic agonist/antagonist, may not be reversed effectively by the opiate analgesic antagonist naloxone (Narcan®).

Notes

1. In Europe, where the sublingual formulation of buprenorphine has been available for over a decade, abusers simply dissolve the sublingual tablet and inject the drug intravenously for its desired actions.

2. In late 2002, FDA approved Suboxone®, a sublingual tablet formulation containing buprenorphine and naloxone, for this indication. The rationale for the use of this combination product was to deter the illegal diversion and illicit intravenous use of buprenorphine. The use of Suboxone® in the treatment of opiate analgesic dependence is usually initiated after the opiate analgesic-dependent person has already initiated buprenorphine maintenance pharmacotherapy. The combination product facilitates outpatient treatment because "take home" doses can be provided with minimal concern about abuse or illegal diversion. The pharmaceutical utility and rationale for this combination have been demonstrated over the past two decades with the combination of pentazocine and naloxone (see Pentazocine monograph).

3. Although used clinically to prevent the opiate analgesic withdrawal syndrome in people who are physically dependent on opiate analgesics, buprenorphine reportedly precipitates an opiate analgesic withdrawal syndrome when consumed in large doses by people who are physically dependent on heroin.

4. An exception is that buprenorphine maintenance programs using the sublingual dosage form may encourage better health for opiate analgesic-dependent women who are pregnant because these programs may (1) reduce risk for infections (e.g., HIV) associated with prostitution and intravenous drug use; (2) provide a means for regular contact with health care providers that enables opiate analgesic-dependent women to obtain prenatal care and to access other needed health resources (e.g., safe shelter, food); and (3) reduce the degree of opiate analgesic withdrawal in neonates (i.e., buprenorphine is associated with a milder neonatal withdrawal [abstinence] syndrome than several other opiate analgesics [e.g., heroin] that are commonly abused by women who are pregnant).

5. Because buprenorphine is a mixed opiate analgesic agonist/antagonist, its administration to a person who is physically dependent on a pure opiate analgesic agonist (e.g., heroin, morphine) will likely precipitate the opiate analgesic withdrawal syndrome.

6. In 1996, buprenorphine became legally available in France as "replacement therapy" (much like methadone maintenance) for the symptomatic treatment of heroin dependence. It is dispensed in sublingual form for this indication. However, many people who are physically dependent on opiate analgesics crush, or simply dissolve, the tablet and inject it intravenously (often in combination with a benzodiazepine). In Europe, over the past decade, several hundred deaths have been directly attributed to buprenorphine overdosage.

References

Barnett, P.G., Zaric, G.S., & Brandeau, M.L. (2001). The cost-effectiveness of buprenorphine maintenance therapy for opiate addiction in the United States. *Addiction, 96*(9), 1267-1278.

Berson, A., Gervais, A., Cazals, D., et al. (2001). Hepatitis after intravenous buprenorphine misuse in heroin addicts. *Journal of Hepatology, 34*(2), 346-350.

Boatwright, D.E. (2002). Buprenorphine and addiction: Challenges for the pharmacist. *Journal of the American Pharmaceutical Association, 42*, 432-438.

Clark, N.C., Lintzeris, N., & Muhleisen, P.J. (2002). Severe opiate withdrawal in a heroin user precipitated by a massive buprenorphine dose. *The Medical Journal of Australia, 176*(4), 166-167.

Comer, S.D., Collins, E.D., & Fischman, M.W. (2002). Intravenous buprenorphine self-administered by detoxified heroin abusers. *The Journal of Pharmacology and Experimental Therapeutics, 301*(1), 266-276.

Dahan, A., Yassen, A., Romberg, R., et al. (2006). Buprenorphine induces ceiling in respiratory depression but not in analgesia. *British Journal of Anaesthesia, 96*(5), 627-632.

Drug Enforcement Administration (DEA), Department of Justice. (2002). Schedules of controlled substances: Rescheduling of buprenorphine from schedule V to schedule III. Final rule. *Federal Register, 67*(194), 62354-62370.

Escher, M., Daali, Y., Chabert, J., et al. (2007). Pharmacokinetic and pharmacodynamic properties of buprenorphine after a single intravenous administration in healthy volunteers: A randomized, double-blind, placebo-controlled, crossover study. *Clinical Therapeutics, 29*(8), 1620-1631.

FDA approves buprenorphine for opiate addiction treatment. (2002, October 14). *Alcoholism & Drug Abuse Weekly, 14*(39), no pagination.

Fiellin, D.A., & O'Connor, P.G. (2002). Office-based treatment of opioid-dependent patients. *New England Journal of Medicine, 347*, 817-823.

Fischer, G., Johnson, R.E., Eder, H., et al. (2000). Treatment of opioid-dependent pregnant women with buprenorphine. *Addiction, 95*(2), 239-244.

Geib, A.J., Babu, K., Ewald, M.B., et al. (2006). Adverse effects in children after unintentional buprenorphine exposure. *Pediatrics, 118*(4), 1746-1751.

Gowing, L., Ali, R., & White, J. (2000). Buprenorphine for the management of opioid withdrawal. *Cochrane Database of Systematic Reviews* (3), CD002025.

Johnson, R.E., Jones, H.E., Jasinski, D.R., et al. (2001). Buprenorphine treatment of pregnant opioid-dependent women: Maternal and neonatal outcomes. *Drug and Alcohol Dependence, 63*(1), 97-103.

Kintz, P. (2001). Deaths involving buprenorphine: A compendium of French cases. *Forensic Science International, 121*(1-2), 65-69.

Muriel, C., Failde, I., Micó, J.A., et al. (2005). Effectiveness and tolerability of the buprenorphine transdermal system in patients with moderate to severe chronic pain: A multicenter, open-label, uncontrolled, prospective, observational clinical study. *Clinical Therapeutics, 27*(4), 451-462.

Nanovskaya, T., Deshmukh, S., Brooks, M., et al. (2002). Transplacental transfer and metabolism of buprenorphine. *The Journal of Pharmacology and Experimental Therapeutics, 300*(1), 26-33.

Obadia, Y., Perrin, V., Feroni, I., et al. (2001). Injecting misuse of buprenorphine among French drug users. *Addiction, 96*(2), 267-272.

Sorge, J., & Sittl, R. (2004). Transdermal buprenorphine in the treatment of chronic pain: Results of a phase III, multicenter, randomized, double-blind, placebo-controlled study. *Clinical Therapeutics, 26*(11), 1808-1820.

Subutex and Suboxone approved to treat opiate dependence. (2002, October 8). *FDA Talk Paper,* US Food and Drug Administration. Available: http://www.fda.gov/bbs/topics/ANSWERS/2002/ANS01165.html.

West, S.L., O'Neal, K.K., & Graham, C.W. (2000). A meta-analysis comparing the effectiveness of buprenorphine and methadone. *Journal of Substance Abuse, 12*(4), 405-414.

BUTABARBITAL (See Barbiturates)

BUTANE

Names

BAN or INN Generic Synonyms: Liquid Petroleum Gas

Brand/Trade: Generally available by generic name

Chemical: N-Butane

Street: Gas; Lighter Fluid

Pharmacologic Classification

Psychodepressant, volatile solvents & inhalants: volatile solvent (aliphatic hydrocarbon)

Brief General Overview

Butane is commercially available for use primarily as a fuel gas or cigarette-lighter fluid.[1] Abuse is primarily limited to school-age children and adolescents, and use is generally of a short-term, experimental nature, usually in the company of friends.

Dosage Forms and Routes of Administration

Butane, a hydrocarbon petroleum distillate, is commonly available in both liquid and gas forms. When abused, butane is obtained from legitimately available commercial products (e.g., cigarette lighter fluid) and is self-administered by inhalation. When available in a pressurized container (e.g., Glade Air Freshener®, which contains both butane and isobutane as hydrocarbon propellants), the butane is administered by simply depressing the valve of the container and directly inhaling the butane gas. The liquid form can be poured onto a rag and the fumes inhaled by placing the rag directly over the mouth and nose. In North America, most users are children and adolescent boys of European descent.

Mechanism of CNS Action

The exact molecular mechanism of butane's general psychodepressant actions has not been determined, but appears to be correlated with its very high lipid solubility.

Pharmacodynamics/Pharmacokinetics

Valid and reliable data are not available. See the Volatile Solvents & Inhalants monograph.

Current Approved Indications for Medical Use

None

Desired Action/Reason for Personal Use

Alcohol-like disinhibitory euphoria or "high" (mild); perceptual distortion(s); sense of weightlessness

Toxicity

Acute: Asphyxia (due to the replacement of arterial oxygen by butane); ataxia; bithalamic injury; cold burn injury to the face, hands, and arms (explosive burns); cardiac dysrhythmias; cough; delusions; disorientation; dizziness; drowsiness; emotional disinhibition; hallucinations; impaired coordination; laryngeal edema (severe); laryngospasm; nausea; numbness; pulmonary irritation; respiratory difficulty; ventricular fibrillation (rare); vomiting

Chronic: Academic impairment; apathy; fatigue; hepatic impairment; memory impairment; mental depression; psychological dependence; pulmonary damage; thirst (constant)

Pregnancy & Lactation: Valid and reliable data are not available. On the basis of knowledge of related petrochemical compounds, the teratogenic potential for butane abuse is expected to be none to low. Butane is not expected to be excreted in human breast milk.

Abuse Potential

Physical dependence: None (USDEA: not a scheduled drug)
Psychological dependence: Low to moderate[2]

Withdrawal Syndrome

A butane withdrawal syndrome has not been reported.

Overdosage

Generally, butane overdosage deaths do not appear to be directly related to use by pulmonary inhalation.[3] However, they may be associated with other "inert" ingredients in commercial butane products. These ingredients were never intended for human pulmonary use. Death also may be due to accidental injuries and burns associated with dizziness, drowsiness, or loss of consciousness. For example, death may rarely be due to suffocation when a butane user loses consciousness with a butane-containing plastic bag in place over the nose and mouth. There is no known antidote for butane overdosage. Additional valid and reliable data are needed.

Notes

1. In Europe, particularly England and Wales, butane-based antiperspirant deodorants (e.g., Radox®), which are available in stores and over the Internet, are the principal sources of butane supply for youth 11 to 15 years of age.
2. Psychological dependence appears to be associated with the IQ and personality characteristics of the butane abuser.
3. A rare exception is death due to ventricular fibrillation, which has been associated in some cases with strenuous muscle exercise following butane use.

References

Davis, G.A., Rudy, A.C., Archer, S.M., et al. (2005). Bioavailability of intranasal butorphanol administered from a single-dose sprayer. *American Journal of Health-System Pharmacy, 62*(1), 48-53.

Doogue, M., & Barclay, M. (2005). Death due to butane abuse—The clinical pharmacology of inhalants. *The New Zealand Medical Journal, 118*(1225), U1732.

Döring, G., Baiumeister, F.A., Peters, J., et al. (2002). Butane abuse associated encephalopathy. *Klinische Padiatrie, 214*(5), 295-298.

Edwards, K.E., & Wenstone, R. (2000). Successful resuscitation from recurrent ventricular fibrillation secondary to butane inhalation. *British Journal of Anaesthesia, 84*(6), 803-805.

Harris, D., & Mirza, Z. (2005). Butane encephalopathy. *Emergency Medicine Journal, 22*(9), 676-677.

Kile, S.J., Camilleri, C.C., Latchaw, R.E., et al. (2006). Bithalamic lesions of butane encephalopathy. *Pediatric Neurology, 35*(6), 439-441.

LoVecchio, F., & Fulton, S.E. (2001). Ventricular fibrillation following inhalation of Glade Air Freshener. *European Journal of Emergency Medicine, 8*(2), 153-154.

Mathew, B., Kapp, E., & Jones, T.R. (2006). Commercial butane abuse: A disturbing case. *Addiction, 84*(5), 563-564.

Sugie, H., Sasaki, C., Hashimoto, H., et al. (2003). Three cases of sudden death due to butane or propane gas inhalation: Analysis of tissues for gas components. *Forensic Science International, 143*(2-3), 211-214.

BUTORPHANOL

Names

BAN or INN Generic Synonyms: None

Brand/Trade: Stadol®; Stadol NS®

Chemical: Morphine-3,14-diol, 17-(cyclobutylmethyl)-,(-), (s-(R*,R*))-2,3-dihydroxybutanediate; (-)-17-(cyclobutylmethyl)morphinan-3,14-diol D

Street: None

Pharmacologic Classification

Psychodepressant, opiate analgesic: mixed agonist/antagonist (synthetic)

Brief General Overview

Butorphanol was first synthesized in 1974. Although the manufacturer claimed in the early 1990s that it had no, or low, potential for abuse because of its mixed action as an opiate analgesic agonist/antagonist, clinical use subsequently demonstrated that these claims were false. Butorphanol has a similar abuse potential to that of the other opiate analgesics (see monograph).

Butorphanol is primarily abused for the self-management of acute severe pain (e.g., migraine headaches). Users include patients who have been prescribed butorphanol by their physicians (e.g., up to 20% of patients who are prescribed butorphanol for the symptomatic management of migraine headache pain reportedly abuse the drug) and health care professionals attempting to self-manage their own pain (often migraine headaches). The intranasal spray formulation reportedly facilitates this pattern of abuse, particularly in users who are not inclined to inject drugs intravenously. In addition, veterinary formulations (i.e., Torbitrol®, an oral solution used for the postoperative management of pain following such surgical procedures as feline neutering) reportedly have been used, primarily by North American adolescent boys of European descent. The oral solution is either ingested orally or retained in the mouth for transmucosal absorption.

Dosage Forms and Routes of Administration

Butorphanol is commercially produced by licit pharmaceutical manufacturers.[1] It is available in both injectable (i.e., intramuscular and intravenous) and intranasal (i.e., nasal spray) formulations.

Mechanism of CNS Action

Butorphanol and its major metabolites act as agonists at kappa-opiate receptors and as mixed agonist/antagonists at mu-opiate receptors. Interaction of butorphanol with these receptors in the CNS apparently mediates most of its pharmacologic actions, including analgesia, cough suppression, miosis, respiratory depression, vomiting, and sedation. Binding to the kappa opiate receptors reportedly mediates the development of tolerance to butorphanol and cross-tolerance to other opiate analgesics. Other actions possibly mediated by non-CNS mechanisms include alteration in bladder sphincter activity, bronchomotor tone, cardiovascular resistance and capacity, and GI secretion and motility. Although butorphanol appears to elicit its analgesic and respiratory depressant actions primarily by binding to the endorphin receptors in the CNS, the exact mechanism of action has not been determined. The partial antagonist activity associated with butorphanol is probably due to competitive inhibition at the receptor sites. See the Opiate Analgesics monograph.

Pharmacodynamics/Pharmacokinetics

Butorphanol is rapidly absorbed after intramuscular injection and attains peak blood concentrations within 20 to 40 minutes. After a 1 mg nasal dose (i.e., as delivered by a single-dose intranasal metered sprayer), mean peak blood concentrations occur within 10 to 60 minutes. The absolute bioavailability of the nasal formulation is 60% to 80%. Bioavailability is unchanged in patients who have allergic rhinitis. In patients using a nasal vasoconstrictor (e.g., oxymetazoline [Dristan Long Lasting Nasal®, Drixoral Nasal®]), the fraction of the dose absorbed reportedly is unchanged, but the rate of absorption is slowed. Peak blood concentrations are approximately half of those achieved in the absence of the vasoconstrictor. After the initial absorption/distribution phase, the single-dose pharmacokinetics of butorphanol administered intramuscularly, intravenously, or nasally have been found to be similar.

Butorphanol's plasma protein binding (~80%) is independent of blood concentration over the range achieved in clinical practice. Its apparent volume of distribution ranges from 4 to 13 L/kg. Butorphanol is transported across the blood–brain and placental barriers and is excreted in breast milk. Butorphanol is extensively metabolized in the liver, with less than 5% excreted unchanged in the urine. A small amount is excreted in feces. The mean elimination half-life is ~5 hours (range 2 to 9 hours).

The analgesic action of butorphanol is influenced by its method of use. Analgesia begins within a few minutes of intravenous injection (i.e., when the drug is used as a preanesthetic). Peak analgesic activity occurs within 30 to 60 minutes after intramuscular injection and within 1 to 2 hours after use of the nasal spray. The duration of analgesia varies, depending on the severity of pain and method of use, but is generally 3 to 4 hours with intramuscular or intravenous injection. Compared with the injectable formulation and other opiate analgesic agonists or agonist/antagonists, butorphanol nasal spray has a longer duration of action (4 to 5 hours).

Current Approved Indications for Medical Use

Pain, acute (moderate to severe)

Desired Action/Reason for Personal Use

Analgesia for self-management of acute pain (moderate to severe, usually migraine headache pain); euphoria (mild); generalized sensation of warmth ("rush"); prevention/self-management of the opiate analgesic withdrawal syndrome

Toxicity

Acute: Cognitive impairment; confusion; constipation; dizziness; drowsiness; dry mouth; dysphoria; fatigue; headache; hypertension (rare); lightheadedness; miosis; nausea; psychomotor impairment; respiratory depression; sedation; somnolence; vomiting

Chronic: Hepatitis (associated with intravenous use); HIV infection (associated with intravenous use); physical dependence; psychological dependence

Pregnancy & Lactation: FDA Pregnancy Category C (see Appendix B). Safety of butorphanol use by adolescent girls and women who are pregnant has not been established. Additional valid and reliable data are needed.

Safety of butorphanol use by adolescent girls and women who are breast-feeding has not been established. Butorphanol has been detected in breast milk. However, the amount that a neonate or an infant would receive from breast-feeding is probably clinically insignificant (estimated as 4 mcg per liter of breast milk for a mother receiving 2 mg intramuscularly four times a day). Although there are no data on use of the nasal spray by adolescent girls and women who are breast-feeding, butorphanol probably is excreted in breast milk in similar amounts after intranasal use. Additional valid and reliable data are needed.

Abuse Potential

Physical dependence: Moderate (USDEA Schedule IV; low potential for abuse)
Psychological dependence: Moderate

Withdrawal Syndrome

A butorphanol withdrawal syndrome has not been reported, most likely because of the mixed opiate analgesic agonist/antagonist action of butorphanol.[2]

Overdosage

Signs and symptoms of butorphanol overdosage are similar to those associated with other opiate analgesic overdosage. The most serious signs are hypoventilation, cardiovascular insufficiency, and coma. Butorphanol overdosage has involved accidental overdosage by young children who ingested the drug after gaining access to it in the home and intentional overdosage by suicidal patients. Although butorphanol is more potent than morphine, it appears to have a ceiling effect in terms of respiratory depression. This ceiling effect is a theoretical advantage because an overdosage involving a large amount of butorphanol should not produce correspondingly excessive respiratory depression. However, suspected or actual butorphanol overdosage requires emergency medical support, with attention to increasing butorphanol elimination. Use of the opiate analgesic antagonist naloxone (Narcan®) may be needed. In these cases, repeated dosing with naloxone is usually required because the duration of butorphanol action exceeds that of naloxone.

Notes

1. Although rarely illicitly synthesized, butorphanol can be chemically derived from thebaine.

2. Butorphanol is a mixed opiate analgesic agonist/antagonist, and its administration to a person who is physically dependent on a pure opiate analgesic agonist (e.g., heroin, morphine) will likely precipitate the opiate analgesic withdrawal syndrome. (See the Opiate Analgesics monograph.)

References

Commiskey, S., Fan, L.W., Ho, I.K., et al. (2005). Butorphanol: Effects of a prototypical agonist-antagonist analgesic on kappa-opioid receptors. *Journal of Pharmacological Sciences, 98*(2), 109-116.

Davis, G.A., Rudy, A.C., Archer, S.M., et al. (2004). Pharmacokinetics of butorphanol tartrate administered from single-dose intranasal sprayer. *American Journal of Health-System Pharmacy, 61*(3), 261-266.

Robbins, L. (2002). Butorphanol nasal spray for headache. Robbins Headache Clinic. Available: http://www.headachedrugs.com/archives/butorphanol.html.

Walker, D.J., Zacny, J.P., Galva, K.E., et al. (2001). Subjective, psychomotor, and physiological effects of cumulative doses of mixed-action opioids in healthy volunteers. *Psychopharmacology, 155*(4), 362-371.

Walsh, S.L., Chausmer, A.E., Strain, E.C., et al. (2008). Evaluation of the mu and kappa opioid actions of butorphanol in humans through differential naltrexone blockade. *Psychopharmacology, 196*(1), 143-155.

CAFFEINE

Names

BAN or INN Generic Synonyms: Methyltheobromine

Brand/Trade: NoDoz®; Stay Awake®; Vivarin®; Wake-Up®

Chemical: 1,3,7-Trimethylxanthine

Street: Caffy; Java; Joe

Pharmacologic Classification

Psychostimulant, miscellaneous: methylxanthine (natural)

Brief General Overview

Chemically, caffeine is a methylated derivative of xanthine (i.e., a methylxanthine). It is found naturally in cocoa beans,[1] cola (kola) nuts,[2] coffee beans (e.g., *Coffea arabica*),[3] *guarana*,[4] *mat* (*yerba mate*),[5] and tea (obtained from the dried leaves of *Camellia [Thea] sinensis*).[6] Caffeine is the most widely used psychoactive substance in the world.

For most North Americans, and others, caffeine consumption is a regular part of their usual social "rituals" (e.g., major component of a favorite morning beverage, ingredient in preferred workday "break" beverage [i.e., coffee, tea, or caffeinated soft drinks]), and a vast majority of North Americans begin each day with a "dose" of caffeine. The dose found in the usual caffeine-containing beverage (i.e., one or two cups of coffee or tea; a can or bottle of caffeine-containing soft drink) can, for most users, result in increased alertness, elevated blood pressure, heightened mood, and increased respiratory rate.[7]

Caffeine affects the cardiovascular system, resulting in increased cardiac contractility and output. Caffeine causes dilation of the coronary arteries, thereby increasing oxygenated blood supply to the myocardium and thus increasing work capacity. By increasing cardiac performance, caffeine also exerts diuretic effects, although it has not demonstrated therapeutic effectiveness or advantage over standard and more efficacious diuretics (e.g., thiazide diuretics). It also produces hypertension and tachycardia. Caffeine decreases blood flow to the brain by constricting the cerebral blood vessels. This action is thought to provide relief for hypertensive headaches and certain types of migraine headaches, conditions for which caffeine has been used medically.

Dosage Forms and Routes of Administration

Caffeine is orally ingested. Although commercially available as an oral tablet formulation (in both single-ingredient products and combination products), it is most frequently consumed as part of a caffeinated beverage (i.e., caffeine-containing cocoa, coffee, cola soft drinks, and tea; see Table 3). It also is ingested in the form of caffeine-containing chocolate candy bars. In a sample of U.S. junior high school students, the average amount of caffeine consumed was about 65 mg/day (range, 0 to 800 mg/day). Boys, on average, consumed significantly more caffeine per day than girls. Increasingly, caffeine is consumed by young adults, particularly men, in "energy drinks" (e.g., Cocaine®, Pimp Juice®, Red Bull®, Spike Shooter®). These energy drinks generally contain 80 to 300 mg of caffeine, as well as 35 grams of sugar (glucose) and varying amounts of ginseng, guarana, and taurine per 8 ounce (240 mL) serving (see related discussion in the Alcohol monograph).

TABLE 3
Caffeine Content of Common Beverages[a]

Product	Caffeine Content
Chocolate candy bar	20 to 30 mg per regular-sized bar
Chocolate drinks	1 to 5 mg per ounce (30 mL) or 8 to 40 mg per 8 ounces (240 mL) or typical beverage cup/glassful
Chocolate milk	1 to 2 mg per ounce (30 mL) or 8 to 16 mg per 8 ounces (240 mL) or typical beverage cup/glassful
Coffee, brewed, regular[b]	30 to 180 mg per 6 ounces (180 mL) or typical coffee cup
Coffee, decaffeinated[c]	2 to 4 mg per 6 ounces (180 mL) or typical coffee cup
Coffee, espresso	100 mg per 2 ounces (60 mL) or typical espresso cup
Coffee, instant	60 to 100 mg per 6 ounces (180 mL) or typical coffee cup
Cola drinks	24 to 48 mg per 12 ounce (360 mL) bottle or can
Jolt Espresso®	120 mg per 12 ounce (360 mL) can
Tea	18 to 80 mg per 6 ounces (180 mL) or typical teacup

[a]These are average values; the actual amount of caffeine may vary significantly by product and manufacturer. Several products have been formulated with higher levels of caffeine (e.g., Jolt® cola contains 71 mg/12 ounces [360 mL]), while others are caffeine free (7 Up® and Sprite® soft drinks; herbal teas).

[b]Depending upon the type of coffee bean used, the amount of ground coffee used, and the method of preparation.

[c]When coffee beans are decaffeinated by the typical "Swiss water process," approximately 98% of the natural caffeine is removed.

Source: Adapted from Pagliaro, L.A., & Pagliaro, A.M. (2004). *Pagliaros' comprehensive guide to drugs and substances of abuse.* Washington, DC: American Pharmacists Association.

Mechanism of CNS Action

Caffeine, as a methylxanthine, is a potent psychostimulant. The cerebral cortex is the most sensitive part of the CNS and is affected first, followed by the brain stem. The spinal cord is stimulated last, but only after extremely large amounts of caffeine are ingested. Initially, the use of caffeine produces increased mental alertness, faster and clearer flow of thought, wakefulness, and restlessness, because the cortex is affected by smaller amounts of caffeine than are necessary to excite the brain stem. These psychostimulant actions may help sustain intellectual effort without disrupting coordinated intellectual or psychomotor performance. Caffeine's actions on the cortex may be observed after ingestion of as little as 100 to 200 mg, or one to two cups of coffee. In usual amounts (i.e., 100 to 500 mg), caffeine potently stimulates the cortex, promoting wakefulness and improving psychomotor performance. Caffeine also may produce nausea and vomiting, effects that probably involve CNS actions, at least in part. In addition to its direct actions on the CNS, caffeine produces direct actions on several other body systems, including the cardiovascular system, the respiratory system, and the musculoskeletal system.

The psychostimulant action of caffeine appears to be modulated by its interaction with adenosine receptors. Specifically, this action appears to be largely due to competitive blockade of A2A and possibly striatal A1 receptors.[8,9] The result is that caffeine causes a range of actions that are the opposite of those caused by adenosine. In addition, it appears that caffeine enhances dopaminergic activity.

Pharmacodynamics/Pharmacokinetics

Caffeine is well absorbed (i.e., 75% to 90%) after oral ingestion. Peak plasma concentrations occur in ~60 to 90 minutes (range, 30 to 120 minutes). It is poorly protein bound (~25%). Caffeine is widely distributed in all body fluids and has an apparent volume of distribution of 0.6 L/kg. It is highly metabolized in the liver, particularly by CYP1A2 isoenzymes, and less than 2% is excreted unchanged in the urine.[10] The mean elimination half-life for caffeine is ~5 hours.

Current Approved Indications for Medical Use

Neonatal respiratory stimulation

Desired Action/Reason for Personal Use

Alertness, vigilance or wakefulness; elevate mood (mild); improve athletic performance[11]; increase energy (feelings of); prevention/self-management of the caffeine withdrawal syndrome; weight loss (similar to nicotine use, and is often used in combination with nicotine); work efficiency/productivity

Toxicity

The adverse effects associated with caffeine use primarily are extensions of its pharmacologic actions. Heavy consumption of caffeine (i.e., 12 or more cups of coffee a day or 1.5 grams of caffeine) can cause more intense stimulant actions marked by agitation, anxiety, cardiac dysrhythmias, heart palpitations, rapid breathing, tachycardia, and tremors. The spinal cord becomes stimulated only after even higher doses of caffeine (i.e., 2 to 5 grams or 20 to 50 cups of coffee) have been consumed; increased stimulation of the spinal reflexes may result. Convulsions and death may occur with massive doses of caffeine (i.e., over 10 grams or 100 cups of coffee). However, because such massive amounts are required, death from caffeine ingestion (i.e., as a consequence of the ingestion of caffeinated beverages) is highly unlikely.

Acute[12]: Anxiety; blood pressure (systolic), increased; diuresis; excitement; heart palpitation; insomnia; irritability; nervousness; plasma free fatty acids, increased; restlessness; tachycardia; tremors

Chronic: Caffeinism[13]; cardiac dysrhythmias; gastric ulceration/irritation; physical dependence; psychological dependence

Pregnancy & Lactation: Reduced birth weight has been associated with maternal consumption of three or more cups of coffee per day during pregnancy.[14] In addition, caffeine consumption during pregnancy has been significantly correlated with fetal loss. Thus, pregnant adolescent girls and women should avoid or minimize caffeine use.

Caffeine is excreted in trace amounts in breast milk. However, the amount excreted in breast milk may be of concern to adolescent girls and women who have high daily caffeine consumption and are breast-feeding premature neonates.[15] Additional valid and reliable data are needed.

Abuse Potential

Physical dependence: Low (USDEA: not a scheduled drug)
Psychological dependence: Moderate

Withdrawal Syndrome

The caffeine withdrawal syndrome has been characterized by drowsiness, fatigue, headache (mild to severe), irritability, lethargy, nervousness, restlessness, sleepiness, and diminished work efficacy/productivity. The etiology of the withdrawal headache is unclear, but most likely it involves reflex dilation of the cerebral vessels in response to increased sensitivity to adenosine.

The syndrome can be ameliorated by a dose of caffeine (i.e., a cup of coffee). The signs and symptoms of caffeine withdrawal generally begin within 12 to 24 hours of last use, peak between 24 and 48 hours after onset, and last for up to 7 days.

Overdosage

Overdosages of caffeine resulting in death are rare, but have been reported. In adults, it is estimated that 10 grams of caffeine may result in cardiac dysrhythmias, convulsions, and respiratory arrest. These effects are generally preceded by excitement, insomnia, mild delirium, rapid respirations, and vomiting. Acute caffeine overdosage requires emergency medical support, with attention to increasing caffeine elimination. There is no known antidote.

Notes

1.   The seeds of *Theobroma cacao* are used to produce cocoa and chocolate.

2. *Cola acuminata* and *Cola nitida*, which are primarily from West Africa.
3. Coffee beans typically contain between 1.1% and 1.4% caffeine, depending on the specific type and variety of bean.
4. *Guarana* is a dried paste made from the seeds of the Brazilian *Paullinia cupana* tree. It has been used as a nutritional supplement and to treat diarrhea.
5. *Mat* is the dried leaves of the South American *Ilex paraguariensis* tree. The leaves are used to make tea, commonly referred to as Bartholomew's tea or Jesuit's tea.
6. *Camellia sinesis* contains theophylline (1,3-dimethylxanthine) in addition to caffeine.
7. The amount of caffeine varies among caffeinated beverages, as shown in the table on page 62.
8. The A2A receptors stimulate GABAergic (i.e., inhibitory) neurons.
9. Caffeine has ergogenic effects (i.e., facilitation of athletic training at greater energy output and for longer periods of time, increased speed and power output in races) that are not primarily related to its psychostimulant action but likely involve the dopamine and cAMP-regulated phosphoprotein (i.e., DARPP-32). For these effects, caffeine appears to create a favorable intracellular environment in active muscle that facilitates force production by each motor unit, particularly in muscle of the upper body. In addition, caffeine can improve athletic performance by improving concentration in a tired athlete. However, psychological factors (or placebo effect) may account for varying results from different studies. The International Olympic Committee (IOC) has removed caffeine from the list of banned substances.
10. Tobacco smoking induces CYP1A2 isoenzymes; thus, tobacco smokers may eliminate caffeine up to twice as fast as nonsmokers. Other factors, such as alcohol use, phase of menstrual cycle, pregnancy, and use of oral contraceptives also can significantly affect the rate of caffeine metabolism by means of alterations in isoenzyme concentrations.
11. Caffeine enhances fatty acid metabolism, leading to glucose conservation. These effects may be of benefit to participants in long-distance endurance events (e.g., marathons, skiing competitions). Thus, although banned by some sporting agencies, the use of caffeine as an ergogenic by athletes is commonly encountered. (Also see Note 9.)
12. Both chocolate and cola, which are common sources of caffeine (particularly for children and adolescents), are included among the most common sources of food allergies.
13. Signs and symptoms of caffeinism (i.e., caffeine intoxication that is generally related to the ingestion by adults of more than 250 mg of caffeine) include agitation, anxiety, headache, hyperreflexia, insomnia, irritability, muscle twitching, nervousness, palpitations, rapid breathing, and tremors.
14. This effect appears to be amplified in women who also smoke tobacco.
15. The elimination half-life of caffeine is increased in premature neonates; thus, the potential for caffeine accumulation exists.

References

Beck, T.W., Housh, T.J., Schmidt, R.J., et al. (2006). The acute effects of a caffeine-containing supplement on strength, muscular endurance, and anaerobic capabilities. *The Journal of Strength & Conditioning Research, 20*(3), 506-510.

Bernstein, G.A., Carroll, M.E., Thuras, P.D., et al. (2002). Caffeine dependence in teenagers. *Drug and Alcohol Dependence, 66*(1), 1-6.

Boozer, C.N., Daly, P.A., Homel, P., et al. (2002). Herbal ephedra/caffeine for weight loss: A 6-month randomized safety and efficacy trial. *International Journal of Obesity and Related Metabolic Disorders, 26*(5), 593-604.

Brice, C.F., & Smith, A.P. (2002). Factors associated with caffeine consumption. *International Journal of Food Sciences and Nutrition, 53*(1), 55-64.

Christensen, M., Tybring, G., Mihara, K., et al. (2002). Low daily 10-mg and 20-mg doses of fluvoxamine inhibit the metabolism of both caffeine (cytochrome P4501A2) and omeprazole (cytochrome P4502C19). *Clinical Pharmacology and Therapeutics, 71*(3), 141-152.

Christian, M.S., & Brent, R.L. (2001). Teratogen update: Evaluation of the reproductive and developmental risks of caffeine. *Teratology, 64*(1), 51-78.

Clauson, K.A., Shields, K.M., McQueen, C.E., et al. (2008). Safety issues associated with commercially available energy drinks. *Journal of the American Pharmacists Association, 48*(3), e55-e63.

Clausson, B., Granath, F., Ekbom, A., et al. (2002). Effect of caffeine exposure during pregnancy on birth weight and gestational age. *American Journal of Epidemiology, 155*(5), 429-436.

Dews, P.B., O'Brien, C.P., & Bergman, J. (2002). Caffeine: Behavioral effects of withdrawal and related issues. *Food and Chemical Toxicology, 40*(9), 1257-1261.

Donovan, J.L., & DeVane, C.L. (2001). A primer on caffeine pharmacology and its drug interactions in clinical psychopharmacology. *Psychopharmacology Bulletin, 35*(3), 30-48.

Forbes, S.C., Candow, D.G., Little, J.P., et al. (2007). Effect of Red Bull energy drink on repeated Wingate cycle performance and bench-press muscle endurance. *International Journal of Sport Nutrition and Exercise Metabolism, 17*(5), 433-444.

George, S.E., Ramalakshmi, K., & Mohan Rao, L.J. (2008). A perception on health benefits of coffee. *Critical Reviews in Food Science and Nutrition, 48*(5), 464-486.

Graham, T.E. (2001). Caffeine and exercise: Metabolism, endurance and performance. *Sports Medicine, 31*(11), 785-807.

Greenway, F.L. (2001). The safety and efficacy of pharmaceutical and herbal caffeine and ephedrine use as a weight loss agent. *Obesity Review, 2*(3), 199-211.

Griffiths, R.R., & Chausmer, A.L. (2000). Caffeine as a model drug of dependence: Recent developments in understanding caffeine withdrawal, the caffeine dependence syndrome, and caffeine negative reinforcement. *Nihon Shinkei Seishin Yakurigaku Zasshi [Japanese Journal of Psychopharmacology], 20*(5), 223-231.

Haller, C.A., Jacob, P. 3rd, & Benowitz, N.L. (2004). Enhanced stimulant and metabolic effects of combined ephedrine and caffeine. *Clinical Pharmacology and Therapeutics, 75*(4), 259-273.

Iancu, I., & Strous, R.D. (2006). Caffeine intoxication: History, clinical features, diagnosis and treatment. *Harefuah, 145*(2), 147-151.

Iyadurai, S.J., & Chung, S.S. (2007). New-onset seizures in adults: Possible association with consumption of popular energy drinks. *Epilepsy & Behavior, 10*(3), 504-508.

Jones, G. (2008). Caffeine and other sympathomimetic stimulants: Modes of action and effects on sports performance. *Essays in Biochemistry, 44*, 109-123.

Kamimori, G.H., Karyekar, C.S., Otterstetter, R., et al. (2002). The rate of absorption and relative bioavailability of caffeine administered in chewing gum versus capsules to normal healthy volunteers. *International Journal of Pharmaceutics, 234*(1-2), 159-167.

Killgore, W.D., Kahn-Greene, E.T., Killgore, D.B., et al. (2007). Effects of acute caffeine withdrawal on Short Category Test performance in sleep-deprived individuals. *Perceptual & Motor Skills, 105*(3, Part 2), 1265-1274.

Klebanoff, M.A., Levine, R.J., Clemens, J.D., et al. (2002). Maternal serum caffeine metabolites and small-for-gestational age birth. *American Journal of Epidemiology, 155*(1), 32-37.

Lane, J.D., & Phillips-Bute, B.G. (1998). Caffeine deprivation affects vigilance performance and mood. *Physiology and Behavior, 65*(1), 171-175.

Leviton, A., & Cowan, L. (2002). A review of the literature relating caffeine consumption by women to their risk of reproductive hazards. *Food and Chemical Toxicology, 40*(9), 1272-1310.

Lopez-Garcia, E., van Dam, R.M., Li, T.Y., et al. (2008). The relationship of coffee consumption with mortality. *Annals of Internal Medicine, 148*(12), 904-914.

Malinauskas, B.M., Aeby, V.G., Overton, R.F., et al. (2007). A survey of energy drink consumption patterns among college students. *Nutrition Journal, 6*, 35.

Mandel, H.G. (2002). Update on caffeine consumption, disposition and action. *Food and Chemical Toxicology, 40*(9), 1231-1234.

Martin, I., López-Vilchez, M.A., Mur, A., et al. (2007). Neonatal withdrawal syndrome after chronic maternal drinking of mate. *Therapeutic Drug Monitoring, 29*(1), 127-129.

McCarthy, D.M., Mycyk, M.B., & DesLauriers, C.A. (2008). Hospitalization for caffeine abuse is associated with abuse of other pharmaceutical products. *American Journal of Emergency Medicine, 26*(7), 799-802.

O'Brien, M.C., McCoy, T.P., Rhodes, S.D., et al. (2008). Caffeinated cocktails: Energy drink consumption, high-risk drinking, and alcohol-related consequences among college students. *Academic Emergency Medicine, 15*(5), 453-460.

Ogawa, N., & Ueki, H. (2007). Clinical importance of caffeine dependence and abuse. *Psychiatry and Clinical Neurosciences, 61*(3), 263-268.

Paluska, S.A. (2003). Caffeine and exercise. *Current Sports Medicine Reports, 2*(4), 213-219.

Shapiro, R.E. (2007). Caffeine and headaches. *Neurological Sciences, 28*(Supplement 2), S179-S183.

Smith, A. (2002). Effects of caffeine on human behavior. *Food and Chemical Toxicology, 40*(9), 1243-1255.

Sökmen, B., Armstrong, L.E., Kraemer, W.J., et al. (2008). Caffeine use in sports: Considerations for the athlete. *The Journal of Strength & Conditioning Research, 22*(3), 978-986.

Watson, J.M., Lunt, M.J., Morris, S., et al. (2000). Reversal of caffeine withdrawal by ingestion of a soft beverage. *Pharmacology, Biochemistry, and Behavior, 66*(1), 15-18.

Williams, A.D., Cribb, P.J., Cooke, M.B., et al. (2008). The effect of ephedra and caffeine on maximal strength and power in resistance-trained athletes. *The Journal of Strength & Conditioning Research, 22*(2), 464-470.

CANNABIS

Names

BAN or INN Generic Synonyms: None

Brand/Trade: None[1]

Chemical: (6αR,10αR)-6α,7,8,10α-Tetrahydro-6,6,9-trimethyl-3-pentyl-6H-dibenzo[b,d,]pyran-1-ol]

Street: 13; 30s; 420[2]; *Abu-Sufian*; Acapulco Gold; Acapulco Red; Ace; *Afgani Indica*; Afi; African; African Black; African Bush; Airplane; AK-47; Al Green; Al Sharpton; Amsterdam; Angola; Arathi; Arathi Highlands; Ashes; Assassin of Youth; Astro Turf; Atshitshi; Aunt Mary; B; Baby; Baby Bad One; Bale; Bamba; Bambalacha; Bammy; *Bangoo*; *Banji*; Bank Head Bud; Banzai Bud; BC Bud; Beasters; Belyando Spruce; *Bhang*; Bio; Bin Laden; Birthday Cake; B-Legit; Black Bart; Black Ganga; Black Gold; Black Gungi; Black Gunion; Black Mo; Black Moat; Black Rope; Blizzies; Blueberry; Blue Sage; Blunts; Bo; Bob Hope; Bobby Brown; Bo-Bo; Bo-Bo Bush; *Boleia*; Boo; Boob; Boo Boo Bama; Boom; Broccoli; Bud; Buddha; Bullyon; Bunk; Burnie; Bush; Butter Flower; *Caca*; *Caca de Chango*; Cambodian Red; Cam Red; Cam Trip; Canadian Black; Canamo; Canappa; Cann; Cannablis; Cannon; Carb; *Cartucho*; Cavite All Star; CD's; Cereal; Cest; *Charas*; Charge; Cheeba; Cheebong; Cheech and Chong; Cheeo; Chicago Black; Chicago Green; Chira; Chocolate Thai; Chro; Chronic; Chucky; Clone; Club; Cochornis; Coconut Rabbi; Coli; Collie Weed; *Coliflor Tostao*; Colorado Cocktail; Colombian; Columbus Black; *Cosa*; Crazy Weed; Creeper; Cripple; Crippy; Crizz; Crying Weed; Cryppie; Cryptonite; Crystal Tea; C.S.; *Dagga*; Dak; Dancouver; Dan K; Dank; Dawamesk; Deaf; Dew; Diambista; Dimba; Ding; Dinkie Dow; Dirt; Dirt Grass; Ditch; Ditch Weed; Djamba; D Nuts; Doctor Kissinger's Crutch; Doggy Nuggz; Domestic; Don Jem; Don Juan; *Dona Juana*; *Dona Juanita*; Doob; Doobee; Doobie; *Dooko*; Dope; *Doshia*; Doug; Draf Weed; Drag Weed; Dry High; Dubbe; Dube; Duby; *Duros*; Dutchie; Dutchies; Earth; Endo; Esra; Fat Stick; Feeling; Fine Stuff; Finger Lid; Fir; Firebush; Flame; Flower; Flower Tops; Food; *Fraho; Frajo*; Friend; *Frios*; Fruit; *Fuma D'Angola*; Gage; Gange; *Ganja*; Gash; Gauge; Gauge Butt; Ghana; Giggle Smoke; Giggle Weed; Goblet of Jam; Gold; Gold Star; Golden; Golden Leaf; Gong; Gonj; Good Butt; Good Giggles; Good Goods; Goody-Goody; Goof Butt; Grapefuit Hydro; Grass; Grass Brownies; Grasshopper; Grata; Green; Green Buds; Green Goddess; Greeter; Gremmies; Greta; Griefo; Griefs; *Grifa*; Griff; Griffa; Griffo; Grim Creeper; Grolid; Gunga; Gunge; Gungeon; Gungun; *Gunja*; Gyve; Haircut; Hairy Ogre; *Hang Liu*; Hanhich; Happy

Cigarette; Happy Smoke; Harry Potter; Has; Hash; Hash Oil; Hashish; Hawaiian Black; Hawaiian Homegrown Hay; Hay; Hay Butt; Haze; Headies; Hemp; Henry; Herb; Herba; Herbalz; Hippie Lettuce; Homegrown; Home Grown; Honey Oil; Hooch; Hydro; Indian Boy; Indian Hay; Indian Hemp; *Indica*; Indo; Indonesian Bud; *Instaga*; *Instagu*; J; Jamaican Gold; Jane; Janjaweed; Jay; Jay Smoke; Jive Stick; Joint; Jolly Green; Jonko; Joy Smoke; Joy Stick; *Juan Valdez*; *Juanita*; Ju-Ju; Jungle; Kabak; Kaff; Kalakit; Kali; Kansas Grass; Kate Bush; Kaya; KB; Kee; Kentucky Blue; Key; KGB; *Khayf*; Ki; Kick Stick; *Kief*; *Kiff*; Killer Green Bud; Kilter; Kind; King Bud; Kona Gold; Krippy; Kryptonite; Kumba; Ladies; Lakbay Diva; Laughing Grass; Laughing Weed; Leaf; LG; Light Stuff; Lima; Lime Green; L.L.; *Llesca*; Loaf; *Lobo*; *Loco*; Loco Weed; Love Weed; L's; Lubage; M; Macaroni; Macon; Maconha; *Mafu*; Magic Smoke; Manhattan Silver; Manitoba Hydro; *Marachuan*; Mari; *Marihuana*; *Marijuana*; *Marimba*; Mary; Mary Ann; Mary Jane; Mary and Johnny; Mary Jonas; Mary Warner; Mary Weaver; Maui Wauie; Maui Wowie; Meg; Megg; Meggie; Messorole; Mexican Brown; Mexican Green; Mexican Locoweed; Mexican Red; Mint; MJ; M.J.; Mo; M.O.; Modams; Mohasky; Mohasty; Monte; Mooca; Moocah; Mooster; Moota; Mooters; Mootie; Mootos; Mor a Grifa; *Mota*; Mother; Mother Mary; *Moto*; Mow the Grass; Mu; M.U.; Muggie; Muggle; Muggles; Murphy; Muta; Mutah; Mutha; Nail; *Neihe*; Nigra; Nordie; Northern Lights; Nug; Nuggets; Number; O.J.; Old Toby; Ontario Hydro; Oregano; *Pakaloco*; *Pakalolo*; Pakistani Black; Panama Cut; Panama Gold; Panama Red; *Panatella*; Paper Blunts; Parsley; *Pasto*; Pat; Phillips; Pin; Pod; Poke; Pot; *Potiguaya*; Potlikker; Potten Bush; P.R.; *Pretendica*; *Pretendo*; Pretties; Puff; Purple; Purple Haze; Purple Kush; Queen Anne's Lace; Ragweed; Railroad Weed; Rainy Day Woman; Rangood; Rasta Weed; Red Bud; Red Cross; Red Dirt; Reef; Reefer; Reefers; Regs; Relish; RGB; Righteous Bush; Rip; *Roacha*; Root; Rope; Rose Marie; Rough Stuff; Rube; *Rubia*; Rugs; Salad; Salt and Pepper; *Santa Marta*; Sasfras; Sativa; Schwag; Schwamp; Scissors; Seeds; Sen; Sensi; Sess; Sezz; Shake; Sheeba; Shwag; Siddi; Sinse; Sinsemilla; Sizzla; Skunk; Skunk Weed; Smoke; Smoke Canada; Snop; Soul Flower; Spliff; Splim; Stack; Stank; Stems; Stick; Sticky; Sticky Black; Stink Weed; Stoney Weed; Straw; Stuff; Sugar Weed; Super Pot; Swag; Swamp Grass; Sweet Leaf; Sweet Lucy; Tack; Taima; *Takkouri*; Tea; Texas Red; Texas Pot; Texas Tea; Tex-Mex; Thai; Thai Sticks; Thaistick Swisher; THC; Thirteen; Thumb; Time; Towels; Tree; Triple A; Tulip; Turtle; Tustin; *Unotque*; Viper's Weed; Wacky Baccy; Wacky Tabacky; Wacky Weed; Wake and Bake; Weed; Weed Oil; Weed Tea; Whackatabacky; Wheat; White-Haired Lady; Winnipeg Wheelchair Weed; Wood; Woodie; *Yaa*; *Yandi*; Yeh; Yellow Submarine; Yen Pop; *Yerba*; *Yerhia*; *Yesca*; *Yesco*; Yoda; Zambi; Zoot

Pharmacologic Classification

Psychodelic, miscellaneous

Brief General Overview

The cannabis plant is a hardy annual that grows well in both tropical and temperate climates. The various species of cannabis include *Cannabis lativa* and *Cannabis sativa* (i.e., Indian hemp). *Cannabis sativa* is the principal variety from which marijuana, hashish, and hashish oil are prepared. There are several varieties of *Cannabis sativa,* including *Cannabis sativa indica, Cannabis sativa ruderalis,* and *Cannabis sativa sativa,*[3] which differ significantly in their concentration of active ingredients.[4] The *indica* variety has the highest concentrations. The concentration of the most prominent ingredient, delta-9-tetrahydrocannabinol (THC), which has been demonstrated to be responsible for virtually all of the mental and physical effects associated with cannabis use, also varies within each cannabis plant. The highest concentrations are found in the bracts or small leaves at the base of the cannabis flowers, and then, in decreasing order, in the flowering tops, upper leaves, large stems, seeds, and roots (lowest concentration). In addition, the female plants tend to have a much higher THC concentration than the male plants.

For over 10,000 years, cannabis has been an integral part of human history. It has been used by different peoples at different times as a cooking oil, a food, a medicine, a religious sacrament, and an intoxicant. Its fibers have been made into clothing, paper, rope, and ship's sails. A timeline of the history of cannabis use is presented in Table 4. Currently, cannabis is the most widely and commonly used illicit drug or substance of abuse in North America.[5] Among North American adolescents, the rates of cannabis use display few ethnic or racial differences. However, by early adulthood (i.e., early 20s) rates of both cannabis use and psychological dependence become significantly higher for those of African descent.

TABLE 4
Historical Timeline of Cannabis Use

8000 BC	Shards of pottery embossed with strips of hemp cord found in archeological debris from a prehistoric community on the island of Taiwan.
6000 BC	Cannabis seeds used for food in China.
4000 BC	Textiles made of hemp first used in China.
3000 BC	First use of cannabis as medicine recorded by Emperor Shen-ung in the Chinese pharmacopoeia Pen-ts'ao Ching for the treatment of absent-mindedness, beri-beri, constipation, "female weakness," gout, malaria, and rheumatism.
1500 BC	Bhang recognized by Hindus as one of the five sacred plants of India. Mentioned in the sacred text *Atharva Veda* and used as a ritual offering to the god Shiva, who is believed to have brought cannabis from the Himalayas for human enjoyment and enlightenment.
700 BC	The Zoroastrians, an ancient Parsee (Persian) religious sect, use cannabis as a central component of their religion. Bhang is described as the "good narcotic" in their holy book, the *Zend-Avesta*.
500 BC	After burial of the dead, the Scythians cleanse themselves with a vapor bath produced by throwing cannabis seeds onto red-hot stones. Cannabis introduced to Europe by the Scythians.
200 BC	Hemp fabrics produced in Europe (in what is now France). The Essenes, an ancient Hebrew sect in Israel, use cannabis medicinally.
70	Pedacius Dioscorides, a Greek physician who traveled with and treated the Roman soldiers for many years, mentions the use of cannabis in his herbal text, *De Materia Medica*, to treat earaches and to diminish sexual desires.
105	First paper created in China by Ts'ai Lun out of pulp produced from hemp fibers and mulberry tree bark.
150	Claudius Galen (AD 130–200), a Greek physician, notes the custom in which rich Romans give a confection made with hemp seed to banquet guests to promote happiness.
600	Jewish Talmud mentions the euphoric properties of cannabis. In the Tantric religion in Tibet, a derivative of Buddhism based on a fear of demons, cannabis use is an integral part of rituals to overcome evil forces and to heighten sensual experience during sexual intercourse.
1000	Hashish eating spreads throughout Arabia.

(continued)

TABLE 4 (continued)
Historical Timeline of Cannabis Use

1300	Cannabis introduced to the east coast of Africa by Arab traders.
	Marco Polo (1254–1324) recounts use of hashish by the followers of Hasan ibn al-Sabbah: The Grand Master of the Assassins, whenever he discovers a young man resolute enough to belong to his murderous legions . . . invites the youth to his table and intoxicates him with the plant "hashish." Having been secretly transported to the pleasure gardens the young man imagines that he has entered the Paradise of Mahomet. The girls, lovely as Houris, contribute to the illusion. After he has enjoyed to satiety all the joys promised by the Prophet to his elect, he falls back to the presence of the Grand Master. Here he is informed that he can enjoy perpetually the delights he has just tasted if he will take part in the war of the infidel as commanded by the Prophet.
1378	Ottoman Emir Soudoun Scheikhouni issues an edict prohibiting the eating of hashish.
1545	Hemp is planted in Chile by the Spanish. Most of the hemp is used to make rope for the Spanish army stationed in Chile. The remainder is used to replace worn-out riggings on sailing ships docked in the harbor at Santiago.
1600s	Various requests made and laws passed throughout this century, both in England and in the New World, that require colonists in the New England colonies (e.g., Connecticut, Maryland, Massachusetts, Virginia) to plant a specified number of hemp plants. Governments reward farmers for producing hemp by offering to trade tobacco for hemp or allowing hemp to be used to pay a farmer's debts. England needed hemp to make ropes and canvas for its sailing ships. The hemp produced in its New World colonies was less expensive than that purchased elsewhere and thus would help England reduce its national foreign debt. The colonies did not meet expectations for hemp production, and most of England's imports of hemp during this century were from France.
1609	Hemp cultivation in Nova Scotia under the supervision of Louis Hébert, a botanist and the first apothecary in New France. France had explorer and politician Samuel de Champlain (1567–1635), co-founder of Montreal, carry hemp seeds with him during his early expeditions to New France. Like England, France had an economic interest in having its New World colonies grow hemp and ship the raw material to Europe.
1753	Indian hemp officially classified as *Cannabis sativa* by the Swedish botanist Carolus Linnaeus (1707–1778).
1762	Colony of Virginia awarded bounties for hemp production.
1765	"Sowed hemp at muddy hole by swamp" (Diary of George Washington [1732–1799], May 12–13, 1765).
1775	The first flag of the United States made by Betsy Ross from hemp cloth.
1800	Napoleon Bonaparte (1769–1821) discovers that much of the Egyptian lower class habitually uses hashish; he prohibits its use by the French army of occupation. However, French soldiers and scientists took hashish back to France when they returned.
1843	*Le Club des Haschischins* (Hash Eater's Club) established in Paris by the French writer Théophile Gautier (1811–1872).
1857	*The Hashish Eater*, by the American writer Fitz Hugh Ludlow (1836–1870), is published. The book was patterned after and strongly influenced by the work on opium by Thomas de Quincey (1822). It was extremely popular and influenced early public opinion on the personal use of cannabis.
1860	*Les Paradis Artificiels* (Artificial Paradise), by the French poet Charles Pierre Baudelaire (1821–1867), published in Paris, describes the experience of hashish use in "Poem of Hashish."
1890	Hashish made illegal in Turkey.
1894	India Hemp Commission Report issued. Several medical uses for cannabis are noted, including the treatment of cholera, diabetes, dysentery, gonorrhea, hay fever, impotence, and urinary incontinence.
1906	U.S. Pure Food and Drug Act passed, regulating the labeling of products that contain, among other ingredients, cannabis.

(continued)

TABLE 4 (continued)
Historical Timeline of Cannabis Use

1910–1930	Mexican migrant laborers commonly bring marijuana with them when they work in the United States.
1914	Marijuana commonly used in Mexico by soldiers of the Mexican general and revolutionary Francisco (Pancho) Villa (1877–1923). A popular Mexican folk song, "La Cucaracha" (the cockroach), which concerns "marihuana" use, supposedly was composed by one of these soldiers during the Mexican revolutions (1909–1914); first noted use of the term "marihuana" for cannabis.
1915	Utah passes first state anti-marijuana law in accordance with Mormon religious prohibitions. California passes anti-marijuana law.
1920s	Many North Americans replace alcohol use, which is prohibited, with marijuana use.
1930s	In North America, marijuana increasingly referred to in both the lay and professional presses as a "menace." States enact laws to restrict or prohibit use.
1937	U.S. Marijuana Tax Act passed by Congress.
1943	Farmers urged to grow hemp for U.S. war effort.
1950–Present	Rastafarians, a contemporary, primarily Jamaican, religious sect, use *ganja* as a sacrament to facilitate communication with god (*Jah*).
1964	THC isolated.
1960–Present	Marijuana use widely popularized among North American youth.
1970	Comprehensive Drug Abuse Prevention and Control Act of 1970 abolishes minimal mandatory sentences for controlled substances (including marijuana) and makes the offense of possession for one's own use a misdemeanor.
1980–Present	"War on drugs" (including cannabis) waged in North America.
1990–Present	Decriminalization and efforts at legalization of cannabis gain increased support in a number of jurisdictions across North America, including several states.[a] Increased public support for medical use of marijuana. Marijuana becomes a major export crop for the Canadian province of British Columbia, with "export" exclusively to the United States.
2004	Federal marijuana laws changed in Canada, making personal possession of less than 15 grams a noncriminal offense.
2008	Federal Court in Canada allows medical marijuana users more freedom in selecting their own growers and allows approved growers to supply medical marijuana to more than one patient.
2009	Marijuana grow-ops increase with youth gang violence, drive-by shootings, and turf war shoot-outs and murders. In Canada, high THC content BC Bud continues to be traded for hand guns and cocaine across the United States–Canada border. California (as well as other states) considers legalization and taxation of marijuana in order to deal with increasing public debt.

[a]However, under U.S. federal law, which supersedes related state laws, possession of cannabis continues to be a criminal offense in all states.
Source: Adapted from Pagliaro, L.A., & Pagliaro, A.M. (2004). *Pagliaros' comprehensive guide to drugs and substances of abuse*. Washington, DC: American Pharmacists Association.

Dosage Forms and Routes of Administration

Although other methods of use have been used (e.g., drinking "marijuana beer," eating "marijuana cookies" or "brownies,"[6] injecting hashish oil intravenously), none of these methods has proved to be as popular among users as pulmonary inhalation ("smoking" or "toking"), which remains the principal, virtually exclusive method of cannabis use.[7] Oral doses of cannabis must be three to five times greater than smoked doses in order to produce equivalent actions (THC is absorbed to a far greater extent from the lungs than from the GI tract, and oral doses have poorer bioavailability), and intravenous injection is associated with such harmful effects as infections and pain and injury at injection sites. Thus, cannabis is prepared in three forms—marijuana, hashish, and hashish oil—for smoking.

Marijuana is the dried plant form of cannabis. Various parts of the plant are dried, chopped, and prepared for smoking. The marijuana is traditionally smoked using a water pipe (e.g., "argileh" or "hookah;" glass pipe, or "bong").[8] More typically, particularly in North America, it is smoked after being rolled into a cigarette (i.e., "joint," "reefer").[9] Each marijuana cigarette usually contains ~750 mg of cannabis. The THC content varies among plants and also varies in regard to the part of the plant that is being used and its sex (female plants have higher THC concentrations than male plants). THC content is highest in the flowering tops and bracts (i.e., small leaves around each bud or flower) and lowest in the stem stock and seeds (i.e., overall range from 0.5% to 10%).[10] However, the amount of THC that reaches the lungs and is absorbed into the bloodstream depends upon the amount smoked, the smoking technique used, and the amount destroyed by pyrolysis. It is important to note that during the 1970s, 1980s, and 1990s, the potency of cannabis increased 5-fold from an average of 2% to 10% THC content. This change in potency occurred as use changed from *Cannabis (sativa) sativa* to *Cannabis (sativa) indica* and as sinsemilla varieties were selectively cultivated. Most of the mid- to high-grade marijuana that is smoked in the United States is grown in Canada and Mexico[11] and is illicitly imported, or smuggled, into the United States from these neighboring countries.

Hashish is the extracted resin and compressed flowers of the cannabis plant, which is dried and sold in "bricks," "cakes," or "slabs." On a weight or volume basis, it has a significantly higher average THC content (i.e., 15% to 30%) than does marijuana. Hashish is often smoked in a "hash pipe." Hashish oil is a refined (purified) derivative of hashish. It has the highest THC concentration (i.e., 30% to 80%), on a weight or volume basis, of all the forms of cannabis. A marijuana joint or tobacco cigarette is often dipped in hashish oil and then smoked.[12,13] Most high-grade hashish is illicitly imported into North America from North Africa, the Middle East, and parts of Asia (e.g., Afghanistan, Morocco,[14] Pakistan, and Turkey).

Mechanism of CNS Action

The exact molecular mechanism of action for cannabis has not been determined, but it appears to involve binding to the cannabinoid receptors (i.e., CB_1 and CB_2) within the CNS.[15,16] CB_1 and its ligands appear to function as a neuromodulatory system. Thus, the first endocannabinoid (i.e., a cannabinoid that occurs naturally in the human body) was named "Anandamide" after the ancient Sanskrit word *ananda*, meaning bliss or happiness. However, individual response to the action of cannabis is not always pleasant, and stimulation of the CB_1 receptor may elicit feelings of anxiety or panic—and even psychosis—in some users. In addition, stimulation of the CB_1 receptor causes feelings of hunger and an increased appetite (i.e., the "munchies"). The cannabinoids also have been demonstrated to inhibit the release of various neurotransmitters in the CNS, including acetylcholine in the hippocampus and noradrenaline in the cerebellum, cortex, and hippocampus.[17] Delta-9-tetrahydrocannabinol has been found to increase dopamine release in the nucleus accumbens and prefrontal cortex.

CB$_2$ receptors are primarily present on immune cells, predominantly outside the CNS. These receptors appear to mediate the activation of mitogen-activated protein kinase and the inhibition of adenylate cyclase. The endocannabinoid activity of these receptors (e.g., enhancement of the physiological response to cytokines) suggests a role in immunosuppression and anti-inflammatory action.

Pharmacodynamics/Pharmacokinetics

Delta-9-tetrahydrocannabinol (THC), the principal psychoactive cannabinoid present in cannabis, is rapidly absorbed and transferred from the lungs to the blood during cannabis smoking. The mean bioavailability of THC from smoked cannabis is 27% (range, 17% to 37%). Oral bioavailability is low (i.e., ~10%) because of extensive first-pass metabolism. Once absorbed into the blood, THC undergoes oxidative metabolism, primarily in the liver, to yield both the active metabolite, 11-hydroxy-delta-9-tetrahydrocannabinol (11-OH-THC),[18] and the inactive metabolite, 11-nor-9-carboxy-delta-9-tetrahydrocannabinol (THCCOOH).[19] THC blood concentrations peak prior to the end of smoking cannabis, 11-OH-THC concentrations peak just after the end of smoking cannabis, and THCCOOH concentrations peak 1.5 to 2 hours after the start of smoking cannabis. THC is ~97% protein bound, while its active metabolite, 11-OH-THC, is highly protein bound (i.e., ~99%). The apparent volume of distribution of THC is ~10 L/kg, primarily because of its high lipid solubility. Some researchers report a mean "initial" (i.e., α or distribution) half-life for THC of ~30 hours.[20] However, the later β-phase elimination half-life is about 3.5 days (because of preferential concentration and storage of THC in the spleen and body fat) (range, 1 to 7 days). Total body clearance of THC generally ranges from 750 to 1200 mL/minute. The elimination half-life of the inactive metabolite, THCCOOH, is 2 to 6 days. Metabolites are excreted in the urine and also secreted back into the gut (by means of enterohepatic recirculation), where they are reabsorbed or excreted in the feces. THC and its two major metabolites, 11-OH-THC and THCCOOH, are present in the urine as glucuronide conjugates. Low concentrations of THC metabolites can often be detected in the feces and urine for more than 5 weeks after cannabis was last used.

Generally, urinary concentrations of THC greater than 1.5 ng/mL are suggestive of cannabis use during the previous 8-hour period. However, significant intersubject variability in THC pharmacokinetics occurs. In addition, during the initial phase of cannabis use (i.e., generally during the first 30 to 45 minutes after "smoking" has begun), hysteresis occurs (i.e., the blood concentrations of THC are "out of phase" with observed mental and physical effects). THC blood concentrations appear to correlate best with observed effects from 1 to 8 hours after use. However, overall, because of pharmacokinetic considerations and resultant extreme interindividual variability, a presumptive blood concentration of THC cannot be reliably related to a specific measurable level of behavior or impairment.

Urine Tests: The urine tests currently used for detecting cannabis use can detect concentrations of both THC and THCCOOH (the major metabolite of cannabis) as low as 1 ng per 1 mL of urine with very good validity and reliability. However, the validity of urine tests per se can be problematic. Urine tests can give false positive results because of the interference of certain other drugs (e.g., ibuprofen) and because the tests cannot differentiate between cannabis that is deliberately smoked and cannabis that is passively inhaled in sidestream smoke (i.e., second-hand smoke). In addition, ingestion of large amounts of hemp seed oil products may produce false positive results if the cutoff values designated by the laboratory for the urine test are too low. Urine tests also can give false negative results. These are much more likely to occur when the urine is deliberately adulterated with an in vitro adulterant (e.g., pyridinium chlorochromate, which is found in "Urine Luck®," a product specifically developed to invalidate urine tests).

False positive or false negative urine tests also may occur as a result of the presence of other drugs and substances that have been used. Usually, these tests can be verified by reanalyzing the urine sample with more specific and sensitive analytical equipment and procedures (e.g., high pressure liquid chromatography [HPLC] or gas chromatography with mass spectrometry [GC–MS]). However, these analytical techniques are much more time consuming and expensive than the urine immunoassays that are generally used, and they can still give false negative results if the urine sample has been deliberately adulterated.

Current Approved Indications for Medical Use[21]

Anorexia and weight loss associated with AIDS (AIDS wasting syndrome); severe nausea and vomiting associated with cancer chemotherapy

Desired Action/Reason for Personal Use

Disinhibition; euphoria; feeling of relaxation; feeling of well-being; pleasure; prevention/self-management of the cannabis withdrawal syndrome; sensory and perceptual distortion

Toxicity[22]

Acute: Abnormal thinking, including paranoia and impaired linear thinking; anxiety; appetite, increased; asthenia; ataxia; attention span, reduced; blood pressure, increased (mild); blurred vision; cognitive impairment, including impaired concentration; confusion; conjunctival redness; delusions; depersonalization (rare); dizziness; drowsiness; dry mouth; hallucinations; headache; heart rate, increased; linear thinking processes, impaired; memory impairment, particularly of short-term memory; motor vehicle crashes[23]; muscle weakness; panic attacks (rare); panic reactions; paranoia; perceptual distortion, including spatial perception and perception of time; psychomotor impairment; psychosis, acute; schizophrenia[24]; sensory stimulation; somnolence; synesthesia; tachycardia; temporal disintegration (i.e., disintegration of sequential thought patterns so that past, present, and future become confused); toxic delirium; visual acuity, decreased; weakness

Chronic: Amotivational syndrome[25]; attentional impairment; conjunctival infections; immunosuppression[26]; lung cancer[27]; lung irritation and disease; memory impairment; physical dependence (relatively mild); psychological dependence; psychosis[28]; respiratory impairment (e.g., bronchitis, chronic cough, irritation of respiratory tract, sore throat, wheezing)[29]

Pregnancy & Lactation: Safety of cannabis use by adolescent girls and women who are pregnant has not been established. The teratogenic potential of cannabis use during pregnancy[30] is considered to be low.[31] Additional valid and reliable data are needed.

Safety of cannabis use by adolescent girls and women who are breast-feeding has not been established. However, significant amounts of THC are excreted in breast milk and expected effects (e.g., drowsiness) can be observed in breast-fed neonates and infants. Therefore, adolescent girls and women who are breast-feeding should not use cannabis.

Abuse Potential

Physical dependence: Low[32] (USDEA Schedule I; use is prohibited)[33]
Psychological dependence: Moderate

Withdrawal Syndrome

Daily users of high dosages of cannabis may experience a relatively mild withdrawal reaction upon abrupt discontinuation of cannabis use. Signs and symptoms, which can last for up to 1 week, may include anorexia, anxiety, chills, insomnia, irritability, nervousness, restlessness, rebound increase in rapid eye movement (REM) sleep, stomach upset, sweating, tremors, and weight loss.

Overdosage

Rarely fatal,[34] severe cannabis overdosages can result in the following signs and symptoms: ataxia, depersonalization, lethargy, panic reactions, postural hypotension, psychomotor impairment, slurred speech, tachycardia, and urinary retention. Most cases of cannabis overdosage may be managed with supportive care provided in a safe, quiet, and reassuring environment. In some cases, diazepam (Valium®) may be required for the medical management of extreme agitation. There is no known antidote currently available. However, antagonists of the cannabinoid receptors have been developed.

Notes

1. The synthetic form of THC is available under the generic name dronabinol (Marinol®). It has been used since 1984 primarily to treat the nausea and vomiting associated with cancer chemotherapy. A related synthetic chemical analogue, nabilone (Cesamet®), also has been produced for similar clinical indications and has been available since 1976.
2. In the United States, April 20 (i.e., 4/20) is the unofficial national "weed smoking holiday" that is commonly referred to as "J-Day." In addition, 4:20 pm is the time that school is let out and, presumably, youth are free to smoke marijuana. The term "420" also is common prison slang for cannabis.
3. Some botanical taxonomies classify *indica*, *ruderalis*, and *sativa* as belonging to different species of cannabis.
4. Over 400 chemicals, including many of the same chemicals found in tobacco smoke (with the notable exception of nicotine), are found in cannabis or are formed (i.e., by means of pyrolysis) when it is burned. Over 60 of these chemicals are unique to cannabis and thus are referred to as cannabinoids (e.g., cannabidiol, cannabinol, delta-8-tetrahydrocannabinol, delta-9-tetrahydrocannabinol [THC]).
5. Cannabis held this distinction for the last several decades of the 20th century, and recent reports suggest that its use is increasing. In addition, as concerns about its use decrease and arguments for decriminalization and legalization continue, cannabis use is expected to increase even more.
6. The oral bioavailability of cannabis is only 5% to 10% (i.e., $F = 0.05$ to 0.1).
7. The heat-generated decomposition (i.e., pyrolysis) of cannabis that occurs during smoking (i.e., burning) results in decarboxylation of the acid derivative of delta-9-tetrahydrocannabinol to its principal active form, delta-9-tetrahydrocannabinol.

8. A more recent and increasingly common method of use involves inhaling a mass of smoke from a "bucket" (i.e., a plastic soft drink or water bottle that has had the top portion or neck cut off). Both marijuana and hashish are "burned" in these "buckets," and the smoke inhaled.

9. Some marijuana smokers, particularly gang members or those who want to be gang members (i.e., "wannabe's"), roll the marijuana in a cigar wrap. These marijuana cigars generally contain significantly more marijuana than do marijuana cigarettes and are commonly referred to as "blunts." Blunts also refer to hollowed-out cigars that are filled with marijuana.

10. Average THC content of commercial grade domestic or Mexican marijuana is 5% to 10%. By comparison, British Columbian marijuana (i.e., "BC Bud"), which is widely available in the northwestern United States, has a current average THC content of 15% to 30%. Sinsemilla varieties of cannabis (i.e., those varieties that are grown without seeds, or only the unfertilized female plants) can have THC concentrations up to twice those listed for marijuana, hashish, and hashish oil (i.e., up to 25% for marijuana, up to 30% for hashish, and up to 80% for hashish oil).

11. Mexico, for example, produced over 15,000 tons of marijuana in 2008.

12. Young men of Hispanic American descent commonly smoke "fry," marijuana cigarettes (i.e., "joints") or marijuana cigars (i.e., "blunts") soaked in "embalming fluid" that has been laced with phencyclidine (PCP). The cannabis and embalming fluid concoction is commonly referred to as "fry" by users because it "fries your brain." (It also is referred to as "wet.") The "fry" is usually smoked with a group of three to five friends (or fellow gang members) who also consume alcoholic beverages (e.g., "Cisco," or fortified wine) while smoking. Delusions, hallucinations, and toxic psychosis occur commonly in relation to the use of "fry." In addition, disorientation, paranoia, and panic frequently occur, and often result in aggressive and violent behavior toward others. Psychomotor impairment also is commonly observed. Regular long-term use has been associated with brain damage, incapacitating mental disorders, and death. (Also see the Phencyclidine monograph.) The combination of marijuana and phencyclidine (see monograph) is often referred to as Happy Sticks; Illies; Love Boat; Wet; Wicky Sticks; or Zoom. If cocaine (see monograph) is added to this combination, it is referred to as "Jim Jones." The combination of marijuana and Crack cocaine is referred to as 3750s, *Diabolitos*, Lace, Oolies, *Primos*, Torpedo, Turbo, or Woolies.

13. During the 1960s an average cannabis cigarette (i.e., "joint," "reefer") contained approximately 10 mg of THC. Currently, a "high grade" cannabis cigarette can contain 150 mg of THC, and up to 300 mg of THC if it is dipped in hashish oil.

14. Hashish is unofficially Morocco's main source of foreign currency.

15. Whereas the CB_1 receptors are found in highest concentrations in the brain (primarily in the amygdala, basal ganglia, brain stem, cerebellum, cerebral cortex, hippocampus, striatum, and thalamus), the CB_2 receptors are found in highest concentrations in the cells of the immune system (i.e., in the spleen and hematopoietic cells).

16. Anandamide (N-arachidonylethanolamide) and 2-arachidonylglycerol have been isolated by researchers and are currently identified as the principal endocannabinoids (i.e., endogenous cannabinoid receptor ligands).

17. The cannabinoids also inhibit the release of noradrenaline at the sympathetic nerve terminals in the peripheral nervous system and inhibit adenylate cyclase.

18. 11-OH-THC is formed by hydroxylation at the 11-position. It is more lipid soluble than THC and, according to some published reports, more potent than THC. Thus, it may play a major role in regard to the observed effects of cannabis use.

19. Also known as 11-nor-delta-9-carboxy-tetrahydrocannabinol-9-carboxylic acid.

20. This mean half-life has often been erroneously reported in the published literature as the value for the elimination half-life.

21. The listed indications have been approved for the synthetic form of THC, dronabinol (see Note 1), and for the synthetic chemical analogue, nabilone. No specific medical uses for natural cannabis products (i.e., marijuana, hashish, hashish oil) currently are globally recognized. However, various states and jurisdictions have increasingly allowed their use for indications including severe nausea and vomiting associated with cancer chemotherapy, chronic pain syndromes, spasticity associated with neurological diseases (e.g., multiple sclerosis), and weight loss associated with debilitating illnesses (e.g., AIDS).

22. The noted effects, their intensity, and their clinical significance depend to a significant degree on the dosage of THC, the environment (circumstances) of use, and the physical, psychological, and social characteristics of the user (i.e., "drug, set, setting").

23. This involves reduced perceptual motor speed and accuracy and is significant enough to markedly contribute to the rate of airplane, car, train, and truck crashes. It is separate and distinct from impairment caused by alcohol consumption, which is common in cannabis users. The effect is significantly augmented when cannabis and alcohol are used concomitantly. However, many studies have indicated that being aware of their cognitive and psychomotor impairment, some marijuana users will make a conscious effort to drive more safely/cautiously (e.g., more slowly) to compensate for the impairment. Conversely, several studies have indicated that when alcohol has also been consumed, a common finding, particularly among young men, is that risk taking increases, as does the incidence of motor vehicle crashes.

24. Can range from precipitation of a first episode of schizophrenia (in a predisposed user) to toxic psychosis (in virtually all users). The use of cannabis can precipitate an acute, sometimes first, episode of schizophrenia in people who have a predisposition for psychotic disorders (i.e., have "preschizophrenia"). It also can exacerbate existing signs and symptoms of schizophrenia or initiate relapse in people who have schizophrenia.

25. This syndrome has been generally recognized since the 1970s. However, supporting evidence is largely anecdotal and derived from uncontrolled studies. Currently, several researchers question the validity of this syndrome and suggest that what actually is observed is simply regular long-term intoxication in cannabis users.

26. Appears to be modulated through interaction with the CB_2 receptor.

27. Lung cancer is an expected adverse effect of regular long-term cannabis smoking because of the presence of known human carcinogens in cannabis smoke in concentrations significantly higher than those found in tobacco cigarette smoke and the method of smoking cannabis (i.e., inhaling into the deepest recesses of the lungs and holding the smoke in the lungs, which is thought to maximize contact with alveoli and, hence, absorption of THC into the capillary system and general bloodstream).

28. Psychosis has been correlated with cannabis use for well over a century. However, the exact nature of this relationship is complex and, for a particular individual, may be (1) a spuriously related coincidence, (2) a result of some other underlying variable or characteristic, (3) an attempt by those with preexisting psychosis to self-medicate, (4) exacerbation or precipitation of frank psychosis when there is an underlying psychopathology (e.g., precipitation of first acute episode of schizophrenia), or (5) actual cannabis-induced psychosis in an otherwise mentally healthy person.

29. This toxicity is associated only with the "smoking" method of cannabis use. Cannabis, when smoked, yields more tar than does tobacco when smoked. In addition, the tar associated with cannabis smoke has higher concentrations of certain carcinogens (e.g., benzpyrene) than are found in the tar from tobacco smoke.

30. Marijuana is the illicit drug or substance of abuse most commonly used by pregnant women in North America.

31. Although THC can cross the placenta, studies of women who have used marijuana infrequently or moderately during pregnancy have not revealed a significant association with teratogenic effects. However, some studies suggest that higher-order cognitive functioning, such as attentional behavior and visual analysis/hypothesis testing in children is negatively correlated with in utero exposure to cannabis. We also note concerns about possible long-term negative effects of in utero exposure on memory processes (e.g., encoding and retrieval mechanisms).

32. Our 35 plus years of clinical experience with patients who have substance use disorders, and our review of the related published literature, indicate that this diagnosis, although previously rarely encountered among North American cannabis users, is increasing. This increase may be due to the higher potency, and hence increased dosage, of the cannabis used today. However, it has, for over 100 years, been noted in published literature on cannabis use in India. The diagnosis of "cannabis dependence with physiological dependence" is included in the *DSM-IV* and *DSM-IV-TR*.

33. Although personal use of cannabis is prohibited throughout Canada and the United States, several states, and the federal government of Canada, have decriminalized the possession of small amounts (generally less than 1 ounce or 30 grams) of cannabis for personal (i.e., recreational) use.

34. Fatalities associated with cannabis overdosage have been reported in the foreign published literature (e.g., professional journals published in India) and invariably involve the consumption of extremely potent forms of cannabis. Several of these fatalities have been associated with the oral consumption of *bhang*. *Bhang* is prepared by wet grinding with water a bolus of cannabis leaves that have a high

THC content. During the Hindu festival of ShivRatri, prayers and offerings are made to the lord Shiva, who is the god of all evils and poisons. *Bhang* is considered to be a special gift on this day and is offered to lord Shiva by means of self-ingestion. As increasing numbers of Hindus migrate to North America, such overdosage incidents may be anticipated, because such traditional beliefs and practices will likely be brought with them.

References

Adlaf, E.M., Paglia, A., Ivis, F.J., et al. (2000). Nonmedical drug use among adolescent students: Highlights from the 1999 Ontario Student Drug Use Survey. *CMAJ: Canadian Medical Association Journal, 162*(12), 1677-1680.

Ashton, C.H. (2001). Pharmacology and effects of cannabis: A brief review. *British Journal of Psychiatry, 178*, 101-106.

Barnes, R.E. (2000). Reefer madness: Legal & moral issues surrounding the medical prescription of marijuana. *Bioethics, 14*(1), 16-41.

Biecheler, M.B., Peytavin, J.F., SAM Group, et al. (2008). SAM survey on "drugs and fatal accidents": Search of substances consumed and comparison between drivers involved under the influence of alcohol or cannabis. *Traffic Injury Prevention, 9*(1), 11-21.

Biegon, A., & Kerman, I.A. (2001). Autoradiographic study of pre- and postnatal distribution of cannabinoid receptors in human brain. *Neuroimage, 14*(16), 1463-1468.

Bolla, K.I., Lesage, S.R., Gamaldo, C.E., et al. (2008). Sleep disturbance in heavy marijuana users. *Sleep, 31*(6), 901-908.

Clark, P.A. (2000). The ethics of medical marijuana: Government restrictions vs. medical necessity. *Journal of Public Health Policy, 21*(1), 40-60.

Cooper, Z.D., & Haney, M. (2008). Cannabis reinforcement and dependence: Role of the cannabinoid CB_1 receptor. *Addiction Biology, 13*(2), 188-195.

Court strikes down restriction in Ottawa's medical marijuana program. *HIV/AIDS Policy & Law Review, 13*(1), 45-46.

Davies, S.N., Pertwee, R.G., & Riedel, G. (2002). Functions of cannabinoid receptors in the hippocampus. *Neuropharmacology, 42*(8), 993-1007.

Ebrahim, S.H., & Gfroerer, J. (2003). Pregnancy-related substance use in the United States during 1996-1998. *Obstetrics and Gynecology, 101*(2), 374-379.

Grekin, E.R., & Ayna, D. (2008). Argileh use among college students in the United States: An emerging trend. *Journal of Studies on Alcohol and Drugs, 69*(3), 472-475.

Gupta, B.D., Jani, C.B., & Shah, P.H. (2001). Fatal 'Bhang' poisoning. *Medicine, Science, and the Law, 41*(4), 349-352.

Harrison, G.P. Jr., Gruber, A.J., Hudson, J.I., et al. (2002). Cognitive measures in long-term cannabis users. *Journal of Clinical Pharmacology, 42*(11, Suppl), 41S-47S.

Hollister, L.E. (2000). An approach to the medical marijuana controversy. *Drug and Alcohol Dependence, 58*(1-2), 3-7.

James, J.S. (2000). Marijuana safety study completed: Weight gain, no safety problems. *AIDS Treatment News, 4*(348), 3-4.

Johns, A. (2001). Psychiatric effects of cannabis. *British Journal of Psychiatry, 178*, 116-122.

Kumar, R.N., Chambers, W.A., & Pertwee, R.G. (2001). Pharmacological actions and therapeutic uses of cannabis and cannabinoids. *Anaesthesia, 56*(11), 1059-1068.

Lange, J.H., & Kruse, C.G. (2008). Cannabinoid CB_1 receptor antagonists in therapeutic and structural perspectives. *The Chemical Record, 8*(3), 156-168.

Leweke, F.M., Gerth, C.W., Klosterkötter, J. (2004). Cannabis-associated psychosis: Current status of research. *CNS Drugs, 18*(13), 895-910.

Lichtman, A.H., & Martin, B.R. (2005). Cannabinoid tolerance and dependence. *Handbook of Experimental Pharmacology, 168*, 691-717.

Lutz, B. (2002). Molecular biology of cannabinoid receptors. *Prostaglandins, Leukotrienes, and Essential Fatty Acids, 66*(2-3), 123-142.

Maccarrone, M., & Finazzi-Agro, A. (2002). Endocannabinoids and their actions. *Vitamins and Hormones, 65*, 225-255.

MacDonald, S., Mann, R., Chipman, M., et al. (2008). Driving behavior under the influence of cannabis or cocaine. *Traffic Injury Prevention, 9*(3), 190-194.

Manno, J.E., Manno, B.R., Kemp, P.M., et al. (2001). Temporal indication of marijuana use can be estimated from plasma and urine concentrations of delta9-tetrahydrocannabinol, 11-hydroxy-delta9-tetrahydrocannabinol, and 11-nor-delta9-tetrahydrocannabinol-9-carboxylic acid. *Journal of Analytical Toxicology, 25*(7), 538-549.

Moreira, F.A., & Lutz, B. (2008). The endocannabinoid system: Emotion, learning and addiction. *Addiction Biology, 13*(2), 196-212.

Nunez, L.A., & Gurpegui, M. (2002). Cannabis-induced psychosis: A cross-sectional comparison with acute schizophrenia. *Acta Psychiatrica Scandinavica, 105*(3), 173-178.

O'Kane, C.J., Tutt, D.C., & Bauer, L.A. (2002). Cannabis and driving: A new perspective. *Emergency Medicine (Fremantle), 14*(3), 296-303.

Pertwee, R.G. (2000). Cannabinoid receptor ligands: Clinical and neuropharmacological considerations relevant to future drug discovery and development. *Expert Opinion on Investigative Drugs, 9*(7), 1553-1571.

Peters, R.J. Jr., Kelder, S.H., Meshack, A., et al. (2005). Beliefs and social norms about cigarettes or marijuana sticks laced with embalming fluid and phencyclidine (PCP): Why youth use "fry." *Substance Use & Misuse, 40*(4), 563-571.

Radwan, M.M., Ross, S.A., Slade, D., et al. (2008). Isolation and characterization of new Cannabis constituents from a high potency variety. *Planta Medica, 74*(3), 267-272.

Reardon, S.F., & Buka, S.L. (2002). Differences in onset and persistence of substance abuse and dependence among whites, blacks, and Hispanics. *Public Health Reports, 117*(Suppl 1), S51-S59.

Sidney, S. (2002). Cardiovascular consequences of marijuana use. *Journal of Clinical Pharmacology, 42*(11, Suppl), 64S-70S.

Skosnik, P.D., Spatz-Glenn, L., & Park, S. (2001). Cannabis use is associated with schizotypy and attentional disinhibition. *Schizophrenia Research, 48*(1), 83-92.

Wachtel, S.R., ElSohly, M.A., Ross, S.A., et al. (2002). Comparison of the subjective effects of delta(9)-tetrahydrocannabinol and marijuana in humans. *Psychopharmacology (Berlin), 161*(4), 331-339.

Wang, T., Collet, J.P., Shapiro, S., et al. (2008). Adverse effects of medical cannabinoids: A systematic review. *CMAJ, Canadian Medical Association Journal, 178*(13), 1669-1678.

CARISOPRODOL (See Meprobamate)

CATHA EDULIS

Names

BAN or INN Generic Synonyms: None

Brand/Trade: None

Chemical: See "Mechanism of CNS Action"

Street: Abyssinia Salad; Abyssinian Tea; African Salad; Cat; Catha; Chat; Clarkie Cat; Feline; *Graba;* Joad; Kat; *Khat; Miraa; Miurung;* Oat; Pootie; *Qat; Quaadka; Quat; Tschat*

Pharmacologic Classification

Psychostimulant, miscellaneous: amphetamine-like (natural)

Brief General Overview

Catha edulis (*khat*) is a flowering shrub that is indigenous to eastern Africa and the Arabian peninsula (e.g., Yemen), where most *khat* users are found. However, immigrants from that area to Europe and North America have brought the tradition of using *khat* with them. In an effort to secure supplies of *khat* for the growing number of users, some of these immigrants have attempted to grow the *Catha edulis* bush in areas of North America that have climates similar to those of the Middle East (e.g., southern California, southwestern United States). These illegal outdoor commercial operations have been generally unsuccessful because they require rather sophisticated irrigation techniques and approaches for growing the plants. At least for now, needed supplies of *khat* are flown into North America daily from Africa and the Middle East.[1]

Generally, groups of immigrant men (from Eritrea, Ethiopia, Somalia, Yemen, or related countries) socially gather to chew moderate quantities (i.e., one bundle weighing approximately 1 pound, although the weight of each bundle can vary significantly) of *khat*. The fresh leaves and roots of the shrub are chewed intermittently and retained in the cheek until all the juices, which contain active alkaloids, have been extracted and absorbed. Tea and cola soft drinks (see Caffeine monograph) also are customarily consumed during these social gatherings, primarily to counter the bitter taste of *khat*.[2] Habitual khat chewers are most likely to be adolescent boys and men, 15 to 35 years of age, of East African or Arabian descent, and Muslim. Despite its illegal status in North America, the use of khat has steadily increased over the past decade.

Dosage Forms and Routes of Administration

Cathinone and cathine are the naturally occurring alkaloids found in the fresh young leaves of the *khat* (*Catha edulis Forsk*) bush and are the source of its psychostimulant properties. The cathinone in *khat* begins to degrade approximately 48 hours after the plant has been harvested. Cathine remains stable in the plant—even after harvesting. The alkaloids are extracted by chewing small bundles of leaves in a manner similar to chewing tobacco. The leaves are chewed and retained in the cheek—so that they can continue to be chewed intermittently to release the active alkaloids for buccal absorption. The spent leaves are then spat out.

Cathinone, legally available in Israel as 200 mg oral capsules (Hagigat®), is marketed as a natural stimulant and aphrodisiac. The capsules are generally ingested orally. However, some users open the capsules and intranasally sniff (i.e., snort) the contents. The Hagigat® capsules are available in North America primarily by purchase over the Internet. A new form of *Catha edulis* is called *graba*. *Graba*, a dried form of *Catha edulis* similar in appearance to marijuana, is produced in Ethiopia and shipped to Ethiopian and Somalian communities in North America.

Mechanism of CNS Action

The psychostimulant actions of *Catha edulis* are primarily due to two naturally occurring alkaloids, cathine and cathinone. Cathinone (alpha-aminopropiophenone)[3] is approximately 10 times more potent as a CNS stimulant than cathine (d-norpseudoephedrine). *Catha edulis* appears to increase dopamine levels in the synaptic cleft in a manner similar to the amphetamines.[4] (See the Amphetamines monograph for general information.)

Pharmacodynamics/Pharmacokinetics

Cathinone and cathine are well extracted (i.e., ~90%) from the chewed *khat* leaves. The mean buccal absorption (i.e., bioavailability) of the extracted cathinone is ~60% and ~85% for the cathine. The elimination half-life of cathinone is reported to be between 0.5 and 3 hours. The elimination half-life of cathine is reportedly between 2 and 8 hours. Effects generally last for 90 minutes to 3 hours.

Current Approved Indications for Medical Use

None

Desired Action/Reason for Personal Use

Alertness, vigilance or wakefulness; appetite or hunger suppression[5]; decrease fatigue; energy; euphoria (mild); pleasurable psychostimulant effects; sociability

Toxicity

Acute: Acute myocardial infarction; anorexia; chest pain; constipation; dyspnea; gastric irritation; headache; hyperactivity; hypertension; insomnia; poor concentration; mania; memory impairment; myalgia; mydriasis; nausea; tachycardia; violent behavior; vomiting

Chronic: Anorexia; cancer (oral); decreased work productivity[6]; gastritis; mental depression[7]; paranoia; periodontal disease[8]; physical dependence; physical exhaustion; psychological dependence; psychosis (rare); weight loss

Pregnancy & Lactation: Safety of *Catha edulis* use by adolescent girls and women who are pregnant has not been established. Regular use of cathinone during pregnancy has not been reported to be associated with a higher incidence of stillbirths or teratogenic effects. However, as might be expected with the use of a psychostimulant, birth weight is generally reduced. Data on the effects of cathine use during pregnancy are not available. Additional valid and reliable data are needed.

Safety of *Catha edulis* use by adolescent girls and women who are breast-feeding has not been established. Valid and reliable data on cathinone excretion in breast milk are unavailable. However, cathine is excreted in significant quantities in breast milk. Therefore, adolescent girls and women who are breast-feeding should not use *Catha edulis*.

Abuse Potential[9]

Physical dependence: Low to moderate (Cathinone is USDEA Schedule I, use is prohibited; Cathine is a USDEA Schedule IV, low potential for abuse.)
Psychological dependence: Moderate

Withdrawal Syndrome

A specific *Catha edulis* withdrawal syndrome has been reported. After discontinuation of regular, long-term *Catha edulis* use, signs and symptoms of withdrawal may include hallucinations, primarily hypnagogic (dreams occurring just before loss of consciousness), lethargy, mental depression (generally mild), nightmares, and tremor (slight).

Overdosage

Valid and reliable data are not available. There is no known antidote.

Notes

1. The fresh leaves are generally packaged in bundles, which are wrapped in plastic bags or banana leaves in order to help preserve their freshness, and air-freighted by courier services, such as FedEx and UPS, to the immigrants' new homeland. This handling method appears to help preserve the potency of the cathinone. Most air courier shipments originate in Ethiopia, Kenya, Somalia, or Yemen.
2. Because the vast majority of *Catha edulis* users are Muslims, alcohol, which their religion prohibits, is not usually consumed at these social gatherings.
3. Its metabolites are norephedrine and norpseudoephedrine.
4. Although the reference is not entirely accurate, *Catha edulis* has been referred to as a "natural amphetamine" because of its observed pharmacologic action, which is quite similar to that of the amphetamines.
5. *Catha edulis* is used as an anorexiant by some Muslims, particularly during the ninth month of the Muslim year (i.e., Ramadan) when fasting from sunrise to sunset is practiced. However, according to interpretation of the Quran in Saudi Arabia, its cultivation and use are strictly forbidden.
6. This can result in significant economic costs for both the individual user and, where users are numerous, the users' community or country.
7. The depression may be severe and may be accompanied by suicidal ideation and actions.
8. Although oral hygiene and periodontal health generally do not appear to be significantly adversely affected by chewing *Catha edulis*, staining of the teeth (similar to that associated with tobacco chewing) and irritation and sores affecting the buccal membranes, lips, salivary glands, and tongue have been reported.
9. Although *Catha edulis* is illegal in North America, it is legal in most Middle Eastern and East African countries, particularly those that are predominantly Muslim. It also is legal in several European countries, including England, where its importation, exportation, distribution, sale, and use all are legal activities.

References

Al-Habori, M. (2005). The potential adverse effects of habitual use of Catha edulis (khat). *Expert Opinion on Drug Safety, 4*(6), 1145-1154.

Al-Motarreb, A., Briancon, S., Al-Jaber, N., et al. (2005). Khat chewing is a risk factor for acute myocardial infarction: A case control study. *British Journal of Clinical Pharmacology, 59*(5), 574-581.

Belew, M., Kebede, D., Kassaye, M., et al. (2000). The magnitude of khat use and its association with health, nutrition and socio-economic status. *Ethiopian Medical Journal, 38*(1), 11-26.

Bentur, Y., Bloom-Krasik, A., & Raikhlin-Eisenkraft, B. (2008). Illicit cathinone ("Hagigat") poisoning. *Clinical Toxicology, 46*(3), 206-210.

Dhaifalah, I., & Santavý, J. (2004). Khat habit and its health effect. A natural amphetamine. *Biomedical Papers of the Medical Faculty of the University of Palacky, Olomouc, Czech Republic, 148*(1), 11-15.

Hassan, N.A., Gunaid, A.A., Abdo-Rabbo, A.A., et al. (2000). The effect of Qat chewing on blood pressure and heart rate in healthy volunteers. *Tropical Doctor, 30*(2), 107-108.

Hassan, N.A., Gunaid, A.A., & Murray-Lyon, I.M. (2007). Khat (Catha edulis): Health aspects of khat chewing. *Eastern Mediterranean Health Journal, 13*(3), 706-718.

Kassie, F., Darroudi, F., Kundi, M., et al. (2001). Khat (Catha edulis) consumption causes genotoxic effects in humans. *International Journal of Cancer, 92*(3), 329-332.

Mwenda, J.M., Arimi, M.M., Kyama, M.C., et al. (2003). Effects of khat (Catha edulis) consumption on reproductive functions: A review. *East African Medical Journal, 80*(6), 318-323.

Patel, N.B. (2000). Mechanism of action of cathinone: The active ingredient of khat (Catha edulis). *East African Medical Journal, 77*(6), 329-332.

Toennes, S.W., Harder, S., Schramm, M., et al. (2003). Pharmacokinetics of cathinone, cathine and norephedrine after the chewing of khat leaves. *British Journal of Clinical Pharmacology, 56*(1), 125-130.

CATHINE (See *Catha edulis*)

CATHINONE (See *Catha edulis*)

CHLORAL HYDRATE

Names

BAN or INN Generic Synonyms: Trichloroacetaldehyde

Brand/Trade: Aquachloral®; Aquachloral Supprettes®; Noctec®; and generally available by generic name

Chemical: Trichloroacetaldehyde

Street[1]**:** Chlorals; Chorals; Coral; Green Frogs; Mickeys; Peter; TCA

Pharmacologic Classification

Psychodepressant, sedative-hypnotic: miscellaneous

Brief General Overview

Chloral hydrate was first synthesized in 1832 and is the oldest of the synthetic sedative-hypnotic drugs. A popular sedative-hypnotic through most of the 19th and 20th centuries, chloral hydrate, like the barbiturates (see Barbiturates monograph), has been virtually completely replaced in clinical practice by the benzodiazepines (see Benzodiazepines monograph). Similarly, its personal use as a psychodepressant is now mostly of historical interest.

Dosage Forms and Routes of Administration

Chloral hydrate is legally available from licit pharmaceutical manufacturers as an oral capsule (soft gelatin), oral syrup, or rectal suppository. People who use chloral hydrate generally orally ingest the oral formulations.

Mechanism of CNS Action

The CNS depressant action of chloral hydrate is due to its active metabolite, trichloroethanol. The mechanism of action appears to be similar to that for alcohol (see monograph). However, the exact mechanism of action has not been determined.

Pharmacodynamics/Pharmacokinetics

Chloral hydrate is rapidly and well absorbed (~100%) from the GI tract after oral or rectal use. It is 70% to 80% plasma protein bound and has an apparent volume of distribution of ~0.6 L/kg. Chloral hydrate is rapidly and extensively metabolized in the liver and erythrocytes by alcohol dehydrogenase to its active metabolite, trichloroethanol. It is widely distributed to all body tissues, including the placenta. It is found in cerebrospinal fluid and breast milk. Trichloroethanol has a mean elimination half-life of 8 hours (range, 4 to 12 hours). Trichloroethanol is variably metabolized, primarily in the liver, but also in the kidneys, to trichloroacetic acid (an inactive metabolite). The half-life of trichloroethanol is prolonged in preterm neonates (37 hours) and children (10 hours). It is also prolonged in adults with impaired capacity for glucuronidation.

After oral or rectal use of a therapeutic dose of chloral hydrate, the onset of sedative action usually occurs in ~30 minutes. Sleep is induced within 60 minutes.

Current Approved Indications for Medical Use[2]

Insomnia

Desired Action/Reason for Personal Use

Alcohol-like disinhibitory euphoria or "high"; anxiety/stress reduction; also, purposely administered to others without their knowledge in the context of perpetration of a drug-facilitated crime (e.g., robbery; sexual assault, including date rape)[3]

Toxicity

Acute: Ataxia; cardiac dysrhythmias; cognitive impairment; confusion; diarrhea; dizziness; drowsiness; dyspepsia; hypotension; intermittent porphyria (acute); memory impairment; respiratory depression (may be severe); vomiting

Chronic: Gastritis; hepatic damage; mental depression; myocardial depression; neurotoxicity[4]; physical dependence; psychological dependence; renal damage; skin rash

Pregnancy & Lactation: FDA Pregnancy Category "not established." Safety of chloral hydrate use by adolescent girls and women who are pregnant has not been established. Chloral hydrate crosses the placenta, and regular long-term maternal use during pregnancy can result in signs and symptoms of the chloral hydrate withdrawal syndrome in neonates. Adolescent girls and women who are pregnant should not use chloral hydrate.

Safety of chloral hydrate use by adolescent girls and women who are breast-feeding has not been established. However, both chloral hydrate and its active metabolite, trichloroethanol, are excreted in significant concentrations in breast milk and may cause drowsiness in breast-fed neonates and infants, who also may become physically dependent. Adolescent girls and women who are breast-feeding should not use chloral hydrate.

Abuse Potential

Physical dependence: Moderate (USDEA Schedule IV; low potential for abuse)
Psychological dependence: Moderate

Withdrawal Syndrome

A specific chloral hydrate withdrawal syndrome has been reported. Available data suggest that the chloral hydrate withdrawal syndrome is relatively mild (in comparison with the alcohol or barbiturate withdrawal syndrome), and is frequently associated with insomnia.

Overdosage

Signs and symptoms of acute chloral hydrate overdosage resemble those of barbiturate overdosage (see monograph). They include cardiac dysrhythmias, CNS depression progressing to deep coma, hypotension, and respiratory depression or arrest. Cardiac dysrhythmias account for most of the chloral hydrate overdosage fatalities. Other signs and symptoms may include cerebral edema, cyanosis, gastritis, hypothermia, kidney damage with albuminuria, liver damage with jaundice, miosis, muscle flaccidity, pulmonary edema, and vomiting. Chloral hydrate overdosage requires emergency medical support of body systems, with particular attention to the management of cardiac dysrhythmias and increasing chloral hydrate elimination. There is no known antidote.

Notes

1. When mixed with alcoholic beverages, chloral hydrate was commonly known as "Knockout Drops" and "Mickey Finn," particularly during the latter half of the 19th century when it was used to "drug" and conscript (i.e., "Shanghai") men into service on sailing ships for long voyages to China or to work on whaling ships or "whalers."
2. Chloral hydrate pharmacotherapy is not generally recommended because of the availability of equally efficacious and significantly less toxic alternatives (e.g., benzodiazepine pharmacotherapy).
3. In this context, chloral hydrate can be considered to be the original (after alcohol) date-rape drug (see also Note 1).
4. Neurotoxicity is associated with the endogenous formation of 1-trichloromethyl-1,2,3,4-tetrahydro-β-carboline (TaClo), a potent dopaminergic neurotoxin. TaClo also can be endogenously formed after exposure to the industrial solvent trichloroethylene.

References

Gaulier, J.M., Merle, G., Lacassie, E., et al. (2001). Fatal intoxications with chloral hydrate. *Journal of Forensic Sciences, 46*(6), 1507-1509.

Merdink, J.L., Robison, L.M., Stevens, D.K., et al. (2008). Kinetics of chloral hydrate and its metabolites in male human volunteers. *Toxicology, 245*(1-2), 130-140.

Riederer, P., Foley, P., Bringmann, G., et al. (2002). Biochemical and pharmacological characterization of 1-trichloromethyl-1,2,3,4-tetrahydro-β-carboline: A biologically relevant neurotoxin? *European Journal of Pharmacology, 442*(1-2), 1-16.

CHLORDIAZEPOXIDE

Names

BAN or INN Generic Synonyms: None

Brand/Trade: Librium®; Novo-Poxide®

Chemical: 7-Chloro-2-(methylamino)-5-phenyl-3H-1,4-benzodiazepine-4-oxide

Street: Gone Time; Goofers; Lib; Liberty; Libs; Libbies; Tranqs; Tranxs

Pharmacologic Classification

Psychodepressant, sedative-hypnotic: benzodiazepine

Brief General Overview

Chlordiazepoxide was the first benzodiazepine to be introduced into clinical practice as a sedative-hypnotic in North America, over 40 years ago. During this time, it also has been personally used for its psychodepressant actions. Chordiazepoxide has been used in higher dosages and for longer periods of time than medically prescribed, and it has been used in combination with other available drugs and substances "on the street." Having a less glamorous "street appeal" than the more popular benzodiazepines (e.g., diazepam [Valium®] and alprazolam [Xanax®]; see monographs) that have a shorter half-life of elimination and a more desirable "high," chlordiazepoxide is still the preferred benzodiazepine for about 5% of benzodiazepine users.

Dosage Forms and Routes of Administration

Chlordiazepoxide is available from licit pharmaceutical manufacturers in both intramuscular and intravenous injectable formulations and oral capsules and tablets. It is almost always used orally.

Mechanism of CNS Action

Chlordiazepoxide has sedative, hypnotic, and muscle relaxant actions. Although the exact mechanisms of its actions have not been determined, they appear to be mediated by the inhibitory neurotransmitter GABA. Chlordiazepoxide acts selectively on polysynaptic neuronal pathways and may inhibit or augment neuronal transmission, depending on the endogenous function of GABA. See also the Benzodiazepines monograph.

Pharmacodynamics/Pharmacokinetics

Chlordiazepoxide is completely absorbed (100%) after oral ingestion and appears in the bloodstream in 30 to 60 minutes. Peak blood concentrations are achieved in 2 to 4 hours. Intramuscular absorption is generally slow and erratic. After intramuscular injection, effects appear within 15 to 30 minutes. Chlordiazepoxide is highly plasma protein bound (95% to 98%) and has an apparent volume of distribution of ~0.3 L/kg. It is extensively metabolized, primarily in the liver, and has several active metabolites, including desmethyldiazepam and oxazepam (see monograph). Less than 2% of chlordiazepoxide is excreted in unchanged form in the urine. The mean elimination half-life is ~10 hours (range, 5 to 30 hours) and the mean total body clearance is ~35 mL/minute.

Current Approved Indications for Medical Use

Anxiety disorders; management of the alcohol withdrawal syndrome

Desired Action/Reason for Personal Use

Anxiety/stress reduction; disinhibition euphoria (mild); prevention/self-management of the benzodiazepine withdrawal syndrome

Toxicity

Acute: Amnesia; ataxia; cognitive impairment; confusion; constipation; dizziness; drowsiness; mental depression; nausea; respiratory depression; syncope; tiredness; weakness

Chronic: Hepatic dysfunction; physical dependence; psychological dependence

Pregnancy & Lactation: FDA Pregnancy Category D (see Appendix B). Safety of chlordiazepoxide use by adolescent girls and women who are pregnant has not been established. Chlordiazepoxide readily crosses the placental barrier. Fetal blood concentrations are approximately equal to maternal blood concentrations. Chlordiazepoxide appears to be relatively safe for the developing embryo and fetus when it is medically prescribed during pregnancy. However, some published studies have suggested increased risk for congenital malformations when chlordiazepoxide is medically or personally used during the first trimester of pregnancy. Regular maternal use of benzodiazepines during pregnancy also may result in the neonatal benzodiazepine withdrawal syndrome, characterized by crying, insomnia, irritability, and poor breast-feeding. Adolescent girls and women who are pregnant should not use chlordiazepoxide.

Safety of chlordiazepoxide use by adolescent girls and women who are breast-feeding has not been established. Chlordiazepoxide is excreted in breast milk. Breast-fed neonates and infants may display drowsiness or lethargy. They also may become physically dependent. Adolescent girls and women who are breast-feeding should not use chlordiazepoxide.

Abuse Potential

Physical dependence: Low to moderate (USDEA Schedule IV; low potential for abuse)
Psychological dependence: Low to moderate

Withdrawal Syndrome

A chlordiazepoxide withdrawal syndrome has been associated with the abrupt discontinuation of regular, long-term chlordiazepoxide pharmacotherapy or personal use. Signs and symptoms of the withdrawal syndrome range from mild dysphoria and insomnia to more severe signs and symptoms, including abdominal and muscle cramps, convulsions, sweating, tremors, and vomiting. The severity of the withdrawal syndrome and its duration appear to be related to the dosage and duration of chlordiazepoxide pharmacotherapy or personal use. (See the Benzodiazepines monograph.)

Overdosage

Signs and symptoms of chlordiazepoxide overdosage include ataxia, confusion, diminished reflexes, drowsiness, and coma. Depression of the cardiovascular and respiratory centers may occur. Chlordiazepoxide overdosage requires emergency medical support of body systems, with attention to increasing chlordiazepoxide elimination. The benzodiazepine antagonist flumazenil (Anexate®, Romazicon®) may be required. Severe cases of chlordiazepoxide overdosage, and those affecting elderly patients, may warrant continuous infusion of flumazenil to prevent resedation and resultant respiratory insufficiency.[1]

Note

1. Caution is required when a person is physically dependent on chlordiazepoxide, because the chlordiazepoxide withdrawal syndrome may be precipitated. The initial use of lower flumazenil dosages, cautious dosage titration, and careful clinical monitoring are recommended.

References

Hardern, R., & Page, A.V. (2005). An audit of symptom triggered chlordiazepoxide treatment of alcohol withdrawal on a medical admissions unit. *Emergency Medicine Journal, 22*(11), 805-806.

Maxa, J.L., Ogu, C.C., Adeeko, M.A., et al. (2003). Continuous-infusion flumazenil in the management of chlordiazepoxide toxicity. *Pharmacotherapy, 23*(11), 1513-1516.

CLONAZEPAM

Names

BAN or INN Generic Synonyms: None

Brand/Trade: Clonopin®; Klonopin®; Rivotril®

Chemical: 5-(o-Chlorophenyl)-1-3-dihydro-7-nitro-2H-1,4-benzodiazepin-2-one

Street: Clo; Klondike Bars; Klonnies; Klons; K-Pins; La Roche; Pins

Pharmacologic Classification

Psychodepressant, sedative-hypnotic: benzodiazepine (anticonvulsant)

Brief General Overview

Clonazepam, synthesized in 1969, continues to be clinically used primarily for its potent anticonvulsant action. It is personally used for its psychodepressant actions, and currently it is among the top three benzodiazepines used in North America.

Dosage Forms and Routes of Administration

Clonazepam is produced by licit pharmaceutical manufacturers and is available in oral tablet form. It is virtually always orally ingested.

Mechanism of CNS Action

The benzodiazepines cause dose-related CNS depression ranging from mild impairment of cognitive and psychomotor functions to hypnosis. The exact mechanism of action for the anticonvulsant action of clonazepam has not been determined, but benzodiazepines appear to act at the benzodiazepine receptors (types 1 and 2 [BZD-1 and BZD-2]). These receptors are found at several sites within the CNS, particularly in the cerebral cortex and limbic system. The benzodiazepine receptors are found primarily in conjunction with the GABA-receptor complex and predominantly in association with the $GABA_A$ receptor. Thus, it appears that the benzodiazepines elicit their pharmacologic actions by potentiating the actions of GABA, a major inhibitory neurotransmitter, in the CNS (see Benzodiazepines monograph).

Pharmacodynamics/Pharmacokinetics

Clonazepam is generally well absorbed from the GI tract after oral ingestion ($F = 0.9$). Onset of action is within 1 hour and peak blood concentrations are achieved within 2 hours. Duration of action ranges from 6 to 12 hours. Clonazepam is moderately protein bound (~86%), with a mean apparent volume of distribution of 3.2 L/kg. It is extensively metabolized in the liver, with only small amounts (<1%) eliminated in unchanged form in the urine. Clonazepam has a mean elimination half-life of 23 hours (range, 10 to 50 hours), and its mean total body clearance is ~90 mL/hour/kg.

Current Approved Indications for Medical Use

Seizure disorders

Desired Action/Reason for Personal Use

Anxiety/stress reduction; disinhibition euphoria; also, purposely administered to intended victims without their knowledge in the perpetration of drug-facilitated crime (e.g., robbery; sexual assault, including date rape)

Toxicity

Acute: Ataxia; blurred vision; cognitive impairment; confusion; dizziness; drowsiness; headache; hypotension; hypotonia; memory impairment; psychomotor impairment; respiratory depression; sedation; seizures (worsening of preexisting seizure disorder in about 5% of people); tiredness; weakness

Chronic: Antisocial behavior, particularly among children; hepatic dysfunction; memory impairment; physical dependence; psychological dependence

Pregnancy & Lactation: FDA Pregnancy Category "not established." Safety of clonazepam use during pregnancy has not been established (see Benzodiazepines monograph). However, because of the potential for the neonatal clonazepam withdrawal syndrome, adolescent girls and women who are pregnant should not use clonazepam.

Safety of clonazepam use by adolescent girls and women who are breast-feeding has not been established. Clonazepam is excreted in breast milk. Although maximal intake of clonazepam by breast-fed infants may be only about 2.5% of the maternal dosage, adolescents and women who are breast-feeding should not use clonazepam.[1]

Abuse Potential

Physical dependence: Moderate (USDEA Schedule IV; low potential for abuse)
Psychological dependence: Moderate

Withdrawal Syndrome

A specific clonazepam withdrawal syndrome has been noted. Abrupt discontinuation of regular, long-term clonazepam pharmacotherapy or personal use may result in status epilepticus, particularly when high dosages have been used. In these cases, clonazepam should be slowly discontinued, with gradual reduction of the dosage according to individual response.

Overdosage

Signs and symptoms of clonazepam overdosage include ataxia, coma, confusion, diminished reflexes, and somnolence. Clonazepam overdosage requires emergency medical support of body systems, with attention to increasing clonazepam elimination. The benzodiazepine antagonist flumazenil (Anexate®, Romazicon®) may be required.[2] Caution is indicated for people whose clonazepam use is for the medical management of seizure disorders. These people may be at increased risk for the occurrence of seizures when treated with flumazenil.

Notes

1. Likewise, if clonazepam is used for the medical management of seizure disorders, these women should avoid breast-feeding.
2. Particular caution is required because flumazenil antagonism may precipitate the clonazepam withdrawal syndrome in people who are physically dependent on clonazepam. Associated signs and symptoms include status epilepticus.

Reference

Dowd, S.M., Strong, M.J., Janicak, P.G., et al. (2002). The behavioral and cognitive effects of two benzodiazepines associated with drug-facilitated sexual assault. *Journal of Forensic Sciences, 47*(5), 1101-1107.

CLORAZEPATE

Names

BAN or INN Generic Synonyms: None

Brand/Trade: Novo-Clopate®; Tranxene®

Chemical: 7-Chloro-2,3-dihydro-2-oxo-5-phenyl-1H-1,4-benzodiazepine-3-carboxylic acid

Street: None

Pharmacologic Classification

Psychodepressant, sedative-hypnotic: benzodiazepine

Brief General Overview

Clorazepate, a prodrug, is personally used for its psychodepressant actions in much the same way as are the other benzodiazepines, particularly chlordiazepoxide (Librium®) and diazepam (Valium®). (See respective monographs and the Benzodiazepines monograph.)

Dosage Forms and Routes of Administration

Clorazepate is produced by licit pharmaceutical manufacturers and is available in oral capsules and tablets. It is almost always orally ingested.

Mechanism of CNS Action

Clorazepate has the chemical characteristics of the benzodiazepines and produces similar psychodepressant actions. Its exact mechanism of action has not been determined, but it appears to be mediated by, or to work in concert with, the inhibitory neurotransmitter GABA. (See also the Benzodiazepines monograph.)

Pharmacodynamics/Pharmacokinetics

Clorazepate is rapidly metabolized in the liver to its active major metabolite, nordiazepam (desmethyldiazepam). There is virtually no circulating parent drug in the blood. Nordiazepam is highly plasma protein bound (~98%) and is extensively metabolized in the liver. Nordiazepam's metabolites are primarily excreted in the urine, with <1% of nordiazepam excreted in unchanged form in the urine. The mean elimination half-life for nordiazepam is 2 to 3 days and the mean total body clearance is ~1 mL/minute. (See also the Benzodiazepines monograph.)

Current Approved Indications for Medical Use

Alcohol withdrawal syndrome (symptomatic management of acute withdrawal); anxiety disorders; seizure disorders

Desired Action/Reason for Personal Use

Anxiety/stress reduction; disinhibition euphoria; prevention/self-management of the clorazepate withdrawal syndrome

Toxicity

Acute: Ataxia; blurred vision; cognitive impairment; dry mouth; dizziness; drowsiness; fatigue; headache; mental depression

Chronic: Anemia (rare); fatigue; hepatic dysfunction; mental depression; physical dependence; psychological dependence

Pregnancy & Lactation: FDA Pregnancy Category C (see Appendix B). Safety of clorazepate use by adolescent girls and women who are pregnant has not been established. Clorazepate, a benzodiazepine derivative, has not been clearly associated with an increased risk of teratogenesis. Additional valid and reliable data are needed.

Safety of clorazepate use by adolescent girls and women who are breast-feeding has not been established. The active metabolite of clorazepate, nordiazepam, is excreted in breast milk. Drowsiness and lethargy may occur in breast-fed neonates and infants, who also may become physically dependent. Adolescent girls and women who are breast-feeding should not use clorazepate.

Abuse Potential

Physical dependence: Low to moderate (USDEA Schedule IV; low potential for abuse)
Psychological dependence: Low to moderate

Withdrawal Syndrome

Abrupt discontinuation of regular, long-term clorazepate use may result in the clorazepate withdrawal syndrome, the signs and symptoms of which may include abdominal cramps, diarrhea, delirium, insomnia, irritability, memory impairment, seizures, sweating, and vomiting. Regular, long-term clorazepate use should be gradually discontinued.

Overdosage

Signs and symptoms of clorazepate overdosage correspond to varying degrees of CNS depression, ranging from slight sedation to coma. Clorazepate overdosage requires emergency medical support of body systems, with attention to increasing clorazepate elimination. The benzodiazepine antagonist flumazenil (Anexate®, Romazicon®) may be required.[1]

Note

1. Caution is required, because flumazenil antagonism may precipitate the clorazepate withdrawal syndrome in people who are physically dependent on clorazepate.

Reference

Pagliaro, L.A., & Pagliaro, A.M. (2004). *Pagliaros' comprehensive guide to drugs and substances of abuse.* Washington, DC: American Pharmacists Association.

COCAINE

Names

BAN or INN Generic Synonyms: None

Brand/Trade: Generally available by generic name

Chemical: [1R-(exo,exo)]-3-(Benzoyloxy)-8-methyl-8-azabicyclo[3.2.1]octane-2-carboxylic acid methylester

Street: 24-7; 151; 256; A1; All American Drug; Angel; Angie; Aspirin; Aunt Nora; Badrock; 8 Ball; Basa; Base; *Baso*; *Basuco*; Batman; Bazulco; Beak; Beam; Bernice; Bernie; Bernie's Flakes; Bernie's Gold Dust; Big Bloke; Big C; Big Flake; Big Rush; Billie Hoke; Bing; Bing Crosby; Biscuits; *Blanca*; Blast; Blizzard; Blow; Bogata; Bolivian; Bolivian Marching Powder; Bolo; Bopper; Boulders; Bouncing Powder; *Boutros*; Boy; Brooke Shields; Bump; Bumper; Burese; Burnese; C; *Cabello*; Cadillac; Caine; Cakes; California Cornflakes; Cane; Candy; Candy C; Candy Sugar; Carnie; Carrie; Carrie Nation; Casper; CDs; C-Dust; Cecil; C-Game; Champagne; *Chandi*; Charlie; Ching; Choe; Cholly; Cloud; Coca; Coconut; Coca-Cola; Co-ca-ee-na; Coke; Cola; Colombian; Columbian Marching Powder; Combol; Cookies; Cornbread; Corrine; Corrinne; Crack; Crumbs; *Dama Blanca*; Devil's Dandruff; Double Bubble; Dream; Dust; Electric Kool-Aid; *Esnortiar*; Fast White Lady; Flake; Flave; Florida Snow; Foo Foo; Foo-Foo Dust; Freebase; Friskie Powder; Gift of the Sun; Gift-of-the-Sun-God; Gin; Girl; Girlfriend; Glad Stuff; Gold Dust; Gravel; Grits; Hail; Hamburger; Happy Dust; Happy Powder; Happy Trails; Hardball; Heaven; Heaven Dust; Henry VIII; Her; Hollywood; Hooter; Hunter; Inca Message; *Jejo*; Jelly; Jessica Simpson; Johnny; Kibbles & Bits; King; King's Habit; Kryptonite; Lady; Lady C; Lady Caine; Lady Snow; Late Night; Line; Liquid Lady; *Llello*; Love Affair; *Ma'a*; Mama Coca; Marching Dust; Marching Powder; Mayo; Merca; Merck; Merk; Mojo; Monster; Moon Rocks; Mosquitos; Movie Star Drug; *Mujer; Nieve*; Night Train; Nose; Nose Candy; Nose Powder; OJ; Oyster Stew; Paradise; Paradise White; Pariba; Pearl; Pebbles; Pepsi; *Percia, Percio; Perico;* Peruvian; Peruvian Flake; Peruvian Lady; Piece; *Piedra*; Pimp; Pimp Dust; *Polvo Blanco*; Powder; Powder Diamonds; Press; Purple Caps; Ready Rock; Real Tops; *Roca*; Rock; Roseanne Barr; Roxanne; Scorpion; Scottie; Serpico 21; Sevenup; Shake; She; Showbiz Sherbert; Sleigh Ride; Snai; Sniff; Snort; Snow; Snow Birds; Snow Cone; Snowcones; Snow Seals; Snow Train; Snow White; Society High; Soda; Squib; Star; Star-Spangled Powder; Stardust; Stones; Street Caviar; Studio Fuel; Sugar Boogers; *Talco*; Tardust; Teenager; Teeth; Tony; Tony Montana; Toot; Trails; Turtle Stuff; *Tutti-Frutti*; Twenty; Twinkie; 7-Up; Up; White; White Devil; White Dragon; White Girl; White Horse; White Lady; White Lion; White Mosquito; White Pony; White Stuff; Yada; Yadidi; Yak; Yale; Yam; Yao; Yay; *Yeyo*; Yiz; Yola; Zing; Zip

Pharmacologic Classification

Psychostimulant, miscellaneous

Brief General Overview

Cocaine is an alkaloid extracted from the leaves of two varieties of the coca plant *Erythroxylon coca*, which is indigenous to the eastern slopes of the Andes mountains in South America. One variety, *Erythroxylon Huano coca*, is a greenish-brown plant that grows 3 to 7 feet in height and has a thick, shiny stem and smooth-edged leaves. The second variety, *Erythroxylon Truxillo coca*, is a pale green plant. Both varieties grow wild in Bolivia and Peru and can be harvested several times each year. The coca leaves from these plants typically contain, by weight, about 1% cocaine. Cocaine use in this region, primarily by chewing the leaves, dates back to antiquity, with records of its use during the time of the Incan empire. Over the past 40 years, the use of cocaine in various forms (e.g., cocaine hydrochloride, crack cocaine) has become inculcated in the North American drug culture.

Currently, well over 200,000 hectares are under coca cultivation in South America, primarily in Bolivia, Colombia, and Peru. Approximately one-third of the total amount of cocaine produced in South America (or about half of the amount that is exported) ends up in North America, primarily in the United States. It has been estimated that in the last 5 years of the 20th century, an average of 300 metric tons of pure cocaine annually reached the U.S. domestic retail market, primarily from Columbia, for personal use. Mexico is the primary transshipment country for the cocaine used in the United States, with more than 90% of the cocaine moving through or stopping in Mexico prior to entering the United States.

Dosage Forms and Routes of Administration

The cocaine extracted from the leaves of the *Erythroxylon coca* bush is made into a crude coca paste.[1] The paste is then used to produce two forms of cocaine, each with its own pharmacologic characteristics and patterns of use: cocaine hydrochloride and cocaine base (i.e., "freebase" or "crack" cocaine).[2]

Cocaine hydrochloride, produced from the further chemical refinement of the coca paste, is an odorless, white, crystalline powder that is highly soluble in water (i.e., 1 gram in 0.5 mL). This form of cocaine has been licitly produced by pharmaceutical manufacturers for over 100 years and is used for such medical purposes as oral or ophthalmic local anesthesia. In regard to illicit or personal use, this form of cocaine can be intravenously injected when diluted, or the undiluted powder can be intranasally sniffed (snorted) because it is readily absorbed from the mucous membranes lining the nasal cavity.[3]

Unlike cocaine hydrochloride, cocaine base is only slightly soluble in water (i.e., 1 gram in 1300 mL); thus, it does not lend itself to intravenous or intranasal use. However—because it dissolves readily in ethanol (i.e., 1 gram in 7 mL), ether (i.e., 1 gram in 4 mL), and chloroform (i.e., 1 gram in 0.5 mL); has a significantly lower melting point (98°C versus 195°C); is highly volatile; vaporizes much more readily; and is involved in less pyrolysis[4]—cocaine base is suitable for pulmonary inhalation by smoking. Smoking cocaine base achieves blood concentrations of cocaine that are equal to those achieved by the intravenous injection of cocaine hydrochloride.[5] In addition, the onset of action is actually more rapid, and a subjectively greater or more intense desired action is achieved than when cocaine is administered by any other route, including intravenous injection. North Americans, in an attempt to increase the amount of cocaine that can be used illicitly without injecting it, have also converted cocaine hydrochloride back to its "base" form for smoking.

Although cocaine is used by people of all ages, genders, races, and socioeconomic levels throughout North America, the highest rate of abuse occurs among urban-dwelling men, 35 years of age and older, of African descent. These men use significantly more crack cocaine by population percentage than those of European descent, who use more cocaine hydrochloride. Another population group in which cocaine use is disproportionately high is the gay and bisexual community, regardless of race. Gay and bisexual men socially use cocaine as one of their five major party or club drugs (i.e., cocaine, gamma-hydroxybutyrate [GHB], ketamine, methamphetamine, and methylenedioxymethamphetamine [MDMA, Ecstasy). Cocaine also is used by many North Americans in combination with other drugs and substances of abuse.[6]

Mechanism of CNS Action

After absorption into the systemic circulation, cocaine is found in virtually all areas of the brain. However, it appears to preferentially accumulate in the caudate nucleus, the nucleus accumbens, and the ventral tegmental area. Cocaine attenuates the efficacy of dopamine transporter (DAT) clearance and thus blocks reuptake of the neurotransmitter dopamine into the presynaptic cells. It also has been demonstrated to block the reuptake of other monoamines, including serotonin and norepinephrine. Consequently, it increases the amount of neurotransmitter(s) present in the synaptic cleft. A simplified, stylized representation of the proposed principal site and mechanism of cocaine's psychostimulant action is shown in Figure 5.

FIGURE 5
Psychostimulant Action of Cocaine

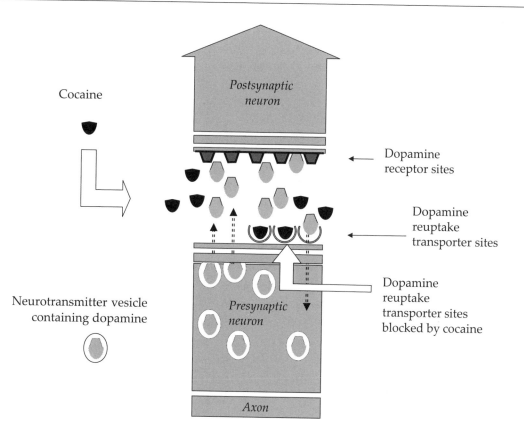

Pharmacodynamics/Pharmacokinetics

The mean oral bioavailability of cocaine is 33%, whereas the mean intranasal bioavailability is 70%.[7] Peak serum concentrations of cocaine occur ~45 minutes after oral ingestion, ~10 minutes after intranasal snorting, and ~1 minute after smoking or intravenous injection. Pulmonary bioavailability of cocaine is high (i.e., $F > 0.9$) when smoked with a glass "crack pipe." However, a small portion of the dose is destroyed by pyrolysis[8] and a larger portion remains in the crack pipe before being delivered to the lungs for absorption.

Cocaine is hydrolyzed and metabolized primarily in the liver to several metabolites, including benzoylecgonine, ecgonine, ecgonine methyl ester, hydroxycocaine, hydroxybenzoylecgonine, and norcocaine. Esterases found in a number of tissues, including hepatocytes, are predominantly responsible for the formation of the major metabolite, benzoylecgonine. The mean elimination half-life of cocaine is 1.25 hours, and elimination appears to be influenced by urinary pH (as with the amphetamines). In addition, the total body clearance of cocaine may be significantly reduced with the concurrent use of alcohol.[9]

Current Approved Indications for Medical Use

Topical local anesthetic used primarily in dental practice

Desired Action/Reason for Personal Use

Alertness, vigilance or wakefulness; appetite or hunger suppression; arouse sexual desires and enhance sexual experiences (particularly, among gay and bisexual men); decreased fatigue; energy (increased); enhance sociability (particularly, among gay and bisexual men); euphoria (intense); sense of well-being, power, and self-confidence (increased)

Toxicity

Acute: Agitation; alveolar damage (associated with smoking crack cocaine); anxiety; asthma or other chronic obstructive pulmonary disease (COPD), acute exacerbation of[10]; cardiovascular collapse; dry mouth; excited delirium (potentially fatal); formication (a tactile hallucination with the sensation of bugs, such as ants, crawling under the skin); frontal lobe deficits in performance; headache; hyperpyrexia; hypertension; impaired concentration; increased risk-taking behavior; insomnia; muscle rigidity; mydriasis; myocardial infarction; nervousness; panic attacks; paranoia; psychosis; seizures; stroke; tachycardia; tachypnea; tremor; violent behavior

Chronic: Agranulocytosis[11]; impaired decision making; inability to control behavior; insomnia; paranoid psychosis; psychological dependence; pulmonary damage[12]; rhabdomyolysis; rhinopalatal erosion and perforation of the nasal septum[13]; necrotic ulcers[14]; sexually transmitted diseases, increased risk for (particularly hepatitis B, hepatitis C, herpes simplex virus-2 [HSV-2], HIV, and syphilis)[15]; suicide, risk for[16]

Pregnancy & Lactation: Cocaine use by pregnant adolescent girls and women is a significant problem in most major cities across North America. Factors correlated with a high rate of cocaine use during pregnancy are African race,[17] low maternal educational attainment, and low maternal socioeconomic status.

Cocaine use during pregnancy has been associated with intrauterine death (including spontaneous abortions), low birth weight, preterm delivery, neonatal seizures, neonatal tachycardia, intrauterine growth retardation (reduced head circumference), and a variety of fetal physical anomalies.[18] In addition, a significantly higher rate of developmental delays and behavioral and learning disorders (e.g., attention-deficit/hyperactivity disorder, mental retardation) is reported for preschoolers and school-age children who were exposed to cocaine in utero. As well, autopsies performed on fetuses exposed to cocaine in utero have often revealed cerebral hemorrhages or infarctions.[19] If large amounts of cocaine are used near term, the neonate may experience CNS excitation (e.g., increased crying, irritability, and tremulousness). Adolescent girls and women who are pregnant should not use cocaine.

Cocaine is excreted in the breast milk of adolescent girls and women who use cocaine. Exposed neonates and infants have displayed characteristic signs and symptoms of CNS excitation, including dilated pupils, irritability, seizures, and tremulousness. Adolescent girls and women who are breast-feeding should not use cocaine.

Abuse Potential

Physical dependence: Low to moderate (USDEA Schedule II; high abuse potential)
Psychological dependence: High

Withdrawal Syndrome

Although there is not a classic withdrawal syndrome such as occurs with physical dependence (i.e., development of tolerance or a need for more drug to achieve the desired actions, and the occurrence of unwanted signs and symptoms with abrupt discontinuation of the drug that are immediately relieved by resumed use of the drug),[20] abrupt discontinuation of regular personal use of cocaine may result in apathy, dysphoria, extreme fatigue, mental depression, psychomotor fatigue, and sleep pattern changes. The signs and symptoms of cocaine withdrawal appear to be most pronounced in cocaine users who also have a history of depression.

Overdosage

Cocaine overdosage can be fatal. Death is generally the result of cardiac dysrhythmias, hyperthermia, intracranial hemorrhage (stroke), respiratory arrest, or status epilepticus. Cocaine use also has been related to fatal accidents, homicides, and suicides. Acute cocaine overdosage requires emergency medical support, with attention to increasing cocaine elimination. There is no known antidote.

Notes

1. The paste form, or *baso*, is made during the production of cocaine hydrochloride. It is virtually identical psychopharmacologically to crack cocaine. *Baso* is widely used, by smoking, in South American countries, and its use has resulted in significant health and social problems.
2. During the late 1990s, the drug cartels in Colombia began exporting a new form of cocaine, "black cocaine." As the name implies, its color is black. However, it is not really a new form of cocaine but rather a new method of concealing cocaine for illicit trafficking. Cocaine hydrochloride is mixed with a red-black powder (iron thiocyanate), rendering it undetectable by most drug detection kits that are

based on color. The presence of iron thiocyanate prevents, or masks, positive readings for cocaine color reaction-based tests (e.g., Becton Dickinson test kits). The potential health risks associated with the presence of iron thiocyanate in black cocaine have not been formally evaluated.

3. The surface area of the nostrils and nasal passages is quite limited and, consequently, so is the amount of cocaine hydrochloride that can be absorbed from this site.

4. Chemical decomposition resulting from an increase in temperature (i.e., heat).

5. The surface area of the lungs is virtually unlimited, in comparison with that of the nostrils and nasal passages. Consequently, so is the amount of cocaine base that can be absorbed from this site.

6. Combined use with heroin is referred to as a "Belushi," "Dynamite," "H & C;" "Murder One," or "Speedball." Adding this combination to a tobacco cigarette results in a "flamethrower." The combination of cocaine, heroin, and LSD is referred to as a "Frisco Special" or a "Frisco speedball."

7. However, the rate of absorption and the total amount absorbed may be significantly reduced by the limited surface area of the nasal mucosa and the local vasoconstricting action of cocaine.

8. The major product of the pyrolysis of crack cocaine is methylecgonidine. The amount of methylecgonidine produced is variable, generally ranging from 1% to 5%, depending upon the temperature and rate of air flow in the crack pipe. Methylecgonidine (i.e., anhydroecgonine methyl ester) has been used as a biological marker to differentiate (e.g., in forensic biological samples) crack cocaine smoking from other methods of cocaine use.

9. Cocaine users often comment that the concomitant use of alcohol appears to enhance or prolong the euphoria associated with cocaine use while also mitigating its associated unpleasant effects. Concomitant use of alcohol and cocaine may result in up to 20% of the systemically available cocaine being converted to cocaethylene, a psychoactive ethyl homologue of cocaine. This interaction exclusively involves alcohol and cocaine.

10. Acute exacerbation of asthma and other COPDs is associated specifically with smoking crack cocaine.

11. Agranulocytosis (i.e., a condition marked by an acute deficit of white blood cells, particularly neutrophils) has been associated with the use of cocaine adulterated with levamisole, a drug used primarily in veterinary medicine to de-worm pigs. Related cases of agranulocytosis have been reported in Alberta (Canada), Delaware, and New Mexico.

12. Chronic alveolar epithelial and microvascular lung damage is associated with habitual crack cocaine smoking. The condition is sometimes referred to as "crack lung."

13. Associated with intranasal sniffing (snorting) of cocaine hydrochloride. As the cocaine base is absorbed from the nasal site, the hydrochloride is left behind to form dilute hydrochloric acid, resulting in local tissue damage, including perforation of the nasal septum, oronasal fistulas, and infections.

14. "Coke burns" associated with repeated inadvertent subcutaneous injection of cocaine by intravenous cocaine users.

15. Associated with both sharing contaminated needles and syringes used to intravenously inject cocaine and being paid with cocaine for sexual favors (i.e., sex-for-drug exchanges), such as unprotected sexual intercourse with multiple partners (a common practice in crack houses). Generally, North American women of African descent who use crack cocaine are significantly more likely than any other group of drug and substance abusers to engage in oral sex for drugs or money (almost always to buy more crack cocaine). This group also has the highest incidence markers for chlamydia, hepatitis, herpes simplex-2, HIV, and syphilis. North American men of African descent who smoke crack cocaine and are HIV positive are the demographic group that is most at risk for having unprotected sex, even when they know that they are HIV positive.

16. Although most health care professionals tend to associate suicide (including failed attempts) with the use of psychodepressants, the use of cocaine has long been recognized as also being associated with suicide. People who have cocaine use disorders—perhaps at least in part because of personal losses and other sequelae related to their cocaine use (e.g., divorce, financial problems, loss of family, loss of job)—are at significant risk for suicide.

17. Crack cocaine use by North American women of African descent who are pregnant has been highly correlated with cocaine use by male family members (e.g., brother, father).

18. A definite causal relationship between cocaine use and the various observed fetal abnormalities has not been established. This lack of a definitive relationship is due, in part, to the observation that women who use cocaine while pregnant are over 50 times more likely to use other drugs and substances of abuse as well, including alcohol and tobacco.

19. Criminal charges have been brought in several cases against women whose fetuses have died as a result of their cocaine use during pregnancy. To date, the cases have almost always ended in acquittal.

20. The use of additional cocaine will **not** relieve the associated signs and symptoms, because the neurotransmitter dopamine is depleted (see "Mechanism of Action").

References

Askin, D.F., & Diehl-Jones, B. (2001). Cocaine: Effects of in utero exposure on the fetus and neonate. *The Journal of Perinatal & Neonatal Nursing, 14*(4), 83-102.

Bada, H.S., Das, A., Bauer, C.R., et al. (2002). Gestational cocaine exposure and intrauterine growth: Maternal lifestyle study. *Obstetrics and Gynecology, 100*(5, Part 1), 916-924.

Baldwin, G.C., Choi, R., Roth, M.D., et al. (2002). Evidence of chronic damage to the pulmonary microcirculation in habitual users of alkaloidal ("crack") cocaine. *Chest, 121*(4), 1231-1238.

Blaho, K., Logan, B., Winbery, S., et al. (2000). Blood cocaine and metabolite concentrations, clinical findings, and outcome of patients presenting to an ED. *The American Journal of Emergency Medicine, 18*(5), 593-598.

Booth, R.E., Kwiatkowski, C.F., & Chitwood, D.D. (2000). Sex related HIV risk behaviors: Differential risks among injection drug users, crack smokers, and injection drug users who smoke crack. *Drug and Alcohol Dependence, 58*(3), 219-226.

Boutros, N.N., Gelernter, J., Gooding, D.C., et al. (2002). Sensory gating and psychosis vulnerability in cocaine-dependent individuals: Preliminary data. *Biological Psychiatry, 51*(8), 683-686.

Boyd, C.J., & Holmes, C. (2002). Women who smoke crack and their family substance abuse problems. *Health Care for Women International, 23*(6-7), 576-586.

Buchanan, D., Tooze, J.A., Shaw, S., et al. (2006). Demographic, HIV risk behavior, and health status characteristics of "crack" cocaine injectors compared to other injection drug users in three New England cities. *Drug and Alcohol Dependence, 81*(3), 221-229.

Bull, S.S., Piper, P., & Rietmeijer, C. (2002). Men who have sex with men and also inject drugs—profiles of risk related to the synergy of sex and drug injection behaviors. *Journal of Homosexuality, 42*(3), 31-51.

Cambell, S. (2003). Prenatal cocaine exposure and neonatal/infant outcomes. *Neonatal Network: NN, 22*(1), 19-21.

Couper, F.J., Pemberton, M., Jarvis, A., et al. (2002). Prevalence of drug use in commercial tractor-trailer drivers. *Journal of Forensic Sciences, 47*(3), 562-567.

Coyer, S.M. (2003). Women in recovery discuss parenting while addicted to cocaine. *MCN. The American Journal of Maternal/Child Nursing, 28*(1), 45-49.

de Azevedo, R.C., Botega, N.J., & Guimarães, L.A. (2007). Crack users, sexual behavior and risk of HIV infection. *Revista Brasileira de Psiquiatria [Brazilian Journal of Psychiatry], 29*(1), 26-30.

Fattinger, K., Benowitz, N.L., Jones, R.T., et al. (2000). Nasal mucosal versus gastrointestinal absorption of nasally administered cocaine. *European Journal of Clinical Pharmacology, 56*(4), 305-310.

Filip, M., Frankowska, M., Zaniewska, M., et al. (2005). The serotonergic system and its role in cocaine addiction. *Pharmacological Reports, 57*(6), 685-700.

Fillmore, M.T., & Rush, C.R. (2002). Impaired inhibitory control of behavior in chronic cocaine users. *Drug and Alcohol Dependence, 66*(3), 265-273.

Halkitis, P.N., & Palamar, J.J. (2008). Multivariate modeling of club drug use initiation among gay and bisexual men. *Substance Use & Misuse, 43*(7), 871-879.

Harris, D.S., Everhart, E.T., Mendelson, J., et al. (2003). The pharmacology of cocaethylene in humans following cocaine and ethanol administration. *Drug and Alcohol Dependence, 72*(2), 169-182.

Helmus, T.C., Downey, K.K., & Wang, L.M., et al. (2001). The relationship between self-reported cocaine withdrawal symptoms and history of depression. *Addictive Behavior, 26*(3), 461-467.

Hwang, L.Y., Ross, M.W., Zack, C., et al. (2000). Prevalence of sexually transmitted infections and associated risk factors among populations of drug abusers. *Clinical Infectious Diseases, 31*(4), 920-926.

Jufer, R.A., Wstadik, A., Walsh, S.L., et al. (2000). Elimination of cocaine and metabolites in plasma, saliva, and urine following repeated oral administration to human volunteers. *Journal of Analytical Toxicology, 24*(7), 467-477.

Kalechstein, A.D., Newton, T.F., & Leavengood, A.H. (2002). Apathy syndrome in cocaine dependence. *Psychiatry Research, 109*(1), 97-100.

Keller, R.W. Jr., & Snyder-Keller, A. (2000). Prenatal cocaine exposure. *Annals of the New York Academy of Sciences, 909*, 217-232.

Kelly, T.M., Cornelius, J.R., & Lynch, K.G. (2002). Psychiatric and substance use disorders as risk factors for attempted suicide among adolescents: A case control study. *Suicide and Life-Threatening Behavior, 32*(3), 301-312.

Klausner, H.A., & Lewandowski, C. (2002). Infrequent causes of stroke. *Emergency Medicine Clinics of North America, 20*(3), 657-670.

Kolbrich, E.A., Barnes, A.J., Gorelick, D.A., et al. (2006). Major and minor metabolites of cocaine in human plasma following controlled subcutaneous cocaine administration. *Journal of Analytical Toxicology, 30*(8), 501-510.

Laizure, S.C., & Parker, R.B. (2009). Pharmacodynamic evaluation of the cardiovascular effects following the coadministration of cocaine and ethanol. *Drug Metabolism and Disposition, 37*, 310-314.

Lason, W. (2001). Neurochemical and pharmacological aspects of cocaine-induced seizures. *Polish Journal of Pharmacology, 53*(1), 57-60.

Lester, B.M., El Sohly, M., Wright, L.L., et al. (2001). The Maternal Lifestyle Study: Drug use by meconium toxicology and maternal self-report. *Pediatrics, 107*(2), 309-317.

Lim, K.O., Choi, S.J., Pomara, N., et al. (2002). Reduced frontal white matter integrity in cocaine dependence: A controlled diffusion tensor imaging study. *Biological Psychiatry, 51*(11), 890-895.

MacDonald, S., Mann, R., Chipman, M., et al. (2008). Driving behavior under the influence of cannabis or cocaine. *Traffic Injury Prevention, 9*(3), 190-194.

Mari, A., Arranz, C., Gimeno, X., et al. (2002). Nasal cocaine abuse and centrofacial destructive process: Report of three cases including treatment. *Oral Surgery, Oral Medicine, Oral Pathology, Oral Radiology, and Endodontics, 93*(4), 435-439.

McCann, B., Hunter, R., & McCann, J. (2002). Cocaine/heroin induced rhabdomyolysis and ventricular fibrillation. *Emergency Medicine Journal, 19*(3), 264-265.

Müller, C.P., Carey, R.J., Huston, J.P. et al. (2007). Serotonin and psychostimulant addiction: Focus on 5-HT1A-receptors. *Progress in Neurobiology, 81*(3), 133-178.

Ross, M.W., Hwang, L.Y., Zack, C., et al. (2002). Sexual risk behaviours and STIs in drug abuse treatment populations whose drug of choice is crack cocaine. *International Journal of STD & AIDS, 13*(11), 769-774.

Savitz, D.A., Henderson, L., Dole, N., et al. (2002). Indicators of cocaine exposure and preterm birth. *Obstetrics and Gynecology, 99*(3), 458-465.

Servoss, S.J., Januzzi, J.L., & Muller, J.E. (2002). Triggers of acute coronary syndromes. *Progress in Cardiovascular Diseases, 44*(5), 369-380.

Singer, L.T., Arendt, R., Minnes, S., et al. (2002). Cognitive and motor outcomes of cocaine-exposed infants. *JAMA, 287*(15), 1952-1960.

Smith, J.C., Kacker, A., & Anand, V.K. (2002). Midline nasal and hard palate destruction in cocaine abusers and cocaine's role in rhinologic practice. *Ear, Nose & Throat Journal, 81*(3), 172-177.

Spittal, P.M., Craib, K.J., Wood, E., et al. (2002). Risk factors for elevated HIV incidence rates among female injection drug users in Vancouver. *CMAJ: Canadian Medical Association Journal, 166*(7), 894-899.

Tashkin, D.P. (2001). Airway effects of marijuana, cocaine, and other inhaled illicit agents. *Current Opinion in Pulmonary Medicine, 7*(2), 43-61.

Timpson, S.C., Williams, M.L., Bowen, A.M., et al. (2003). Condom use behaviors in HIV-infected African American crack cocaine users. *Substance Abuse, 24*(4), 211-220.

Vilela, R.J., Langford, C., McCullagh, L., et al. (2002). Cocaine-induced oronasal fistulas with external nasal erosion but without palate involvement. *Ear, Nose & Throat Journal, 81*(8), 562-563.

Warner, A., & Norman, A.B. (2000). Mechanisms of cocaine hydrolysis and metabolism in vitro and in vivo: A clarification. *Therapeutic Drug Monitoring, 22*(3), 266-270.

Weber, J.E., Shofer, F.S., Larkin, G.L., et al. (2003). Validation of a brief observation period for patients with cocaine-associated chest pain. *The New England Journal of Medicine, 348*(6), 510-517.

Zaas, D., Brock, M., & Yang, S., et al. (2002). An uncommon mimic of an acute asthma exacerbation. *Chest, 121*(5), 1707-1709.

CODEINE

Names

BAN or INN Generic Synonyms: Methylmorphine

Brand/Trade: Codeine Contin®; Paveral®; and generally available by generic name

Chemical: (5α,6α)-7,8-Didehydro-4,5-epoxy-3-methoxy-17-methylmorphinan-6-ol

Street: AC/DC; Captain; Cement; Cod; Co-Dine; Cods; Codys; Cough Syrup; Deens; Lean & Dean; Purple Drink; Schoolboy; T3

Pharmacologic Classification

Psychodepressant, opiate analgesic: pure agonist (natural)

Brief General Overview

Codeine, methylmorphine, is a naturally occurring opiate analgesic produced by the opium poppy (*Papaver somniferum*). It is used personally for its analgesic and other psychodepressant actions.

Dosage Forms and Routes of Administration

Codeine is produced by licit pharmaceutical manufacturers and is available in a wide variety of injectable (i.e., intravenous, intramuscular, subcutaneous) and oral (i.e., elixirs, solutions, syrups, tablets) dosage formulations. Codeine can be obtained legally from physicians and pharmacists, with or without a medical prescription, depending on the dosage. It also can be obtained over the Internet without prescription. It is commonly used by young and old alike.

The most frequently abused prescriptions for codeine are obtained from family physicians, medi-centers or walk-in clinics, and emergency rooms. These prescriptions usually are used to obtain codeine for one's personal use, but they also are commonly obtained for use by one's adult children. Most people who abuse codeine are poly-drug and substance users[1] whose prescriptions are paid for by welfare or Medicaid. Although they generally use the codeine themselves, they also trade it for money, goods, or services.[2]

Over the past decade, increasing numbers of high school and college or university students have practiced "pharming" (i.e., going through the family medicine cabinet to obtain whatever is available to get "high"). Pharming is often done with friends while listening to "screw," a form of hip-hop music associated with this pattern of drug use. Very often, one of the drugs found in the medicine cabinet is codeine, a common ingredient in several combination analgesic products (e.g., 222®; Tylenol with Codeine®) and cough and cold products (e.g., Cheracol® with Codeine Syrup; Robitussin A-C® Syrup). Codeine also is available alone in prescription strength formulations that contain 30 mg or more of codeine per dosage unit, and in nonprescription (over-the-counter [OTC]) products that contain 15 mg or less of codeine per dosage unit.

Mechanism of CNS Action

Codeine appears to elicit its opiate analgesic action primarily by binding to endorphin receptors in the CNS. This binding is thought to result in the inhibition of neurotransmission in the ascending pain pathways and in diminished pain perception. However, the exact mechanism of action has not been determined.

Similar to other opiate analgesics, codeine produces other actions in addition to analgesia. These actions are mediated by both central and peripheral mechanisms of action and include (1) cough reduction associated with suppression of the central cough center, (2) constipation associated with decreased GI motility, (3) nausea and vomiting associated with stimulation of the chemoreceptor trigger zone in the medulla, and (4) respiratory depression associated with decreased responsiveness of the central respiratory center to stimulation by carbon dioxide. See also the Opiate Analgesics monograph.

Pharmacodynamics/Pharmacokinetics

The oral availability of codeine varies (range, 40% to 70%; mean, 53%). Codeine is only slightly (7%) bound to plasma protein and has an apparent volume of distribution of 2 to 3 L/kg. The onset of action is generally within 30 minutes after oral ingestion, intramuscular injection, or subcutaneous injection. The duration of action is 4 to 6 hours, or ~12 hours for the extended-release formulation. Codeine is metabolized in the liver to several active metabolites, including morphine, which accounts for about 10% of these metabolites (see Morphine monograph). Less than 5% of codeine is excreted in unchanged form in the urine. The mean elimination half-life is ~2 to 3 hours and the total body clearance is ~800 mL/minute.

Current Approved Indications for Medical Use

Cough, nonproductive; pain, mild to moderate

Desired Action/Reason for Personal Use[3]

Drowsy "high"; euphoria (mild); prevention/self-management of the codeine, or other opiate analgesic, withdrawal syndrome

Toxicity

Acute: Anorexia; ataxia; blurred vision; bronchospasm; chills; cognitive impairment; constipation; diplopia; dizziness; drowsiness; dry mouth; fatigue; flushing; headache; intestinal cramping; laryngospasm; lightheadedness; loss of coordination; mental depression; miosis; nausea; nystagmus; perspiration, excessive; sedation; urinary retention; vomiting

Chronic: Constipation, chronic; mental depression; miosis; physical dependence; psychological dependence; reduced sex drive; respiratory impairment

Pregnancy & Lactation: FDA Pregnancy Category C (see Appendix B). Safety of codeine use by adolescent girls and women who are pregnant has not been established. Generally, codeine is not recommended for adolescent girls or women who are pregnant because it crosses the placenta. However, it is unlikely that codeine is a teratogen. If it is, its potency and incidence as a teratogen are extremely low. Codeine is widely used during pregnancy, particularly as a combination analgesic and as a cough and cold product. Only a few cases of possible teratogenic effects (e.g., cleft lip and palate) have been reported in the published literature. Regular, long-term maternal use of codeine during pregnancy may result in the neonatal codeine withdrawal syndrome. Maternal use near term may result in neonatal depression, which is associated with the expected actions of an opiate analgesic. Adolescent girls and women who are pregnant should not use codeine.

Safety of codeine use by adolescent girls and women who are breast-feeding has not been established. The active metabolites of codeine (e.g., morphine) are excreted in low concentrations in breast milk. Codeine use by adolescent girls or women who are breast-feeding may result in expected pharmacologic effects in their neonates and infants. For example, after several days (i.e., 4 or 5 days) of breast-feeding, respiratory depression was observed in neonates whose mothers used codeine. Drowsiness and lethargy also may occur in breast-fed neonates and infants. In addition, these neonates and infants may become physically dependent. Adolescent girls and women who are breast-feeding should not use codeine.

Abuse Potential

Physical dependence: Moderate (USDEA Schedule II; high abuse potential)
Psychological dependence: Moderate to high

Withdrawal Syndrome

A specific codeine withdrawal syndrome has been reported. It can occur after the abrupt discontinuation of regular, long-term high-dosage codeine use. The withdrawal syndrome is similar to that for morphine and other opiate analgesics, but generally is less severe. Signs and symptoms, which begin approximately 8 hours after the last use of codeine, can last for up to 1 week and include anorexia, anxiety, muscle aches and twitching, mydriasis, nasal discharge, restless sleep, sweating, tremors, watery eyes, and yawning.

Overdosage

Signs and symptoms of codeine overdosage may include respiratory depression with reduced respiratory rate and tidal volume, Cheyne-Stokes respirations, cyanosis, extreme somnolence progressing to stupor or coma, skeletal muscle flaccidity, cold clammy skin, and, sometimes, hypotension and bradycardia. Severe overdosage may result in apnea, circulatory collapse, cardiac arrest, and death. Mydriasis may occur with terminal narcosis or severe hypoxia.

Codeine overdosage requires emergency medical support, with attention to codeine elimination. Naloxone (Narcan®), a pure opiate analgesic antagonist, is a specific antidote for the respiratory depression associated with codeine and other opiate analgesic overdosage. However, use of the opiate analgesic antagonist should be avoided if possible, because the usual dose will precipitate the opiate analgesic withdrawal syndrome in people who are physically dependent on codeine. The severity of the withdrawal syndrome depends on the severity of physical dependence and the dose of the antagonist that is administered. If an opiate analgesic antagonist is required for the medical management of serious respiratory depression and other signs and symptoms of codeine overdosage when a person is physically dependent, lower dosages, cautious dosage titration, and careful clinical monitoring are recommended.

Notes

1. Other drugs and substances of abuse that are frequently used by illicit codeine users, in descending order, are alcohol, benzodiazepines, cannabis, and heroin. It is interesting to note that psycho-stimulants (e.g., amphetamines, cocaine) are not included in this list.

2. Many poly-drug users, particularly those who are subject to mandatory urine testing for illicit drug use (e.g., users being screened for a new job or being monitored on the job, users enrolled in opiate dependence maintenance programs [e.g., methadone maintenance programs], or users who are on parole), are increasingly buying adulterant products available on the Internet. One such product, Stealth®, is particularly effective for avoiding the detection of codeine and morphine use by gas chromatography with mass spectrometry (GC-MS); however, urine samples usually still test positive by immunoassay.

3. Most self-identified heroin addicts view codeine as "crap" or "garbage" and would only use it to prevent or treat the opiate analgesic withdrawal syndrome when no other opiate analgesic was readily available.

References

Cody, J.T., Valtier, S., & Kuhlman, J. (2001). Analysis of morphine and codeine in samples adulterated with Stealth. *Journal of Analytical Toxicology, 25*(7), 572-575.

Elwood, W.N. (2001). Sticky business: Patterns of procurement and misuse of prescription cough syrup in Houston. *Journal of Psychoactive Drugs, 33*(2), 121-133.

Kim, I., Barnes, A.J., Oyler, J.M., et al. (2002). Plasma and oral fluid pharmacokinetics and pharmacody-namics after oral codeine administration. *Clinical Chemistry, 48*(9), 1486-1496.

Peters, R.J. Jr., Kelder, S.H., Markham, C.M., et al. (2003). Beliefs and social norms about codeine and promethazine hydrochloride cough syrup (CPHCS). Use and perceived addiction among urban Houstonian adolescents: An addiction trend in the city of lean. *Journal of Drug Education, 33*(4), 415-425.

Peters, R.J. Jr., Williams, M., Ross, M.W., et al. (2007). Codeine cough syrup use among African-American crack cocaine users. *Journal of Psychoactive Drugs, 39*(1), 97-102.

Peters, R. Jr., Yacoubian G.S. Jr., Rhodes, W., et al. (2007). Beliefs and social norms about codeine and promethazine hydrochloride cough syrup (CPHCS) use and addiction among multi-ethnic college students. *Journal of Psychoactive Drugs, 39*(3), 277-282.

CRACK (See Cocaine)

DEXTROAMPHETAMINE

Names

BAN or INN Generic Synonyms: Dexamfetamine; Dexamphetamine; d-α-Methylphenethylamine

Brand/Trade: Dexedrine®; Dextrostat®

Chemical: (+)-α-Methylphenethylamine

Street: Blues; Browns; Co-Pilots; Dex; Dexies; Dexo; Dexy; Greenies; Hearts; Oranges; Peaches

Pharmacologic Classification

Psychostimulant, amphetamine

Brief General Overview

After the synthesis of methamphetamine by the Japanese in 1919, dextroamphetamine was synthesized as a replacement drug for ephedrine because of concern that increased medical use of ephedrine as an alternative to epinephrine pharmacotherapy for the management of nasal congestion and bronchoconstriction would deplete its supply. Dextroamphetamine's psychostimulant actions were well recognized, and it was used by the both Axis and Allied forces during WW II (1939–1945), particularly to enable pilots to fly long distances without fatigue. Large quantities were stockpiled during the postwar years, and it was increasingly abused.

By the 1950s, dextroamphetamine was prescribed for a variety of medical disorders, including mild depression, narcolepsy, and obesity. By the early 1960s, it also was prescribed for the management of attention-deficit/hyperactivity disorder (ADHD), which was then known as "minimal brain dysfunction."[1] During this time, the oral dosage formulations of dextroamphetamine (tablets and spansules) were commonly used by (1) women whose physicians prescribed them for weight control, (2) college and university students using them to stay awake to study for examinations, and (3) truck drivers wanting to complete "long hauls" without falling asleep. In addition, population groups that were considered socially marginalized abused dextroamphetamine-containing inhalers purchased from pharmacies without a prescription. However, little attention was given to the potential physical and psychological dependence associated with dextroamphetamine and other amphetamines.

In 1965, FDA initiated measures to control and severely restrict the availability of dextroamphetamine in the United States. For the next 25 years illicit use continued, but at a significantly lower level. However, during the 1990s, dextroamphetamine prescriptions, clinical use, and abuse more than doubled. Today, dextroamphetamine, like other amphetamines (see Amphetamines monograph), continues to be widely used in North America for its psychostimulant actions. However, its illicit use generally has been reduced by the increased illicit production and use of methamphetamine (Crystal Meth) (see monograph).

Dosage Forms and Routes of Administration

Dextroamphetamine is legally produced by pharmaceutical companies in North America. It is available in oral capsule and oral tablet formulations. Most people who abuse dextroamphetamine orally ingest these dosage formulations. However, some users dissolve them and inject the dextroamphetamine intravenously. Rarely, the oral tablets are ground into a fine powder that is intranasally sniffed (snorted).

Mechanism of CNS Action

Dextroamphetamine causes indirect effects at both α-adrenergic and β-adrenergic receptors. It has a marked stimulant effect on the CNS, particularly the cerebral cortex. Peripheral actions include elevation of systolic and diastolic blood pressure and weak bronchodilator and respiratory stimulant actions. Dextroamphetamine appears to elicit its psychostimulant action primarily by increasing the release of norepinephrine from presynaptic storage vesicles in adrenergic neurons. A direct effect on α- and β-adrenergic receptors, inhibition of the enzyme amine oxidase and release of the neurotransmitter dopamine, also may be involved. However, the exact mechanism of dextroamphetamine's psychostimulant action has not been determined. (Also see the Amphetamines monograph.)

Pharmacodynamics/Pharmacokinetics

Dextroamphetamine appears to be fairly well absorbed after oral ingestion. Peak blood concentrations occur within ~3 hours. The mean elimination half-life is ~12 hours. Additional valid and reliable data are not available.

Current Approved Indications for Medical Use

Attention-deficit/hyperactivity disorder; sleep disorders: narcolepsy

Desired Action/Reason for Personal Use

Alertness, vigilance or wakefulness; appetite or hunger suppression and weight loss; decreased fatigue; euphoria; exhilaration (intense); general feeling of well-being; increased mental activity; mood elevation

Toxicity

Acute: Aggressive behavior; anorexia; anxiety; blood pressure, increased; blurred vision; dizziness; dry mouth; hallucinations; headache; impotence; insomnia; nausea; nervousness; palpitations; respirations, increased; restlessness; seizures; sexual desire (change in); tachycardia; talkativeness; Tourette's disorder (verbal tics), precipitation of (in predisposed people); tremor; violent behavior, precipitation of (in predisposed people); vomiting

Chronic: Cardiomyopathy; growth suppression in children; physical dependence; psychological dependence; psychosis, generally with paranoia; stereotypic behavior (e.g., picking at the skin); weight loss

Pregnancy & Lactation: FDA Pregnancy Category C (see Appendix B). Safety of dextroamphetamine use by adolescent girls and women who are pregnant has not been established. Studies on the maternal use of dextroamphetamine during the first trimester of pregnancy have provided mixed results concerning the potential for congenital malformations and are thus inconclusive. Pregnant women who are physically dependent on the amphetamines are at increased risk for premature delivery and delivery of a low birth weight neonate. Neonates exposed to dextroamphetamine in utero may display signs and symptoms of the neonatal amphetamine withdrawal syndrome, including agitation and lassitude. Adolescent girls and women who are pregnant should not use dextroamphetamine. (See also the Amphetamines monograph.)

Safety of dextroamphetamine use by adolescent girls and women who are breast-feeding has not been established. Amphetamines are excreted in breast milk. Expected pharmacologic actions and effects may be observed in breast-fed neonates and infants, who also may become physically dependent. Adolescent girls and women who are breast-feeding should not use dextroamphetamine.

Abuse Potential

Physical dependence: High (USDEA Schedule II; high potential for abuse)
Psychological dependence: High

Withdrawal Syndrome

A true dextroamphetamine withdrawal syndrome has not been reported. However, the abrupt discontinuation of regular, long-term or high-dose dextroamphetamine use may result in the replacement of desired euphoric and other effects with feelings of depression and lethargy. (See the Amphetamines monograph.)

Overdosage

Signs and symptoms of acute dextroamphetamine overdosage include cardiovascular reactions (e.g., dysrhythmias, hypertension or hypotension, and circulatory collapse), combativeness, confusion, GI complaints (e.g., abdominal cramps, diarrhea, nausea and vomiting), dilated and reactive pupils, hallucinations, hyperpyrexia, hyperreflexia, panic, restlessness, rhabdomyolysis (i.e., marked destruction of skeletal muscle), seizures, tachypnea, tremor, and urine discoloration (dark red or cola colored). Depression and fatigue usually follow the central stimulation. Fatal overdosages usually terminate in convulsions and coma. Dextroamphetamine overdosage requires emergency medical support of body systems, with attention to increasing dextroamphetamine elimination. There is no known antidote.

Note

1. Dextroamphetamine continues to be indicated for the medical management of ADHD. Two salt forms of dextroamphetamine (as well as two salt forms of amphetamine) are included in the mixed amphetamines product Adderall® (i.e., amphetamine aspartate, amphetamine sulfate, dextroamphetamine saccharate, and dextroamphetamine sulfate), which is used to treat ADHD (see Mixed Amphetamines monograph).

Reference

Strakowski, S.M., Sax, K.W., Rosenberg, H.L., et al. (2001). Human response to repeated low-dose d-amphetamine: Evidence for behavioral enhancement and tolerance. *Neuropsychopharmacology*, 25(4), 548-554.

DEXTROMETHORPHAN

Names

BAN or INN Generic Synonyms: Demorphan

Brand/Trade: Balminil DM®; Benylin DM®; Koffex DM®; Novahistex DM®; Novahistine DM®; Robitussin Children's Cough DM®

Chemical: 3-Methoxy-17-methylmorphinan

Street: CCC; Cough Syrup; Crystal Dex; Dexter; Dextro; DM; DXM; Red Baron; Robo; Robo-Cop; Rojo; Rome; Skittles; Syrup; Triple C (for Coricidin HBP Cough & Cold Tablets®); Tussin; Velvet; X

Pharmacologic Classification

Psychodepressant, opiate derivative: antitussive (synthetic)

Brief General Overview

Dextromethorphan is structurally related to the opiate analgesics (i.e., it is a structural analogue of codeine and the d-isomer of the opiate analgesic levorphanol). It was developed in an attempt to provide opiate-type cough suppression without opiate-type physical and psychological dependence. Dextromethorphan is largely successful in this regard. However, the use of high oral dosages (i.e., typically 3 to 10 times the recommended daily antitussive dosage) is capable of causing both physical and psychological dependence.

Dosage Forms and Routes of Administration

Dextromethorphan, the most widely used antitussive in North America, is available as the principal active ingredient in several nonprescription cough suppressants and as a component of many more combination cough and cold products. It is available in various oral dosage formulations (capsules, solutions, syrup) and is usually orally ingested. Dextromethorphan is licitly produced by pharmaceutical manufacturers and is widely available in virtually every pharmacy, large food store, and convenience store across North America. It also is available in pure powder form over the Internet. The powder form is intranasally sniffed (snorted) and also can be heated and the fumes inhaled (i.e., "chasing the dragon"). With the popularity of these latter methods of use over the past 5 years, a simple acid–base extraction technique was developed to extract relatively pure dextromethorphan from the unwanted alcohol, coloring agents, guaifenesin, sweeteners, and other ingredients found in the various cough and cold products. This technique is published on the Internet.

People who use dextromethorphan for anything other than the symptomatic management of nonproductive cough are typically older adolescent boys, 16 to 20 years of age, of European descent. In order to get "high," they consume many times (i.e., generally 5 to 10 times) the amount recommended for the symptomatic management of a nonproductive cough.[1] Case studies also have been published of elderly chronic abusers of dextromethorphan.

Mechanism of CNS Action

The exact mechanism of CNS action of dextromethorphan has not been determined. Dextromethorphan is a glutaminergic N-methyl-d-aspartate (NMDA) receptor antagonist, which may play a role in its actions. Dextromethorphan does have an active metabolite, dextrophan, which is produced in variable amounts depending on the endogenous action of cytochrome P450 isoenzyme 2D6 in dextromethorphan users.

Pharmacodynamics/Pharmacokinetics

Dextromethorphan is well absorbed after oral ingestion and has an onset of action within 30 minutes. The duration of effects is generally 3 to 6 hours. Dextromethorphan is metabolized by demethylation in the liver to several metabolites, including dextrophan, an active metabolite. Metabolic clearance may be reduced in the elderly. Additional valid and reliable data are not available.

Current Approved Indications for Medical Use

Cough suppression

Desired Action/Reason for Personal Use

Alcohol-like disinhibitory euphoria or "high"[2] (more likely to occur at *lower* dosages); hallucinations (auditory, tactile, and visual; more likely to occur at *higher* dosages)

Toxicity

Acute: Aggression; ataxia; dizziness; drowsiness (mild); excitability; hypertension; impaired judgment; lethargy; lightheadedness; mood changes; nausea; nervousness; nystagmus; psychomotor impairment; psychosis (particularly in rapid metabolizers with high levels of cytochrome P450 isoenzyme 2D6); restlessness; slurred speech; stomach pain; sweating; vomiting

Chronic: Global cognitive deterioration; physical dependence; psychological dependence

Pregnancy & Lactation: Safety of dextromethorphan use by adolescent girls and women who are pregnant has not been established. However, on the basis of the lack of published negative reports and the known pharmacology of dextromethorphan, risk for significant harm to the developing fetus and neonate is expected to be minimal. Valid and reliable data are needed.

Safety of dextromethorphan use by adolescent girls and women who are breast-feeding has not been established. Valid and reliable data are needed.

Abuse Potential[3]

Physical dependence: Low (USDEA: not a scheduled drug)
Psychological dependence: Moderate

Withdrawal Syndrome

A mild dextromethorphan withdrawal syndrome has been noted upon abrupt discontinuation of regular, long-term high-dosage use. Associated signs and symptoms reportedly include dysphoria and difficulty sleeping.

Overdosage[4]

Overdosage solely involving dextromethorphan is generally mild and self-limiting.[5] However, it rarely can be fatal. Signs and symptoms of dextromethorphan overdosage include ataxia, lethargy, nausea, nystagmus, visual disturbances, vomiting, and urinary retention. Severe signs and symptoms can vary from profound sedation, or coma, for which medical management with attention to the support of body systems and the use of the opiate analgesic antagonist naloxone (Narcan®) may be required, to seizures, which may require additional medical management with intravenous benzodiazepine pharmacotherapy (e.g., diazepam [Valium®]; see monograph).

Notes

1. Usually, homeless people who "live on the street" and are regular long-term users of drugs and substances of abuse use whatever drug or substance of abuse is readily available to them, including cough and cold products containing dextromethorphan. However, these users are generally more interested in the possible alcohol content of these cough and cold products than in the effects of the dextromethorphan.
2. The effects of dextromethorphan appear to be greater in users who have a positive personal or genetic history of alcohol abuse.
3. The abuse potential may be increased to a moderate level in users who have a positive personal or family history of alcohol abuse.
4. Because dextromethorphan is commonly available in a wide variety of cough and cold products, overdosage may also involve the toxic effects of alcohol and other product ingredients, most notably antihistamines and decongestants. In addition, because abuse of dextromethorphan often takes place in the context of "pharming" (i.e., using whatever drug may be found in the home medicine cabinet, as described in the Codeine monograph), the likelihood of multiple poisons is significantly increased.
5. This may be due, in part, to the neuroprotective action that is observed with high dosages of dextromethorphan. The observed neuroprotective actions of dextromethorphan have been linked to low affinity, non-competitive N-methyl-D-aspartate (NMDA) receptor antagonism (i.e., dextromethorphan's basic mechanism of action).

References

Banerji, S., & Anderson, I.B. (2001). Abuse of Coricidin HBP cough & cold tablets: Episodes recorded by a poison center. *American Journal of Health-System Pharmacy, 58*(19), 1811-1814.

Bryner, J.K., Wang, U.K., Hui, J.W., et al. (2006). Dextromethorphan abuse in adolescence: An increasing trend: 1999-2004. *Archives of Pediatrics & Adolescent Medicine, 160*(12), 1217-1222.

Chyka, P.A., Erdman, A.R., Manoguerra, A.S., et al. (2007). Dextromethorphan poisoning: An evidence-based consensus guideline for out-of-hospital management. *Clinical Toxicology, 45*(6), 662-677.

Cochems, A., Harding, P., & Liddicoat, L. (2007). Dextromethorphan in Wisconsin drivers. *Journal of Analytical Toxicology, 31*(4), 227-232.

Desai, S., Aldea, D., Daneels, E., et al. (2006). Chronic addiction to dextromethorphan cough syrup: A case report. *The Journal of the American Board of Family Medicine, 19*(3), 320-323.

Hendrickson, R.G., & Cloutier, R.L. (2007). "Crystal dex:" Free-base dextromethorphan. *The Journal of Emergency Medicine, 32*(4), 393-396.

Lessenger, J.E., & Feinberg, S.D. (2008). Abuse of prescription and over-the-counter medications. *The Journal of the American Board of Family Medicine, 21*(1), 45-54.

Levine, D.A. (2007). "Pharming": The abuse of prescription and over-the-counter drugs in teens. *Current Opinion in Pediatrics, 19*(3), 270-274.

Martin, N., Kurani, A., Kennedy, C.A., et al. (2007). Dextromethorphan-induced near-fatal suicide attempt in a slow metabolizer at cytochrome P450 2D6. *The American Journal of Geriatric Pharmacotherapy, 5*(2), 162-165.

Schwartz, R.H., (2005). Adolescent abuse of dextromethorphan. *Clinical Pediatrics, 44*(7), 565-568.

Shin, E.J., Lee, P.H., Kim, H.J., et al. (2008). Neuropsychotoxicity of abused drugs: Potential of dextromethorphan and novel neuroprotective analogs of dextromethorphan with improved safety profiles in terms of abuse and neuroprotective effects. *Journal of Pharmacological Sciences, 106*(1), 22-27.

Soyka, M., Bondy, B., Eisenburg, B., et al. (2000). NMDA receptor challenge with dextromethorphan—subjective response, neuroendocrinological findings and possible clinical implications. *Journal of Neural Transmission, 107*(6), 701-714.

Werling, L.L., Lauterbach, E.C., & Calef, U. (2007). Dextromethorphan as a potential neuroprotective agent with unique mechanisms of action. *The Neurologist, 13*(5), 272-293.

DEXTROPROPOXYPHENE (See Propoxyphene)

DIACETYLMORPHINE (See Heroin)

DIAZEPAM

Names

BAN or INN Generic Synonyms: None

Brand/Trade: Diastat®; Diazemuls®; Diazepam Intensol®; Valium®; Valrelease®; Vivol®

Chemical: 7-Chloro-1,3-dihydro-1-methyl-5-phenyl-2H-1,4-benzodiazepin-2-one

Street: Ardins; Blues; French Blues; Mother's Little Helper; Pami; Vallies; Vals; Vees; Vs; Whitshire Blues; Yellows

Pharmacologic Classification

Psychodepressant, sedative-hypnotic: benzodiazepine

Brief General Overview

Diazepam, which was synthesized in 1963, was one of the first available benzodiazepines and, together with chlordiazepoxide (see monograph), has the longest history of clinical use in North America. Since its introduction, it has been personally used for its psychodepressant actions by both men and women and by both those receiving legitimate prescriptions and those using illicitly diverted diazepam from hospital supplies or other sources (e.g., "double-doctoring," pharmacy burglaries). Currently, diazepam is among the top three benzodiazepines used in North America.

Dosage Forms and Routes of Administration

Diazepam is synthesized by licit pharmaceutical manufacturers in North America. It is available in a variety of dosage formulations, including injectable (intramuscular or intravenous), oral (capsules, solutions, tablets), and rectal (gel). People who abuse diazepam that has been obtained by legitimate prescription usually ingest the oral dosage formulations. Other people who illicitly use diazepam usually inject it intravenously. Most of these users may substitute diazepam when their usual psychodepressant of choice (e.g., heroin) is unavailable, or when its cost exceeds what they are able to pay. When used in combination with other drugs, diazepam is most frequently used with other psychodepressants, usually alcohol or opiate analgesics.

Mechanism of CNS Action

The exact mechanism of action of diazepam has not been determined. However, it appears to be primarily mediated by, or to work in concert with, the inhibitory neurotransmitter GABA. Thus, diazepam appears to act by binding to the benzodiazepine receptors (types I and II [BZD-1 and BZD-2]) within the GABA complex. (See the Benzodiazepines monograph.)

Pharmacodynamics/Pharmacokinetics

Diazepam is virtually completely absorbed after oral ingestion ($F \cong 1$) and achieves peak blood concentrations within 1 to 2 hours. After intravenous injection, peak blood concentrations are achieved within 15 minutes and, although absorption may be erratic depending on blood flow to the muscle injected, peak absorption after intramuscular injection usually occurs within 2 hours. Once absorbed, diazepam is highly plasma protein bound (~98%) and has an apparent volume of distribution of ~1 L/kg. It is extensively metabolized in the liver to both active (e.g., desmethyldiazepam [also known as nordazepam and nordiazepam], oxazepam) and inactive metabolites. Less than 1% of diazepam is excreted in unchanged form in the urine. The mean elimination half-life is 43 hours, and the mean total body clearance is 28 mL/minute.

Current Approved Indications for Medical Use

Anxiety disorders; prevention/management of the alcohol withdrawal syndrome; prevention/management of the diazepam and other benzodiazepine withdrawal syndromes; seizure disorders; skeletal muscle spasm

Desired Action/Reason for Personal Use

Alcohol-like disinhibitory euphoria or "high"; anxiety/stress reduction; prevention/self-management of the diazepam withdrawal syndrome; self-management of the opiate analgesic withdrawal syndrome (i.e., when the opiate is unavailable or unaffordable)

Toxicity

Acute: Ataxia; blurred vision; bradycardia; cognitive impairment; confusion; dizziness; drowsiness; dry mouth; fatigue; headache; hypotension; mental depression; slurred speech; tremor; weakness

Chronic: Physical dependence; psychological dependence

Pregnancy & Lactation: FDA Pregnancy Category D (see Appendix B). An increased risk for congenital malformations (e.g., cleft lip and palate, limb and digit malformations) has been associated with diazepam pharmacotherapy and regular personal use during the first trimester of pregnancy. However, data are inconclusive. Maternal use near term has been associated with expected pharmacologic actions in neonates, including hypotonia, low Apgar scores, poor feeding, and signs and symptoms of the benzodiazepine withdrawal syndrome. Adolescent girls and women who are pregnant should not use diazepam.

Diazepam is excreted in breast milk in sufficient quantities to cause sedation and physical dependence in breast-fed neonates and infants. Adolescent girls and women who are breast-feeding should not use diazepam.

Abuse Potential

Physical dependence: Low (USDEA Schedule IV; low abuse potential)
Psychological dependence: Moderate

Withdrawal Syndrome

Abrupt discontinuation of regular, long-term high-dosage diazepam use has been associated with a diazepam withdrawal syndrome, which is similar to the alcohol withdrawal syndrome. Signs and symptoms of the diazepam withdrawal syndrome include abdominal and muscle cramps, convulsions, sweating, tremor, and vomiting. Milder signs and symptoms, such as dysphoria and insomnia, have been associated with abrupt discontinuation of benzodiazepine pharmacotherapy in patients who were receiving recommended dosages over several months. Abrupt discontinuation of diazepam use should be avoided, particularly when higher dosages are used and use has extended over several months. In these cases, diazepam use should be discontinued slowly, with a gradual reduction in dosage.

Overdosage

Signs and symptoms of diazepam overdosage include confusion, somnolence, coma, and diminished reflexes. Although diazepam is rarely fatal when used alone,[1] diazepam overdosage requires emergency medical support, with attention to increasing diazepam elimination. The benzodiazepine antagonist flumazenil (Anexate®, Romazicon®) may be required.

Note

1. Diazepam overdosage often occurs in the context of alcohol consumption, which significantly increases CNS depression and the resultant risk of death.

References

Singh, R.K., Jain, R., Ray, R., et al. (2001). Abuse liability of diazepam through different routes. *Indian Journal of Physiology and Pharmacology, 45*(2), 181-190.

Smith, T.A. (2001). Type A gamma-aminobutyric acid (GABAA) receptor subunits and benzodiazepine binding: Significance to clinical syndromes and their treatment. *British Journal of Biomedical Science, 58*(2), 111-121.

DIETHYLPROPION

Names

BAN or INN Generic Synonyms: Amfepramone; Diethylcathinone

Brand/Trade: Tenuate®; Tenuate Dospan®

Chemical: 1-Phenyl-2-diethylamino-1-propanone

Street: None

Pharmacologic Classification

Psychostimulant, miscellaneous: amphetamine derivative

Brief General Overview

Diethylpropion is derived from the amphetamines. It is personally used for its psychostimulant actions. Regular, long-term diethylpropion use may result in physical and psychological dependence because diethylpropion is chemically and pharmacologically related to the amphetamines, which have high abuse potential. Diethylpropion use has been associated with the development of tolerance when users for whom it is medically prescribed increase their dosages to many times those recommended or use the drug more often than recommended. Signs and symptoms of this pattern of use include hyperactivity, irritability, insomnia, personality changes, and severe dermatoses. Psychosis that is often clinically indistinguishable from schizophrenia also has been associated with diethylpropion abuse.

Dosage Forms and Routes of Administration

Diethylpropion is produced by licit pharmaceutical manufacturers. It is commercially available in oral tablet formulations and is virtually always orally ingested. Most North Americans who develop problematic patterns of diethylpropion use are middle-aged women of European descent who have been prescribed diethylpropion by their physicians for weight management but exceed the dosage guidelines and recommendations for short-term use.

Mechanism of CNS Action

The exact mechanism of diethylpropion's psychostimulant action has not been determined. However, diethylpropion appears to directly stimulate the CNS. Metabolic or other actions also may be involved.

Pharmacodynamics/Pharmacokinetics

Diethylpropion is rapidly and well absorbed following oral ingestion. It is extensively metabolized in the liver, primarily by N-dealkylation and reduction, to several active and inactive metabolites. Additional valid and reliable data are not available.

Current Approved Indications for Medical Use

Exogenous obesity, short-term adjunctive pharmacotherapy

Desired Action/Reason for Personal Use

Appetite suppression and weight loss; euphoria; feelings of increased energy

Toxicity

Acute: Abdominal discomfort; agitation; anxiety; anorgasmia; blurred vision; dizziness; dry mouth; dyskinesia; gynecomastia; headache; hallucinations (rare with higher dosages); hyperactivity; hypertension; irritability; insomnia; muscle pain; mydriasis; nausea; nervousness; palpitations; restlessness; seizures (increased in people with epilepsy); tachycardia

Chronic: Physical dependence; psychological dependence; primary pulmonary hypertension (rare, but potentially fatal)[1]; psychosis[2]; tolerance

Pregnancy & Lactation: FDA Pregnancy Category B (see Appendix B). Safety of diethylpropion use by adolescent girls and women who are pregnant has not been established. Regular, long-term diethylpropion use by adolescent girls and women during pregnancy may result in the neonatal diethylpropion withdrawal syndrome. Signs and symptoms of this syndrome resemble those of the neonatal amphetamine withdrawal syndrome (see Amphetamines monograph). Adolescent girls and women who are pregnant should not use diethylpropion.

Safety of diethylpropion use by adolescent girls and women who are breast-feeding has not been established. Diethylpropion and its metabolites are excreted in breast milk. Therefore, adolescent girls and women who are breast-feeding should not use diethylpropion.

Abuse Potential

Physical dependence: Moderate (USDEA Schedule IV; low potential for abuse)
Psychological dependence: Moderate

Withdrawal Syndrome

Abrupt discontinuation of regular, long-term diethylpropion use has been associated with an amphetamine-like withdrawal syndrome that includes signs and symptoms of extreme fatigue and mental depression. Electroencephalographic changes also have been reported. Users should be cautioned against abrupt discontinuation of regular, long-term diethylpropion use. Gradual tapering of the dosage is recommended.

Overdosage

Signs and symptoms of acute diethylpropion overdosage include aggressiveness/combativeness, confusion, convulsions, diarrhea, drowsiness, exhaustion, hallucinations, hyperreflexia, hyperventilation, insomnia, irritability, mydriasis, nervousness, panic, restlessness, tachycardia, tremor, and vomiting. The initial stimulatory phase is usually followed by drowsiness, exhaustion, fatigue, and CNS depression. Diethylpropion overdosage may be fatal and requires emergency medical support, with attention to increasing diethylpropion elimination. There is no known antidote.

Notes

1. Risk appears to be directly associated with a duration of use in excess of 3 months.
2. Often clinically indistinguishable from schizophrenia, but generally abates with the discontinuation of diethylpropion use.

References

Bray, G.A. (2000). A concise review on the therapeutics of obesity. *Nutrition, 16*(10), 953-960.
Glazer, G. (2001). Long-term pharmacotherapy of obesity 2000: A review of efficacy and safety. *Archives of Internal Medicine, 161*(15), 1814-1824.

DIHYDROCODEINE (See Hydrocodone)

DIHYDROHYDROXYCODEINONE (See Oxycodone)

DIHYDROMORPHINONE (See Hydromorphone)

DIMENHYDRINATE (See Diphenhydramine)

2,5-DIMETHOXY-4-METHYLAMPHETAMINE

Names

BAN or INN Generic Synonyms: 4-Methyl-2,5-dimethoxyamphetamine

Brand/Trade: None

Chemical: 2,5-Dimethoxy-α,4-dimethylphenethylamine

Street: DOM; STP[1]

Pharmacologic Classification

Psychodelic, amphetamine-like psychodelic: phenethylamine

Brief General Overview

2,5-Dimethoxy-4-methylamphetamine (DOM) is a 3,4-methylenedioxyamphetamine-like (see monograph) chemical analogue (i.e., phenylisopropylamine). It was first synthesized in 1964 by Alexander Shulgin and was a popular psychodelic during the 1960s and 1970s. However, the use of DOM declined precipitously during the late 1970s when it was found that (1) higher dosages could produce psychodelic actions (e.g., hallucinations) that persisted for up to 3 days, despite the contrary wishes of the user, (2) the prolonged experiences were difficult to manage, and (3) other, more "user friendly," psychodelics were becoming available. Currently, its use is rare.[2]

Dosage Forms and Routes of Administration

DOM is produced in tablet form for oral ingestion by illicit chemical laboratories. It is rarely intravenously injected. DOM is rarely used today and, because of the low demand, is not generally available for purchase from illicit suppliers. Most users synthesize DOM themselves from recipes that are available on the Internet.

Mechanism of CNS Action

The exact mechanism of DOM's action has not been determined. It appears to be mediated by activation of serotonin receptors, specifically 5-HT2A and 5-HT2C.

Pharmacodynamics/Pharmacokinetics

Psychodelic actions generally persist for 16 to 24 hours. Additional valid and reliable data are not available.

Current Approved Indications for Medical Use

None

Desired Action/Reason for Personal Use

Euphoria (mild with lower dosages); hallucinations (primarily visual; potent); rush of energy (particularly with higher doses); self-insight

Toxicity

Acute: Anorexia; anxiety; blurred vision; dry mouth; elevated body temperature; flushing; hallucinations, auditory and visual; inability to control thought processes; inattention (inability to concentrate); increased blood pressure; mydriasis; nausea; panic; paresthesia; psychosis; sweating; tremor; vomiting

Chronic: Valid and reliable data are not available.

Pregnancy & Lactation: Valid and reliable data are not available.

Abuse Potential

Physical dependence: None to low (USDEA Schedule I; use is prohibited)
Psychological dependence: Low

Withdrawal Syndrome

A specific DOM withdrawal syndrome has not been reported. However, tolerance (i.e., tachyphylaxis) reportedly occurs in regard to the subjective effects of DOM over as few as 3 days of use.

Overdosage

Valid and reliable data are not available.

Notes

1. STP is the acronym for "Serenity, Tranquility, and Peace," a name used for 2,5-dimethoxy-4-methylamphetamine during the 1960s by the hippies. Other abbreviations and acronyms associated with "STP" are the motor oil product STP and acronyms for "Stop the Police" and "Super Terrific Psychodelic."
2. DOM is occasionally combined with lysergic acid diethylamide (LSD), methamphetamine, and strychnine. This combination is referred to as "four ways" or "orange cupcakes."

Reference

Eckler, J.R., Greizerstein, H., Rabin, R.A., et al. (2001). A sensitive method for determining levels of 2,5-dimethoxy-4-methylamphetamine in brain tissue. *Journal of Pharmacological and Toxicological Methods, 46*(1), 37-43.

N,N-DIMETHYLTRYPTAMINE

Names

BAN or INN Generic Synonyms: Desoxybufotenine; Nigerine

Brand/Trade: None

Chemical: 3-[2-(Dimethylamino)ethyl]indole

Street: 45 Minute Psychosis; 45 Minute Trip; Businessman's LSD; Businessman's Lunch; Businessman's Special; Businessman's Trip; Dimitri; Disneyland; Disneyworld; DMT; Fantasia; Instant Psychosis; Psychosis; Special LSD

Pharmacologic Classification

Psychodelic, LSD-like psychodelic: indole/tryptamine

Brief General Overview

N,N-dimethyltryptamine (DMT), an ultra-short-acting psychodelic, occurs naturally in several plant species.[1] These species include *Anadenanthera peregrina* and *Virola calophylla*, which are indigenous to the West Indies and parts of South America. South American Indians have used the psychodelic for religious, ceremonial, and other social purposes for over 500 years.[2]

Dosage Forms and Routes of Administration

Botanical sources of DMT have been used for centuries by indigenous South Americans in the form of snuff (known commonly as *cohoba*, *yakee*, *yato*, or *yupa*), which is usually intranasally sniffed (i.e., snorted).[3] DMT was first synthesized in 1931 and since 1954 has been synthesized in illicit chemical laboratories.[4] It is available in pure crystalline form for intramuscular, intravenous, or subcutaneous injection; intranasal sniffing (snorting); or pulmonary inhalation (i.e., smoking).

Mechanism of CNS Action

The exact mechanism of the CNS action of DMT has not been determined. However, its action appears to be largely related to its affinity for the serotonin (5-hydroxytryptamine) receptors, particularly 5-HT2.[5] Dopamine D_2-receptor agonism also appears to mediate the CNS actions of DMT.

Pharmacodynamics/Pharmacokinetics

Oral availability is generally low because of catabolic deamination.[6] Onset of action is rapid: within 10 seconds after pulmonary inhalation (smoking) or 5 minutes after intramuscular injection. The duration of action is relatively brief, with an absence of residual effects generally within 10 minutes after smoking or within 60 minutes after intramuscular injection. Additional valid and reliable data are not available.

Current Approved Indications for Medical Use

None

Desired Action/Reason for Personal Use

Euphoria; dissociation; hallucinations (primarily LSD-like, with bright-colored visual imagery); sensations of warmth ("rush"); sensitivity to tactile sensations

Toxicity

Acute: Agitation; anxiety; ataxia; depersonalization; difficulty concentrating; dizziness; dry mouth; hypertension; hyperthermia; mydriasis; nausea; nystagmus; panic reactions (relatively common); paranoid psychosis; seizures; tachycardia

Chronic: Bradycardia

Pregnancy & Lactation: Valid and reliable data are not available.

Abuse Potential

Physical dependence: None to low (USDEA Schedule I; use is prohibited)
Psychological dependence: Low

Withdrawal Syndrome

A DMT withdrawal syndrome has not been reported.

Overdosage

Coma and respiratory arrest have been reported with higher dosages. There is no known antidote. Additional valid and reliable data are needed.

Notes

1. DMT also naturally occurs in minute quantities in the human body. However, its biological site of origin and its function(s) have not been determined. It has been hypothesized that DMT has a neuromodulating role, a role involved in the regulation of REM sleep, or both.
2. The first record of such use was noted during Christopher Columbus's second voyage to the West Indies in 1496.
3. When orally ingested, DMT causes minimal pharmacologic effects because of its poor oral bioavailability. A noted exception occurs when it is combined with the harmala alkaloids (see monograph).
4. The synthesis, production, possession, and use of DMT were legal in North America until 1970.
5. This proposed mechanism of action is very similar to that of lysergic acid diethylamide (LSD), with which DMT shares most of its CNS actions.
6. Oral bioavailability of DMT may be significantly increased by concurrent ingestion of selective peripheral monoamine oxidase inhibitors, such as the harmala alkaloids (see monograph). Both of these psychodelic compounds are found in the Amazonian ceremonial tea *ayahuasca*, which is also known as *Hoasca* or *Yajè*.

References

Gouzoulis-Mayfrank, E., Heekeren, K., Neukirch, A., et al. (2005). Psychological effects of (S)-ketamine and N,N-dimethyltryptamine (DMT): A double-blind, cross-over study in healthy volunteers. *Pharmacopsychiatry, 38*(6), 301-311.

Kärkkäinen, J., Forsström, T., Tornaeus, J., et al. (2005). Potentially hallucinogenic 5-hydroxytryptamine receptor ligands bufotenine and dimethyltryptamine in blood and tissues. *Scandinavian Journal of Clinical and Laboratory Investigation, 65*(3), 189-199.

Ott, J. (2001). Pharmepena-Psychonautics: Human intranasal, sublingual and oral pharmacology of 5-methoxy-N,N-dimethyl-tryptamine. *Journal of Psychoactive Drugs, 33*(4), 403-407.

Riba, J., Anderer, P., Morte, A., et al. (2002). Topographic pharmaco-EEG mapping of the effects of the South American psychoactive beverage ayahuasca in healthy volunteers. *British Journal of Clinical Pharmacology, 53*(6), 613-628.

Szára, S. (2007). DMT at fifty. *Neuropsychopharmacologia Hungarica, 9*(4), 201-205.

DIPHENHYDRAMINE

Names

BAN or INN Generic Synonyms: None

Brand/Trade: Allerdryl®; Allernix®; Benadryl®; Benylan®; Benylin®; Diphenhist®; Nytol®; Simple Sleep®; Sominex®; Unisom®; Vicks Formula 44®

Chemical: 2-(Diphenylmethoxy)-N,N-dimethylethylamine

Street: Ben; Pink Panther

Pharmacologic Classification

Psychodepressant, sedative-hypnotic: miscellaneous (ethanolamine-type antihistamine)

Brief General Overview

Diphenhydramine is an antihistamine with antiemetic and antispasmodic activity. It is produced by licit pharmaceutical manufacturers in North America and is widely available, generally without prescription, being sold over-the-counter in many pharmacies, including those within grocery stores. It was introduced into clinical practice in North America in 1946 and over the past 60 years has been one of the most widely used drugs in allergy treatment.

Dimenhydrinate (i.e., Dramamine®; Gravol®) is a closely related 8-chlorotheophyllinate salt form of diphenhydramine and shares its same principal active metabolite, but dimenhydrinate is 50% less potent on a milligram per milligram basis. In addition to being commonly available without a prescription in pharmacies and major food stores, both diphenhydramine and its related salt, dimenhydrinate, are widely available through Internet sites.

Dosage Forms and Routes of Administration

Diphenhydramine is licitly produced by a number of different pharmaceutical manufacturers in North America. It is available in a wide variety of dosage formulations (e.g., injectable; oral caplet, capsule, tablet, chewable tablet; oral elixir, solution, and syrup; topical cream, spray, and stick) reflective of its wide spectrum of clinical applications in the management of allergy and related mild to moderate hypersensitivity reactions. Young adolescent boys, mostly of European descent, are the primary users of diphenhydramine. These adolescents usually orally ingest diphenhydramine in the context of "pharming" (i.e., taking whatever drugs are available in the home from their family medicine cabinet and experimenting with them to get "high"). (See the Codeine monograph; see also the Heroin monograph for combined use.)

Mechanism of CNS Action

Diphenhydramine is an antihistamine H_1-receptor antagonist that elicits its effects both centrally and peripherally by actively displacing histamine from its receptor binding sites.

It also displays anticholinergic activity that results in its antiemetic and antiparkinsonian actions.

Pharmacodynamics/Pharmacokinetics

Diphenhydramine is rapidly absorbed after oral ingestion, with maximal action occurring within 1 hour. It is highly plasma protein bound (e.g., 99%). Diphenhydramine undergoes extensive first-pass hepatic metabolism following oral ingestion. Cytochrome P450 isoenzymes 2D6 and 3A4 are involved in its metabolism. Two major metabolites are desmethyldiphenhydramine, which is rapidly produced, and diphenylmethoxyacetic acid, which is more slowly produced through several metabolic steps. The mean elimination half-life of diphenhydramine is 4 hours (range, 2 to 7 hours).

Current Approved Indications for Medical Use

Motion sickness prophylaxis; sleep disorders: insomnia (short-term management); symptomatic management of allergic reactions (e.g., allergic rhinitis, contact dermatitis, hay fever, pruritus, urticaria); symptomatic management of extrapyramidal signs and symptoms associated with Parkinson's disease; vomiting

Desired Action/Reason for Personal Use

Delirium[1] ; dissociation (with very realistic delusions); hallucinations and illusions; also, purposely administered to others without their knowledge in the context of perpetration of a drug-facilitated crime (e.g., robbery; sexual assault, including date rape)[2]

Toxicity

Acute: Ataxia; blurred vision; delirium; dizziness; drowsiness; dry mouth and mucous membranes; epigastric distress; excitement (particularly in children); memory impairment; sedation; tachycardia; urinary retention

Chronic: Hypersomnolence; lethargy; psychological dependence; social withdrawal

Pregnancy & Lactation[3]: FDA Pregnancy Category B (see Appendix B). Safety of diphenhydramine use by adolescent girls and women who are pregnant has not been established. There is no evidence of teratogenic risk in humans, despite such adverse findings in animals. The chance of fetal harm appears to be remote. However, maternal use near term has resulted in signs of toxicity (i.e., diarrhea and restlessness) in the neonate. These signs of toxicity may actually be signs of a neonatal diphenhydramine withdrawal syndrome. Additional valid and reliable data are needed.

Safety of diphenhydramine use by adolescent girls and women who are breast-feeding has not been established. However, diphenhydramine appears to have low potential for toxicity in breast-fed neonates and infants. Additional valid and reliable data are needed.

Abuse Potential

Physical dependence: None to low (USDEA: Not a scheduled drug; low potential for abuse)
Psychological dependence: Low

Withdrawal Syndrome

A diphenhydramine withdrawal syndrome has not been reported. See comments in "Pregnancy & Lactation."

Overdosage

Signs and symptoms of diphenhydramine overdosage can be quite varied and include agitation, coma, confusion, delirium, drowsiness, dry mucous membranes, flushing, mydriasis, psychomotor impairment, tachycardia, and tremor. Diphenhydramine overdosage may be fatal. Major pathology contributing to death includes cardiac dysrhythmias, pulmonary congestion/hypertension, and seizures. Acute overdosage requires emergency medical support and monitoring of body systems with attention to increasing diphenhydramine elimination. There is no known antidote.

Notes

1. Diphenhydramine is commonly referred to as a "deliriant" by users.
2. Diphenhydramine seldom or rarely appears to be used in this context, in comparison with other drugs and substances of abuse such as flunitrazepam and gamma-hydroxybutyrate (see respective monographs). However, this use has been documented in a number of cases in the published literature.
3. The alcohol content of diphenhydramine elixir formulations is significant (~15%) and can pose a teratogenic risk for the developing embryo and fetus when these formulations are used on a regular basis by mothers during pregnancy. (See the Alcohol monograph.)

References

Baker, A.M., Johnson, D.G., Levisky, J.A., et al. (2003). Fatal diphenhydramine intoxication in infants. *Journal of Forensic Sciences 48*(2), 425-428.

Centers for Disease Control and Prevention (CDC). (2007). Infant deaths associated with cough and cold medications—Two states, 2005. *Morbidity and Mortality Weekly Report (MMWR), 56*(1), 1-4.

Garcia-Bournissen, F., Finkelstein, Y., Rezvani, M., et al. (2006). Exposure to alcohol-containing medications during pregnancy. *Canadian Family Physician, 52*(9), 1067-1068.

Griffiths, R.R., & Johnson, M.W. (2005). Relative abuse liability of hypnotic drugs: A conceptual framework and algorithm for differentiating among compounds. *Journal of Clinical Psychiatry, 66* (Supplement 9), 31-41.

Jaffe, J.H., Bloor, R., Crome, I., et al. (2004). A postmarketing study of relative abuse liability of hypnotic sedative drugs. *Addiction, 99*(2), 165-173.

Kintz, P., Evans, J., Villain, M., et al. (2007). Hair analysis for diphenhydramine after surreptitious administration to a child. *Forensic Science International, 173*(2-3), 171-174.

Marinetti, L., Lehman, L., Casto, B., et al. (2005). Over-the-counter cold medications—Postmortem findings in infants and the relationship to cause of death. *Journal of Analytical Toxicology, 29*(7), 738-743.

Nine, J.S., & Rund, C.R. (2006). Fatality from diphenhydramine monointoxication: A case report and review of the infant, pediatric, and adult literature. *The American Journal of Forensic Medicine and Pathology, 27*(1), 36-41.

Pragst, F., Herre, S., & Bakdash, A. (2006). Poisonings with diphenhydramine—A survey of 68 clinical and 55 death cases. *Forensic Science International, 161*(2-3), 189-197.

Rimsza, M.E., & Newberry, S. (2008). Unexpected infant deaths associated with use of cough and cold medications. *Pediatrics, 122*(2), e318-e322.

Scharmen, E.J., Erdman, A.R., Wax, P.M., et al. (2006). Diphenhydramine and dimenhydrinate poisoning: An evidence-based consensus guideline for out-of-hospital management. *Clinical Toxicology, 44*(3), 205-223.

Sundararaghavan, S., & Suarez, W.A. (2004). Oral benadryl and central venous catheter abuse—A potentially "lethal combination." *Pediatric Emergency Care, 20*(9), 604-606.

Thundiyil, J.G., Kearney, T.E., & Olson, K.R. (2007). Evolving epidemiology of drug-induced seizures reported to a Poison Control Center System. *Journal of Medical Toxicology, 3*(1), 15-19.

Traynor, K. (2007). Nonprescription cold remedies unsafe for young children, FDA advisers say. *American Journal of Health-System Pharmacy, 64*(23), 2408-2410.

Vernacchio, L., Kelly, J.P., Kaufman, D.W., et al. (2008). Cough and cold medication use by U.S. children, 1999-2006: Results from the Slone Survey. *Pediatrics, 122*(2), e323-e329.

DRONABINOL (See Cannabis)

EPHEDRA (See Ephedrine)

EPHEDRINE

Names

BAN or INN Generic Synonyms: None

Brand/Trade: Generally available by generic name[1]

Chemical: α-[l-(Methylamino)ethyl]benzene-methanol

Street: Black Beauties[2]; Blasting Caps; Brigham Tea; Chewa; Chinese Ephedra; Chi Powder; Desert Herb; Desert Tea; Diet Max; Diet Pep; Herbal Fuel; Horsetail; Joint Fir; *Ma Huang*; Mao; Mao-Kon; Mexican Tea; Mormon Tea; Natural Ecstasy; Sea Grape; Shrubby; Squaw Tea; Teamster's Tea; Yellow Astringent; Yellow Horse; Yellow Jackets[3]

Pharmacologic Classification

Psychostimulant, miscellaneous: naturally occurring sympathomimetic

Brief General Overview

Ephedrine and related alkaloids are naturally derived from the *Ephedra* genus of shrublike plants.[4] Ephedrine also can be chemically synthesized. The drug was isolated from the plant during the 1800s, but its stimulant actions were not recognized until the early 1920s, when it was used as a bronchodilator and a nasal decongestant. More recently, ephedrine was rediscovered by university students who wanted to stay awake to study for examinations. It is found in many nonprescription cough and cold products, and these and other ephedrine-containing products are increasingly being marketed and used for ergogenic purposes (e.g., to increase athletic performance) and to promote weight loss.[5]

Herbal products containing ephedrine also are being marketed to adolescents, primarily over the Internet, as street drug alternatives, with claims that they produce euphoria, heightened awareness, increased energy, and increased sexual sensations. There is no typical ephedrine user or abuser, because the drug is widely used by many segments of society (e.g., bodybuilders, high school and college students, professional athletes, truck drivers) for a variety of reasons.

Dosage Forms and Routes of Administration

Ephedrine is available in oral capsule and tablet formulations, as well as in an injectable formulation, from a number of licit pharmaceutical manufacturers. In addition, it is available in a variety of licit and illicit dietary products and herbal remedies or supplements that are widely available without prescription in food markets, health food stores, and pharmacies. These products also are widely available by mail order in North America, and worldwide through purchase over the Internet.

Mechanism of CNS Action

Ephedrine acts both directly by stimulating adrenergic receptors (i.e., α, β_1, and β_2) in the CNS and indirectly by stimulating the release of norepinephrine from storage vesicles in the parasympathetic nervous system.[6]

Pharmacodynamics/Pharmacokinetics

Ephedrine is generally well absorbed after oral ingestion. Peak blood concentrations are achieved in ~1 hour. Ephedrine also is well absorbed after metered intranasal spray administration. The apparent volume of distribution is ~3 L/kg. A minor percentage of ephedrine is metabolized in the liver, but the majority (70% to 80%) is excreted in unchanged form in the urine. The mean elimination half-life for ephedrine is ~6 hours (usual range, 3 to 6 hours) and is pH dependent.

Current Approved Indications for Medical Use[7]

Nasal decongestion

Desired Action/Reason for Personal Use

Decrease fatigue[8]; feeling of well-being; maintain or lose body weight

Toxicity

Acute: Anorexia; anxiety; cardiac dysrhythmias; dizziness; GI upset; hallucinations (rare); headache; hypertension; hypoglycemia; insomnia; irritability; myocardial infarction (rare)[9]; nausea; nervousness; nephrolithiasis; orthostatic hypotension; palpitations; restlessness; sudden death (rare); stroke (rare); tachycardia; tension; tremor; urinary hesitancy; vomiting

Chronic: Hypertension; psychological dependence; weight loss

Pregnancy & Lactation: FDA Pregnancy Category C (see Appendix B). Safety of ephedrine use by adolescent girls and women who are pregnant has not been established. No teratogenic effects have been reported to date in the published literature. However, ephedrine crosses the placenta and can increase fetal heart rate. In addition, ephedra has been demonstrated to induce uterine contractions. Therefore, adolescent girls and women who are pregnant should not use ephedrine.

Ephedrine appears to be excreted in breast milk and has reportedly been associated with crying, insomnia, and irritability in breast-fed neonates and infants whose mothers use ephedrine. Additional valid and reliable data are needed.

Abuse Potential

Physical dependence: Low (USDEA: not a scheduled drug)
Psychological dependence: Moderate

Withdrawal Syndrome

An ephedrine withdrawal syndrome has not been reported.

Overdosage

Overdosages involving ephedrine or ephedra herbal products have been fatal. Death is usually due to associated myocardial infarction or stroke. Severe hypertension and tachycardia may be treated with an appropriate β-adrenergic blocker (pretreatment with a vasodilator is generally necessary to prevent paradoxic worsening of the blood pressure). Acute ephedrine overdosage requires emergency medical support of body systems. There is no known antidote.

Notes

1. Also commonly available in combination cold products and herbal remedies.
2. In the 1960s, 1970s, and 1980s, "Black Beauties" referred to combination amphetamine-containing capsules (i.e., Biphetamine®), and "Yellow Jackets" referred to barbiturate-containing capsules (i.e., pentobarbital [Nembutal®]).
3. As noted elsewhere in this text, associating street names with generic names must always be considered in context. For example, "Yellow Jackets" also is a common street name for pentobarbital capsules (see monograph). See also Note 2.
4. The *Ephedra* genus is indigenous worldwide and has more than 50 species, including *Ephedra equisetina*, *Ephedra intermedia*, *Ephedra sinica* (*Ma Huang*), and *Ephedra vulgaris*; however, it appears that ephedrine is found only in Eurasian species.
5. Although ephedrine is popularly used for bodybuilding and weight loss, neither indication has been clearly established in the clinical literature. However, ephedrine continues to be found in many related herbal products despite a federal ban on the sale of dietary supplements containing ephedrine alkaloids that was issued by FDA in 2004.
6. The reduced efficacy of ephedrine that is observed with repeated use occurs, in large part, because of the depletion of norepinephrine.
7. Ephedrine has a long history of use in traditional Chinese medicine and in the traditional folk medicine of many other cultures. It has been used to treat a number of conditions and diseases, including arthritis, colds, cough, depression, diabetes, edema, enuresis, fatigue, fever, flu, gonorrhea, liver spots, joint pain, narcolepsy, nephritis, and syphilis. It also has been used as an upper respiratory and uterine stimulant.

8. For example, a significant percentage of commercial tractor-trailer drivers in North America use licit and illicit psychostimulants, including ephedrine, to decrease fatigue and to stay awake while driving for long periods of time.

9. Risk for myocardial infarction may be increased with intravenous injection.

References

Avois, L., Robinson, N., Saudan, C., et al. (2006). Central nervous system stimulants and sport practice. *British Journal of Sports Medicine, 40*(Supplement 1), i16-i20.

Berlin, I., Warot, D., Aymard, G., et al. (2001). Pharmacodynamics and pharmacokinetics of single nasal (5 mg and 10 mg) and oral (50 mg) doses of ephedrine in healthy subjects. *European Journal of Clinical Pharmacology, 57*(6-7), 447-455.

Boroda, A., & Akhter, R. (2008). Hallucinations in a child: A case demonstrating the pitfalls of urine dipstick drug testing. *Journal of Forensic and Legal Medicine, 15*(3), 198-199.

Couper, F.J., Pemberton, M., Jarvis, A., et al. (2002). Prevalence of drug use in commercial tractor-trailer drivers. *Journal of Forensic Sciences, 47*(3), 562-567.

FDA issues cyber letter to yellow jackets promoter. (2002, October 7). *FDA News*.

Guidance for industry: Street drug alternatives. (2000, March). U.S. Department of Health and Human Services, Food and Drug Administration. Center for Drug Evaluation and Research.

Haller, C.A., Jacob, P. 3rd, & Benowitz, N.L. (2002). Pharmacology of ephedra alkaloids and caffeine after single-dose dietary supplement use. *Clinical Pharmacology and Therapeutics, 71*(6), 421-432.

Jones, W.K. (2000, August 8–9). Safety of dietary supplements containing ephedrine alkaloids. Public meeting on Safety of Ephedrine Alkaloids. Report. U.S. Food and Drug Administration Center for Food Safety and Applied Nutrition.

Kanayama, G., Gruber, A.J., & Pope, H.G. Jr. (2001). Over-the-counter drug use in gymnasiums: An underrecognized substance abuse problem? *Psychotherapy and Psychosomatics, 70*(3), 137-140.

Morgenstern, L.B., Viscoli, C.M., Kernan, W.N., et al. (2003). Use of ephedra-containing products and risk for hemorrhagic stroke. *Neurology, 60*(1), 132-135.

Peterson, E., Stoebner, A., Weatherill, J., et al. (2008). Case of acute psychosis from herbal supplements. *South Dakota Medicine, 61*(5), 173-177.

Rome, E.S. (2001). It's a rave new world: Rave cultures and illicit drug use in the young. *Cleveland Clinic Journal of Medicine, 68*(6), 541-550.

Samenuk, D., Link, M.S., Homoud, M.K., et al. (2002). Adverse cardiovascular events temporally associated with ma huang, an herbal source of ephedrine. *Mayo Clinic Proceedings, 77*(1), 12-16.

Schaneberg, B.T., Crockett, S., Bedir, E., et al. (2003). The role of chemical fingerprinting: Application to ephedra. *Phytochemistry, 62*(6), 911-918.

Secretary Thompson urges strong warning labels for ephedra. (2002, October 8). *FDA News*.

EPHEDRONE (See Methcathinone)

ESTAZOLAM

Names

BAN or INN Generic Synonyms: None

Brand/Trade: ProSom®

Chemical: 8-Chloro-6-phenyl-4H-s-triazolo[4,3-α][1,4]benzodiazepine

Street: None

Pharmacologic Classification

Psychodepressant, sedative-hypnotic: benzodiazepine

Brief General Overview

Estazolam is clinically used in North America for its hypnotic actions. Its abuse is virtually exclusively restricted to people for whom it was medically prescribed. (See the Benzodiazepines monograph.)

Dosage Forms and Routes of Administration

Estazolam is available from licit pharmaceutical manufacturers in the United States. It is produced as an oral tablet formulation that is orally ingested.

Mechanism of CNS Action

The exact mechanism of estazolam's hypnotic action has not been determined. It appears to be mediated by, or to work in concert with, the inhibitory neurotransmitter GABA. Thus, estazolam's action appears to be accomplished by binding to benzodiazepine receptors within the GABA complex. (See also the Benzodiazepines monograph.)

Pharmacodynamics/Pharmacokinetics

Estazolam is well and extensively absorbed after oral ingestion ($F > 0.9$). Peak blood concentrations generally are achieved within 2 hours. Estazolam is ~93% bound to plasma proteins and is widely distributed in body tissues and fluids. It is extensively metabolized in the liver. Estazolam and its metabolites are primarily excreted in the urine. Less than 5% of estazolam is excreted in unchanged form. The mean elimination half-life is ~18 hours (range, 13 to 35 hours).

Current Approved Indications for Medical Use

Insomnia

Desired Action/Reason for Personal Use[1]

Alcohol-like disinhibitory euphoria or "high" (mild); anxiety/stress reduction

Toxicity

Acute: Ataxia; cognitive impairment; constipation; dizziness; drowsiness; dry mouth; fatigue; hypokinesia; memory impairment; pruritus

Chronic: Agranulocytosis (rare); mental depression; physical dependence; psychological dependence

Pregnancy & Lactation: FDA Pregnancy Category X (see Appendix B). Safety of estazolam use by adolescent girls and women who are pregnant has not been established. However, on the basis of animal studies and the teratogenic effects associated with other benzodiazepines, the FDA has contraindicated estazolam use during pregnancy. Adolescent girls and women who are pregnant should not use estazolam.

Safety of estazolam use by adolescent girls and women who are breast-feeding has not been established. Additional valid and reliable data are needed. (Also see the Benzodiazepines monograph.)

Abuse Potential

Physical dependence: Moderate (USDEA Schedule IV; low potential for abuse)
Psychological dependence: Moderate

Withdrawal Syndrome

Short-term or regular, long-term estazolam pharmacotherapy or personal use may result in physical and psychological dependence. Abrupt discontinuation of use may result in an estazolam withdrawal syndrome similar to the withdrawal syndrome associated with other benzodiazepines and to the alcohol withdrawal syndrome. Signs and symptoms may be mild, and include dysphoria and insomnia. They may also be more severe and include abdominal and muscle cramps, convulsions, sweating, tremor, and vomiting. Signs and symptoms may occur after several months of medically recommended dosages when estazolam pharmacotherapy is abruptly discontinued. To avoid withdrawal in these cases, estazolam use should be slowly discontinued, with a gradual reduction in dosage.

Overdosage

Signs and symptoms of estazolam overdosage include confusion, somnolence, coma, and diminished reflexes. Estazolam overdosage requires emergency medical support of body systems, with attention to increasing estazolam elimination. The benzodiazepine antagonist flumazenil (Anexate®, Romazicon®) may be required.[2]

Notes

1. Estazolam has been smuggled into some Asian countries (e.g., China) for illicit use. It also has been used in some European countries (e.g., France) for the perpetration of drug-facilitated sexual assaults.
2. Caution is required because flumazenil antagonism may precipitate the estazolam withdrawal syndrome in people who are physically dependent on estazolam.

Reference

Marc, B., Baudry, F., Vaquero, P., et al. (2000). Sexual assault under benzodiazepine submission in a Paris suburb. *Archives of Gynecology and Obstetrics, 263*, 193-197.

ESZOPICLONE

Names

BAN or INN Generic Synonyms: S-zopiclone; (+) zopiclone

Brand/Trade: Estorra®; Lunesta®

Chemical[1]**:** (+)-(5S)-6-(5-Chloropyridin-2-yl)-7-oxo-6,7-dihydro-5H-pyrrolo[3,4-b]pyrazin-5yl-4-methylpiperazine-1-carboxylate

Street: None

Pharmacologic Classification

Psychodepressant, sedative-hypnotic: miscellaneous (cyclopyrrolone)

Brief General Overview

Eszopiclone is the levorotatory isomer of zopiclone (see monograph) and was approved for use in the United States in 2004.[2] It is a short-acting cyclopyrrolate-derivative hypnotic. Although its chemical structure is unrelated to those of the benzodiazepines, its spectrum of pharmacologic action is virtually identical. It is one of the most frequently prescribed hypnotics in North America. Eszopiclone is personally used for its psychodepressant actions.

Dosage Forms and Routes of Administration

Eszopiclone is produced in North America by licit pharmaceutical manufacturers and is available in oral tablet form. People who use eszopiclone generally ingest the tablets orally.

Mechanism of CNS Action

The exact mechanism of eszopiclone's psychodepressant action has not been determined. However, eszopiclone appears to work in concert with the inhibitory neurotransmitter GABA in a manner very similar to, if not identical to, that of the benzodiazepines (see Benzodiazepines monograph). Binding of eszopiclone (i.e., [+]-zopiclone) to benzodiazepine receptors is approximately 50-fold higher than is the binding of zopiclone (i.e., [±]-zopiclone), and binding to the $GABA_A$ receptor complexes has been reported to be up to 1000 times greater.

Pharmacodynamics/Pharmacokinetics

Eszopiclone is rapidly absorbed following oral ingestion ($T_{max} \cong 1$ hour). The ingestion of food may delay absorption by 1 to 2 hours but does not reduce absorption. Eszopiclone is weakly bound to plasma proteins (i.e., ~55%) and has an apparent volume of distribution of ~90 L. Eszopiclone is extensively metabolized in the liver, primarily by oxidation and demethylation to inactive metabolites (s)-desmethylzopiclone and (N)-oxide–zopiclone.

The metabolism is principally mediated by hepatic microsomal isoenzymes CYP3A4 and CYP2E1. Less than 10% is eliminated in unchanged form in the urine (as racemic zopiclone). The mean elimination half-life of eszopiclone is 6 hours.[3]

Current Approved Indications for Medical Use

Sleep disorders: insomnia (short-term, symptomatic management)

Desired Action/Reason for Personal Use

Alcohol-like disinhibitory euphoria or "high"[4]

Toxicity

Acute: Cognitive impairment; dizziness; dry mouth; dysmenorrhea; headache; somnolence; unpleasant taste; unusual dreams

Chronic: Mental depression; physical dependence; psychological dependence

Pregnancy & Lactation: FDA Pregnancy Category C (see Appendix B). Safety of eszopiclone use by adolescent girls and women who are pregnant has not been established. Caution is warranted because of its pharmacologic similarity to the benzodiazepines (see Benzodiazepines monograph). Additional valid and reliable data are needed.

Safety of eszopiclone use by adolescent girls and women who are breast-feeding has not been established. However, its racemic form (i.e., zopiclone, see monograph) is excreted in significant concentrations in breast milk. Additional valid and reliable data are needed.

Abuse Potential

Physical dependence: Low (USDEA Schedule IV; low potential for abuse)
Psychological dependence: Low to moderate

Withdrawal Syndrome

An eszopiclone withdrawal syndrome, similar to the withdrawal syndrome associated with alcohol and the benzodiazepines, has been observed upon abrupt discontinuation of regular, long-term eszopiclone pharmacotherapy or regular long-term personal use. This syndrome is characterized by agitation, anxiety, confusion, delirium, hallucinations, headache, irritability, nightmares, palpitations, rebound insomnia, seizures (rare), tachycardia, and tremor. Regular, long-term use of eszopiclone should be gradually discontinued in order to avoid the occurrence of this syndrome.

Overdosage

Eszopiclone overdosage is generally not life threatening when the overdosage solely involves eszopiclone. Signs and symptoms of overdosage include ataxia, coma,[5] hypotension, hypoxia, lethargy, and respiratory depression. Eszopiclone overdosage requires emergency medical support of body systems, with attention to maintaining cardiac and respiratory function. The benzodiazepine antagonist flumazenil (Anexate®; Romazicon®) may be of some assistance.[6]

Notes

1. A mixed (i.e., racemic) formulation of eszopiclone (i.e., zopiclone, see monograph) also is available.
2. It has been approved for use in Europe since 1992.
3. The mean elimination half-life is generally increased in the elderly to 9 hours.
4. Reportedly, very similar to that experienced with diazepam (see monograph).
5. Coma may be prolonged for up to 48 hours.
6. Caution is required because flumazenil antagonism may precipitate the eszopiclone withdrawal syndrome in people who are physically dependent on eszopiclone.

References

Boyle, J., Trick, L., Johnsen, S., et al. (2008). Next-day cognition, psychomotor function, and driving-related skills following nighttime administration of eszopiclone. *Human Psychopharmacology, 23*(5), 385-397.

Eszopiclone: Esopiclone, estorra, S-zopiclone, zopiclone—Sepracor. (2005). *Drugs R D, 6*(2), 111-115.

Eszopiclone (Lunesta), a new hypnotic. (2005). *The Medical Letter on Drugs and Therapeutics, 47*(1203), 17-19.

Forrester, M.B. (2007). Eszopiclone ingestions reported to Texas poison control centers, 2005–2006. *Human & Experimental Toxicology, 26*(10), 795-800.

Griffiths, R.R., & Johnson, M.W. (2005). Relative abuse liability of hypnotic drugs: A conceptual framework and algorithm for differentiating among compounds. *Journal of Clinical Psychiatry, 66* (Supplement 9), 31-41.

Hales, C.J. (2006). Eszopiclone. *American Journal of Health-System Pharmacy, 63*(1), 41-48.

Jaffe, J.H., Bloor, R., Crome, I., et al. (2004). A postmarketing study of relative abuse liability of hypnotic sedative drugs. *Addiction, 99*(2), 165-173.

Krystal, A.D., Walsh, J.K., Laska, E., et al. (2003). Sustained efficacy of eszopiclone over 6 months of nightly treatment: Results of a randomized, double-blind, placebo-controlled study in adults with chronic insomnia. *Sleep, 26*(7), 793-799.

McCall, W.V., Erman, M., Krystal, A.D., et al. (2006). A polysomnography study of eszopiclone in elderly patients with insomnia. *Current Medical Research and Opinion, 22*(9), 1633-1642.

McCrae, C.S., Ross, A., Stripling, A., et al. (2007). Eszopiclone for late-life insomnia. *Clinical Interventions in Aging, 2*(3), 313-326.

Melton, S.T., Wood, J.M., & Kirkwood, C.K. (2005). Eszopiclone for insomnia. *The Annals of Pharmacotherapy, 39*(10), 1659-1666.

Najib, J. (2006). Eszopiclone, a nonbenzodiazepine sedative-hypnotic agent for the treatment of transient and chronic insomnia. *Clinical Therapeutics, 28*(4), 491-516.

Roth, T., Walsh, J.K., Krystal, A., et al. (2005). An evaluation of the efficacy and safety of eszopiclone over 12 months in patients with chronic primary insomnia. *Sleep Medicine, 6*(6), 487-495.

Scharf, M. (2006). Eszopiclone in the treatment of insomnia. *Expert Opinion on Pharmacotherapy, 7*(3), 345-356.

Scharf, M., Erman, M., Rosenburg, R., et al. (2005). A 2-week efficacy and safety study of eszopiclone in elderly patients with primary insomnia. *Sleep, 28*(6), 720-727.

Walsh, J.K., Krystal, A.D., Amato, D.A., et al. (2007). Nightly treatment of primary insomnia with eszopiclone for six months: Effect on sleep, quality of life, and work limitations. *Sleep, 30*(8), 959-968.

Zammit, G.K., McNabb, L.J., Caron, J., et al. (2004). Efficacy and safety of eszopiclone across 6 weeks of treatment for primary insomnia. *Current Medical Research and Opinion, 20*(12), 1979-1991.

ETHANOL (See Alcohol)

ETHCHLORVYNOL

Names

BAN or INN Generic Synonyms: None

Brand/Trade: Placidyl®[1]

Chemical: 1-Chloro-3-ethyl-1-penten-4-yn-3-ol; ethyl-2-chlorovinyl ethinyl carbinol

Street: Dyls; Mickies; Plastivil; Zonker

Pharmacologic Classification

Psychodepressant, sedative-hypnotic: miscellaneous (carbinol derivative)

Brief General Overview

Ethchlorvynol was introduced in the middle of the 20th century as a safe and reliable sedative-hypnotic alternative to the barbiturates. However, it proved to be very similar to the barbiturates in terms of abuse potential and toxicity, particularly in relation to overdosage causing death. Its clinical use has been completely replaced by the equally efficacious, but much safer, benzodiazepines[2]. So too, over the past 20 years, the personal use of ethchlorvynol for its psychodepressant actions has steadily decreased.

Dosage Forms and Routes of Administration

Ethchlorvynol is available in North America from illicit foreign pharmaceutical manufacturers. It is produced in oral capsules that are orally ingested.

Mechanism of CNS Action

The exact mechanism of action of ethchlorvynol has not been determined.

Pharmacodynamics/Pharmacokinetics

Ethchlorvynol has a rapid onset of action that is short in duration. It has adequate bioavailability after oral ingestion and produces sleep within 15 to 60 minutes. Peak blood concentrations are achieved within 1 to 1.5 hours. Ethchlorvynol is 35% to 50% bound to plasma proteins and has an apparent volume of distribution of 3 to 4 L/kg. Ethchlorvynol is metabolized in the liver. Both ethchlorvynol and its metabolites undergo extensive enterohepatic recirculation. Its elimination half-life ranges from 10 to 32 hours.

Current Approved Indications for Medical Use

None[3]

Desired Action/Reason for Personal Use

Alcohol-like disinhibitory euphoria or "high"; anxiety/stress reduction

Toxicity

Acute: Blurred vision; cognitive impairment; dizziness; headache; hives; nausea; vomiting[4]

Chronic: Physical dependence; psychological dependence

Pregnancy & Lactation: FDA Pregnancy Category C (see Appendix B). Safety of ethchlorvynol use by adolescent girls and women who are pregnant has not been established. Cases have been reported in the literature of the occurrence of a neonatal ethchlorvynol withdrawal syndrome in neonates whose mothers used ethchlorvynol during the last trimester of pregnancy. Adolescent girls and women who are pregnant should not use ethchlorvynol.

Safety of the use of ethchlorvynol by adolescent girls and women who are breast-feeding has not been established. Additional valid and reliable data are needed.

Abuse Potential

Physical dependence: Moderate (USDEA Schedule, formerly IV; low potential for abuse)
Psychological dependence: Moderate

Withdrawal Syndrome

Regular, long-term ethchlorvynol use may result in physical and psychological dependence and should be avoided. Abrupt discontinuation of regular, long-term use may result in an ethchlorvynol withdrawal syndrome, characterized by signs and symptoms similar to those associated with the alcohol withdrawal syndrome. Abrupt discontinuation of ethchlorvynol use at dosages as low as 1000 mg daily has been associated with a severe withdrawal syndrome that includes delirium and seizures. Regular, long-term ethchlorvynol use should be slowly discontinued, with a gradual reduction in dosage.

Overdosage

Signs and symptoms of ethchlorvynol overdosage include sedation and coma. Some patients have recovered from overdosages involving ethchlorvynol after coma lasting approximately 1 week. Although fatal blood concentrations are usually in the range of 20 to 50 mcg/mL, blood concentrations of approximately 14 mcg/mL (i.e., 10 times the maximal concentration achieved after ingestion of 1000 mg) have been fatal. Because ethchlorvynol overdosage has often proved fatal, all cases of overdosage require emergency medical support and careful monitoring of body systems, with attention to increasing ethchlorvynol elimination. There is no known antidote.

Notes

1. Formerly a popular brand name for ethchlorvynol capsules produced in North America.
2. Ethchlorvynol is no longer available for clinical use in North America.
3. Formerly, ethchlorvynol was medically prescribed for the short-term (i.e., up to 1 week) management of insomnia.
4. Ethchlorvynol has a pungent, pear-like odor.

Reference

Pagliaro, L.A., & Pagliaro, A.M. (2004). *Pagliaros' comprehensive guide to drugs and substances of abuse.* Washington, DC: American Pharmacists Association.

FENTANYL

Names

BAN or INN Generic Synonyms: None

Brand/Trade: Actiq®; Duragesic®; Fentanyl Ora-Vescent®; Fentora®; ratio-Fentanyl®; Sublimaze®

Chemical: N-Phenyl-N-(1-(2-phenylethyl)-4-piperidinyl) propanamide

Street: Apache; Bear; China Girl; China Town; China White; Dance Fever; Fen; Friend; Goodfella; Great Bear; He-Man; Jackpot; King Ivory; Lollipop; Murder; Murder 8; Perc-O-Pop; Persian White; Poison; Synthetic Heroin; Tango & Cash; TNT

Pharmacologic Classification

Psychodepressant, opiate analgesic: pure agonist (synthetic)

Brief General Overview

Fentanyl is a potent opiate analgesic (i.e., for intravenous doses, 0.1 mg fentanyl provides equivalent analgesia to ~10 mg of morphine). It was developed as an intravenous anesthetic and was introduced to North America in the 1960s under the trade name of Sublimaze®. Several chemical analogues of fentanyl have been developed for clinical use, including alfentanil (Alfenta®; see monograph), carfentanil (Wildnil®), remifentanil (Ultiva®), and sufentanil (Sufenta®). Fentanyl is personally used for its analgesic and other psychodepressant actions.

Dosage Forms and Routes of Administration

Fentanyl is available in four dosage formulations from licit pharmaceutical manufacturers: (1) an injectable formulation for intramuscular or intravenous use, (2) a transdermal delivery system for continuous drug delivery over a period of 72 hours (i.e., Duragesic®),[1] (3) a transmucosal lozenge for buccal absorption, Fentanyl "lollipops" (i.e., Actiq®), and (4) an effervescent buccal tablet (i.e., Fentora®) that uses the OraVescent® drug delivery system. In addition, illicitly manufactured nonpharmaceutical fentanyl (NPF) is available "on the streets" of several states, including Delaware, Illinois, Maryland, Michigan, Missouri, New Jersey, Pennsylvania, and Virginia.

Actiq®, the "fentanyl lollipop," is formulated as a solid drug matrix on a handle that facilitates easy removal from the mouth should signs and symptoms of excessive opiate analgesic action occur during use. Reported cases of both personal use and overdosage have increasingly involved the Duragesic® transdermal delivery system (i.e., the fentanyl patch).[2] The fentanyl transdermal delivery system provides a specific dosage at a constant rate. However, even after the prescribed application time has elapsed, enough fentanyl remains within a patch to provide a potentially lethal dose.

Personal use of fentanyl occurs among health care providers (who use all dosage forms) because of its relative accessibility to them in the work setting. Increasingly, other users have found discarded fentanyl transdermal delivery systems, or patches, to be a ready source of supply and have used them transdermally and in a variety of unapproved ways. These methods of use include (1) oral transmucosal use, in which the transdermal fentanyl delivery system is simply held in the mouth and chewed, releasing the fentanyl into the mouth where it is buccally absorbed,[3] (2) intravenous injection of the fentanyl extracted from the transdermal patch, (3) volatilization and inhalation of the patch contents, and (4) oral ingestion of the patch (i.e., in some cases, the patch is just swallowed).

Mechanism of CNS Action

Fentanyl, as an opiate analgesic, has actions similar to those of morphine and meperidine. However, it is much more potent. A 100 mcg dose of fentanyl is approximately equivalent in analgesic action to 10 mg of morphine or 75 mg of meperidine. Fentanyl elicits its analgesic, psychodepressant, and respiratory depressant actions primarily by binding to the endorphin mu receptors in the CNS. The exact mechanism of action has not been determined. (See the Opiate Analgesics monograph.)

Pharmacodynamics/Pharmacokinetics

Fentanyl's onset of action is virtually immediate after intravenous injection. However, its maximal analgesic and respiratory depressant actions may not occur for several minutes. The usual duration of analgesia is 30 to 60 minutes after a single intravenous dose of up to 100 mcg. After intramuscular injection, onset of action is in 7 to 8 minutes and duration of action is 1 to 2 hours. Fentanyl is ~85% plasma protein bound. Its mean apparent volume of distribution is ~4 L/kg. It is extensively metabolized in the liver, primarily by N-dealkylation to norfentanyl and other inactive metabolites. Less than 10% is excreted in unchanged form in the urine. The mean elimination half-life is ~7 hours (range, 3 to 12 hours).[4] The mean total body clearance is ~1 L/minute. Impairment of fentanyl's hepatic metabolism occurs in people who are homozygous for cytochrome P450 3A5*3 variant. This impairment places these individuals at higher risk for toxicity and overdosage.

Current Approved Indications for Medical Use

Adjunct to anesthesia; pain, severe

Desired Action/Reason for Personal Use

Euphoria; prevention/self-management of the opiate analgesic withdrawal syndrome

Toxicity

Acute: Abdominal pain; amblyopia; anorexia; apnea; asthenia; bradycardia; bronchoconstriction; cognitive impairment; confusion; constipation; diarrhea; dizziness; dry mouth; fatigue; hallucinations; headache; hypotension; laryngospasm; memory impairment; mental depression; miosis; muscle weakness; nausea; orthostatic hypotension; pruritus; psychomotor impairment; respiratory depression; sexual dysfunction; skeletal muscle rigidity; somnolence; sweating, excessive; syncope, postural; urinary retention; vomiting. In addition, acute local effects may occur at the application site of the fentanyl transdermal delivery system, including blisters, irritation, pruritus (itching), skin redness, and swelling.

Chronic: Physical dependence; psychological dependence

Pregnancy & Lactation: FDA Pregnancy Category C (see Appendix B). Safety of fentanyl use by adolescent girls and women who are pregnant has not been established. Fentanyl can cross the placental barrier, and use during labor or delivery may result in neonatal respiratory depression. Fentanyl should not be used by adolescent girls and women who are pregnant.

Safety of fentanyl use by adolescent girls and women who are breast-feeding has not been established. Fentanyl is excreted in breast milk. Pharmacologic effects (e.g., drowsiness, lethargy) may be expected in breast-fed neonate and infants, who also may become physically dependent. Adolescent girls and women who are breast-feeding should not use fentanyl.

Abuse Potential

Physical dependence: High (USDEA Schedule II; high potential for abuse)
Psychological dependence: High

Withdrawal Syndrome

Regular, long-term personal use of fentanyl is associated with both physical and psychological dependence. Abrupt discontinuation of use may result in the opiate analgesic withdrawal syndrome.[5] Signs and symptoms of this syndrome include abdominal pain, anorexia, body aches, chills, diarrhea, difficulty sleeping, fever, nervousness, piloerection (gooseflesh), restlessness, rhinitis, shivering, sneezing, stomach cramps, sweating (excessive), tachycardia, tremors, weakness, and yawning. The opiate analgesic withdrawal syndrome is not usually life threatening, and signs and symptoms can be generally managed with or without medical support (i.e., regular, long-term fentanyl and other opiate analgesic users have managed withdrawal without medical assistance). Gradual discontinuation of regular, long-term personal use may help to prevent or minimize the signs and symptoms of withdrawal.

Overdosage

Fentanyl, because it is a potent opiate analgesic (i.e., 30 to 50 times more potent than heroin), is associated with many fatal overdosages. Signs and symptoms of fentanyl overdosage are variable but are generally extensions of its CNS and respiratory depressant actions, and include coma, confusion, difficulty breathing, dizziness, and miosis (pinpoint pupils). Fentanyl overdosage requires emergency medical support of body systems, with attention to increasing fentanyl elimination. The opiate antagonist naloxone (Narcan®) is usually required to manage the severe respiratory depression associated with fentanyl overdosage.[6] The duration of respiratory depression may be longer than the duration of action of the opiate analgesic antagonist, and repeated administration of naloxone over the recovery period may be required.

Notes

1. Fentanyl transdermal delivery systems (i.e., patches) are designed to precisely deliver a specific and constant amount of fentanyl across the skin layers to the systemic circulation. Each fentanyl patch is formulated to deliver a specific amount of fentanyl, ranging from 12 mcg to 100 mcg per hour (i.e., 0.3 mg to 2.4 mg per 24 hours).

2. Some regular, long-term users of fentanyl or other opiate analgesics (i.e., street addicts) dissolve the fentanyl remaining in discarded patches and intravenously inject the resultant solution. When new, unused patches are available, users often heat the patch and simply inhale the fentanyl vapors. This creative means of overcoming the rate-limited delivery of fentanyl inherent in the transdermal delivery system allows users to rapidly achieve significant fentanyl blood concentrations and associated desired effects.

3. In some cases, users freeze the patch, cut it into pieces, and then place the pieces in the cheek pocket or under the tongue, where the fentanyl can be buccally or sublingually absorbed.

4. The mean half-life of elimination may appear longer (i.e., ~17 hours) in people who use the fentanyl transdermal delivery system because fentanyl may continue to be absorbed from the application site after the system has been removed, because of drug residue left in or on the skin.

5. A fentanyl opiate analgesic withdrawal syndrome has been documented both in intensive care patients whose fentanyl pharmacotherapy was abruptly discontinued and in other patients whose fentanyl transdermal delivery system was abruptly discontinued.

6. Particular caution is indicated because naloxone may precipitate the opiate analgesic withdrawal syndrome in people who are physically dependent on fentanyl.

References

Anderson, D.T., & Muto, J.J. (2000). Duragesic transdermal patch: Postmortem tissue distribution of fentanyl in 25 cases. *Journal of Analytical Toxicology, 24*(7), 627-634.

Baylon, G.J., Kaplan, H.L., Somer, G., et al. (2000). Comparative abuse liability of intravenously administered remifentanil and fentanyl. *Journal of Clinical Psychopharmacology, 20*(6), 597-606.

Centers for Disease Control. (2008). Nonpharmaceutical fentanyl-related deaths multiple states, April 2005-March 2007. *Morbidity and Mortality Weekly Reports (MMWR), 57*(29), 793-796.

Han, P.K., Arnold, R., Bond, G., et al. (2002). Myoclonus secondary to withdrawal from transdermal fentanyl: Case report and literature review. *Journal of Pain and Symptom Management, 23*(1), 66-72.

Inturrisi, C.E. (2002). Clinical pharmacology of opioids for pain. *The Clinical Journal of Pain, 18*(4 Suppl), S3-S13.

Jin, M., Gock, S.B., Jannetto, P.J., et al. (2005). Pharmacogenomics as molecular autopsy for forensic toxicology: Genotyping cytochrome P450 3A4*1B and 3A5*3 for 25 fentanyl cases. *Journal of Analytical Toxicology, 29*(7), 590-598.

Kuhlman, J.J. Jr., McCaulley, R, Valouch, T.J., et al. (2003). Fentanyl use, misuse, and abuse: A summary of 23 postmortem cases. *Journal of Analytical Toxicology, 27*(7), 499-504.

Lilleng, P.K., Mehlum, L.I., Bachs, L., et al. (2004). Deaths after intravenous misuse of transdermal fentanyl. *Journal of Forensic Sciences, 49*(6), 1364-1366.

Lugo, R.A., MacLaren, R., Cash, J., et al. (2001). Enteral methadone to expedite fentanyl discontinuation and prevent opioid abstinence syndrome in the PICU. *Pharmacotherapy, 21*(12), 1566-1573.

Martin, T.L., Woodall, K.L., & McLellan, B.A. (2006). Fentanyl-related deaths in Ontario, Canada: Toxicology findings and circumstances of death in 112 cases (2002-2004). *Journal of Analytical Toxicology, 30*(8), 603-610.

Messina, J., Darwish, M., & Fine, P.G. (2008). Fentanyl buccal tablet. *Drugs Today, 44*(1), 41-54.

Schumann, H., Erickson, T., Thompson, T.M., et al. (2008). Fentanyl epidemic in Chicago, Illinois and surrounding Cook County. *Clinical Toxicology, 46*(6), 501-506.

Teske, J., Weller, J.P., Larsch, K., et al. (2007). Fatal outcome in a child after ingestion of a transdermal fentanyl patch. *International Journal of Legal Medicine, 121*(2), 147-151.

Tharp, A.M., Winecker, R.E., & Winston, D.C. (2004). Fatal intravenous fentanyl abuse: Four cases involving extraction of fentanyl from transdermal patches. *The American Journal of Forensic Medicine and Pathology, 25*(2), 178-181.

Thomas, S., Winecker, R., & Pestaner, J.P. (2008). Unusual fentanyl patch administration. *The American Journal of Forensic Medicine and Pathology, 29*(2), 162-163.

Thompson, J.G., Baker, A.M., Bracey, A.H., et al. (2007). Fentanyl concentrations in 23 postmortem cases from the Hennepin County Medical Examiner's Office. *Journal of Forensic Sciences, 52*(4), 978-981.

Woodall, K.L., Martin, T.L., & McLellan, B.A. (2008). Oral abuse of fentanyl patches (Duragesic): Seven case reports. *Journal of Forensic Sciences, 53*(1), 222-225.

Yassen, A., Olofsen, E., Romberg, R., et al. (2007). Mechanism-based PK/PD modeling of the respiratory depressant effect of buprenorphine and fentanyl in healthy volunteers. *Clinical Pharmacology & Therapeutics, 81*(1), 50-58.

FLUNITRAZEPAM

Names

BAN or INN Generic Synonyms: None

Brand/Trade: None[1]

Chemical: 5-(o-Fluorophenyl)-1,3-dihydro-l-methyl-7-nitro-2H-1,4-benzodiazepin-2-one

Street: 542s; Circles; Date Rape Drug; *Dulcitas*; Forget Me Drug; Forget Me Pill; Forget Pill; *La Rocha*; La Roche; Lunch Money Drug; Mexican Valium; Mind Eraser; *Papas*[2]; *Pappas*; Pingas; Pingus; R-2; R-25; Reynolds; Rib; Rick James Biatch; Ro; Roach-2; Roacha; Roaches; Roachies; Roapies; Robutal; *Rochas Dos*; Roche; *Roche Das*; Roofies; Roofinol; Roopies; Rope; Rophies; Rophy; Ropies; Roples; Row-Shay; Ruffies; Ruffles; Trip and Fall; Wolfies

Pharmacologic Classification

Psychodepressant, sedative-hypnotic: benzodiazepine

Brief General Overview

Flunitrazepam is a potent benzodiazepine sedative-hypnotic that has gained wide notoriety as a popular party drug. It has commonly been used to perpetrate sexual assaults (see later discussion) and is widely known "on the street" as a date-rape drug (see also the Gamma-hydroxybutyrate [GHB] monograph). Although it is illicitly available throughout North America, the availability and use of flunitrazepam currently is particularly prevalent across the entire southern United States, from California to Florida.

Dosage Forms and Routes of Administration

Flunitrazepam is licitly produced by pharmaceutical manufacturers in over 70 countries (primarily for the treatment of insomnia) and is smuggled into the United States, particularly from Mexico and South America. It is generally available in its original blister packs of tablets and is orally ingested.[3] Flunitrazepam is primarily used by adolescent boys, often in combination with beer and cannabis, and by young adults of European and Hispanic descent who use flunitrazepam primarily at bars, nightclubs, and raves. If used to perpetrate a date rape, the tablet is secretly dissolved in the victim's alcoholic drink.[4] Of concern is the increased use of flunitrazepam by sexually active adolescent girls and young women who use it in combination with alcohol and other drugs and substances of abuse, particularly the psychodelics, in order to decrease inhibitions and enhance sexual experiences. A significant number of these adolescent girls and young women have reportedly been physically or sexually assaulted while under the influence of flunitrazepam.[5]

Mechanism of CNS Action

See the Benzodiazepines monograph.

Pharmacodynamics/Pharmacokinetics

The psychodepressant action of flunitrazepam generally begins within 30 minutes after oral ingestion, peaks within 2 hours, and may persist for up to 8 hours. Additional valid and reliable data are not available.

Current Approved Indications for Medical Use

None[6]

Desired Action/Reason for Personal Use

Alcohol-like disinhibitory euphoria or "high"; disinhibition (e.g., increase or enhance sexual experiences in association with decreased inhibitions); feelings of power (higher dosages); reduce feelings of fear and insecurity (higher dosages); also, purposely administered to others without their knowledge in the context of the perpetration of a drug-facilitated crime (e.g., robbery; sexual assault, including date rape).[7]

Toxicity

Acute: Aggressive and violent behavior (similar to that associated with alcohol), particularly when combined with alcohol; ataxia; cognitive impairment; confusion; dizziness; drowsiness; GI upset; headache; hypotension; impulsive decision making; increased risk-taking behavior; loss of consciousness; memory impairment (anterograde amnesia); nightmares; psychomotor impairment; respiratory depression; sedation; slurred speech; urinary retention; visual impairment

Chronic: Learning impairment; physical dependence; psychological dependence

Pregnancy & Lactation: Valid and reliable data are not available. (See the Benzodiazepines monograph.)

Abuse Potential

Physical dependence: Moderate (USDEA Schedule IV; low abuse potential)[8]
Psychological dependence: Moderate

Withdrawal Syndrome

A specific flunitrazepam withdrawal syndrome has been reported. Signs and symptoms include anxiety, confusion, headache, hypertension, insomnia, irritability, muscle pain, restlessness, and tremor. In more severe cases, cardiovascular collapse, delirium, hallucinations, seizures (including status epilepticus), and shock may occur. Withdrawal-related seizures may occur a week or more after the discontinuation of regular, long-term flunitrazepam use. To prevent or minimize the occurrence of withdrawal, the flunitrazepam dosage should be gradually reduced to zero over 1 or 2 weeks. Alternatively, the flunitrazepam dosage can be replaced with a long-acting benzodiazepine, such as diazepam (Valium®), and the dosage gradually reduced to zero over a few weeks.

Overdosage

Several hundred deaths have been reported in association with overdosage of flunitrazepam alone—and over a thousand deaths with flunitrazepam overdosage in combination with other drugs and substances of abuse, particularly alcohol. Severe, acute overdosage requires emergency medical support, with attention to increasing the elimination of flunitrazepam. Although available clinical data are limited, the use of the benzodiazepine antagonist flumazenil (Anexate®, Romazicon®) should be attempted.[9]

Notes

1. Flunitrazepam is legally available in over 70 countries worldwide. A common brand name in these countries is Rohypnol®.
2. *Papas* is Spanish for potatoes. This term is used pejoratively by Hispanic American youth, but it aptly describes the mental capabilities of someone who has ingested a sufficient dose of flunitrazepam.
3. The tablet also is commonly crushed and intranasally sniffed (snorted), often in combination with heroin.
4. Flunitrazepam readily dissolves in alcohol, and once in solution is colorless, odorless, and tasteless. The European and Latin American manufacturer of Rohypnol® (Hoffmann-La Roche) recently reformulated the tablets with a dye that will discolor beverages if a tablet is slipped into a drink.
5. Flunitrazepam is one of the most commonly used date-rape or "predatory" drugs. During the 1990s, its use to facilitate the perpetration of sexual assault by adolescent boys and young men increased significantly. Flunitrazepam is a potent benzodiazepine with a relatively rapid onset of action that is accompanied by significant anterograde amnesia. The product package insert reads, "Some patients may have no recollection of any awakenings occurring during the 6 to 8 hours the drug exerts its actions." Thus, not only is sexual assault facilitated by the use of flunitrazepam, but prosecution of these drug-facilitated rapes is extremely difficult because the victim usually has no memory of the event (or memory is insufficiently clear to provide reliable evidence).
6. Flunitrazepam is widely available in other countries (e.g., United Kingdom), primarily for the symptomatic management of insomnia.
7. The sedative-hypnotic action of flunitrazepam generally begins approximately 15 minutes after ingestion and lasts for approximately 4 to 6 hours. Anterograde amnesia during this period is usually significant. These pharmacologic actions of flunitrazepam contribute to its use as a date-rape drug.
8. Several states, including Florida, Idaho, Minnesota, New Hampshire, New Mexico, North Dakota, Oklahoma, and Pennsylvania, have rescheduled flunitrazepam to Schedule I (use is prohibited).
9. Particular caution is required because flumazenil antagonism may precipitate the flunitrazepam withdrawal syndrome in people who are physically dependent on flunitrazepam.

References

Bechtel, L.K., & Holstege, C.P. (2007). Criminal poisoning: Drug-facilitated sexual assault. *Emergency Medicine Clinics of North America, 25*(2), 499-525.

Beynon, C.M., McVeigh, C., McVeigh, J., et al. (2008). The involvement of drugs and alcohol in drug-facilitated sexual assault: A systematic review of the evidence. *Trauma, Violence, & Abuse, 9*(3), 178-188.

Daderman, A.M., & Edman, G. (2001). Flunitrazepam abuse and personality characteristics in male forensic psychiatric patients. *Psychiatric Research, 103*(1), 27-42.

Daderman, A.M., Fredriksson, B., Kristiansson, M., et al. (2002). Violent behavior, impulsive decision-making, and anterograde amnesia while intoxicated with flunitrazepam and alcohol or other drugs: A case study in forensic psychiatric patients. *Journal of the American Academy of Psychiatry and Law, 30*(2), 238-251.

Diehl, J.L., Guillibert, E., Guerot, E., et al. (2000). Acute benzodiazepine withdrawal delirium after a short course of flunitrazepam in an intensive care patient. *Annales de Medicine Interne (Paris), 151*(Suppl A), A44-A46.

Dowd, S.M., Strong, M.J., Janicak, P.G., et al. (2002). The behavioral and cognitive effects of two benzodiazepines associated with drug-facilitated sexual assault. *Journal of Forensic Sciences, 47*(5), 1101-1107.

Druid, H., Holmgren, P., & Ahlner, J. (2001). Flunitrazepam: An evaluation of use, abuse and toxicity. *Forensic Science International, 122*(2-3), 136-141.

ElSohly, M.A. (2001). Drug-facilitated sexual assault. *Southern Medical Journal, 94*(6), 655-656.

Fitzgerald, N., & Riley, K.J. (2000, April). Drug-facilitated rape: Looking for the missing pieces. *National Institute of Justice Journal*, 8-15.

Forrester, M.B. (2006). Flunitrazepam abuse and malicious use in Texas, 1998-2003. *Substance Use & Misuse, 41*(3), 297-306.

Gatzonis, S.D., Angelopoulos, E.K., Daskalopoulou, E.G., et al. (2000). Convulsive status epilepticus following abrupt high-dose benzodiazepine discontinuation. *Drug and Alcohol Dependence, 59*(1), 95-97.

Lane, S.D., Cherek, D.R., & Nouvion, S.O. (2008). Modulation of human risky decision making by flunitrazepam. *Psychopharmacology, 196*(2), 177-188.

Mintzer, M.Z., & Griffiths, R.R. (2005). An abuse liability comparison of flunitrazepam and triazolam in sedative drug abusers. *Behavioural Pharmacology, 16*(7), 579-584.

Smith, K.M., Larive, L.L., & Romanelli, F. (2002). Club drugs: Methylenedioxymethamphetamine, flunitrazepam, ketamine hydrochloride, and gamma-hydroxybutyrate. *American Journal of Health-System Pharmacy, 59*(11), 1067-1076.

FLURAZEPAM

Names

BAN or INN Generic Synonyms: None

Brand/Trade: Dalmane®; Somnol®

Chemical: 7-Chloro-1-[2-(diethylamino)ethyl]-5-(o-fluorophenyl)-1,3-dihydro-2H-1,4 benzodiazepin-2-one

Street: None

Pharmacologic Classification

Psychodepressant, sedative-hypnotic: benzodiazepine

Brief General Overview

Flurazepam is a benzodiazepine that was widely used by North Americans particularly during the 1970s, 1980s, and 1990s. It continues to be personally used for its psychodepressant actions.

Dosage Forms and Routes of Administration

Flurazepam is available in oral capsules from licit pharmaceutical manufacturers in North America. Oral ingestion is the major method of use for the typical users: women for whom flurazepam was initially medically prescribed but who use increasingly higher dosages and for longer periods of time than recommended.

Mechanism of CNS Action

The exact mechanism of action of flurazepam has not been determined. However, flurazepam appears to act through, or work in concert with, the inhibitory neurotransmitter GABA. This action appears to be accomplished by binding to benzodiazepine receptors within the GABA complex. (See the Benzodiazepines monograph.)

Pharmacodynamics/Pharmacokinetics

Flurazepam is rapidly absorbed after oral ingestion. Initially, it undergoes rapid and pronounced metabolism to two pharmacologically active metabolites, flurazepam aldehyde and hydroxyethylflurazepam. Peak plasma concentrations of these two metabolites are achieved within 60 minutes after a single oral dose. The metabolites are highly plasma protein bound (~97%) and have a mean apparent volume of distribution of 22 L/kg. They are rapidly further metabolized in the liver and are excreted primarily in the urine, with less than 1% in unchanged form. The mean elimination half-life of these metabolites is ~2 hours.

Flurazepam appears to be increasingly effective on the second and third nights of consecutive use because of the formulation and accumulation of active metabolites, including the final active and principal metabolite, desalkylflurazepam. Desalkylflurazepam has a mean elimination half-life of 75 hours (range, 50 to 100 hours). Thus, after discontinuation of flurazepam use, both sleep latency and total wake time may continue to be decreased for one or two nights.

Current Approved Indications for Medical Use

Sleep disorders: Insomnia (short-term use)

Desired Action/Reason for Personal Use

Alcohol-like disinhibitory euphoria or "high"

Toxicity

Acute: Abnormal thinking (rare); ataxia; blurred vision; cognitive impairment; confusion;

daytime sedation; disorientation; dizziness; drowsiness; fall-related injuries and hospitalizations; flushing; headache; heartburn; hypotension; lethargy; lightheadedness; pruritus; psychomotor impairment; psychosis (rare); syncope; vomiting; weakness

Chronic: Mental depression; physical dependence; psychological dependence; reduction in number of functional synaptic GABA$_A$ receptors

Pregnancy & Lactation: FDA Pregnancy Category "not established." Safety of flurazepam use by adolescent girls and women who are pregnant has not been established. However, flurazepam crosses the placenta and depression has been reported in neonates of women who used flurazepam during the last trimester of pregnancy. A neonate whose mother received 30 mg of flurazepam every evening for 10 days prior to delivery appeared hypotonic and inactive during the first 4 days of life. Adolescent girls and women who are pregnant should not use flurazepam. Additional valid and reliable data are needed.

Safety of flurazepam use by adolescent girls and women who are breast-feeding has not been established. Flurazepam is excreted in breast milk. Adolescent girls and women who are breast-feeding should not use flurazepam. (See the Benzodiazepines monograph.)

Abuse Potential

Physical dependence: Moderate (USDEA Schedule IV; low potential for abuse)
Psychological dependence: Moderate

Withdrawal Syndrome

A specific flurazepam withdrawal syndrome has been reported. It is generally transient and includes anxiety and insomnia.

Overdosage

Signs and symptoms of flurazepam overdosage include confusion, disorientation, lethargy, severe sedation or somnolence, and coma. Flurazepam overdosage requires emergency medical support, with attention to increasing flurazepam elimination. The benzodiazepine antagonist flumazenil (Anexate®, Romazicon®) may be required.

Reference

Martello, S. Oliva, A., De Giorgio, F., et al. (2006). Acute flurazepam intoxication: A case report. *The American Journal of Forensic Medicine and Pathology, 27*(1), 55-57.

FREON

Names
BAN or INN Generic Synonyms: Chlorodifluoromethane

Brand/Trade: None[1]

Chemical: Monochlorodifluoromethane

Street: FC22; Gas

Pharmacologic Classification
Psychodepressant, volatile solvents & inhalants: inhalant gas (chlorofluorocarbon)

Brief General Overview
Freon (fluorinated carbons)[2] was previously one of the most frequently abused volatile inhalants in North America and was commonly found as a propellant in the pressurized aerosol cans of several common household products (e.g., computer dust removal spray, hair spray, spray paints, room air fresheners or deodorizers) and in fire extinguishers during the latter half of the 20th century. However, the commercial use of freon was largely phased out during the 1990s because of general concerns that it would deplete the ozone layer, and its availability decreased significantly.[3] Freon continues to be used commercially in cooling units, such as air conditioners and refrigerators, and it continues to be abused, particularly by adolescents who personally use it for its psychodepressant actions.

Dosage Forms and Routes of Administration
Freon is available today primarily as a pressurized gas found in refrigerators and air conditioners.[4] Typically, adolescents, generally in a group of three to five friends, disconnect the cooling tube to a building's air conditioning unit and simply inhale the freon gas to "get high." Alternatively, an adolescent, alone or with one other friend, fills a large plastic bag with freon gas from a home air conditioning unit, covers his or her nose and mouth with the open end of the bag, and inhales the freon gas directly from the bag, sometimes placing his or her entire head into the bag. This method of freon use has resulted in death by suffocation that occurs when the adolescent loses consciousness with the bag covering the nose and mouth, thus blocking his or her air supply.

The typical freon user is an adolescent boy of European descent.[5] However, the use of freon by adolescent girls increased significantly during the 1990s, and girls are closing the gender gap in regard to the use of freon and other inhalants. Another change is that during the 1990s, use increased among 20- to 30-year-old men who, as air conditioning repairmen and mechanics, had access to and used freon gas on their job sites.

Mechanism of CNS Action
The exact mechanism of freon's psychodepressant actions has not been determined.

Pharmacodynamics/Pharmacokinetics

Volatilized freon gas is well and rapidly absorbed from the lungs. Following inhalation, psychodepressant actions last for ~15 to 60 minutes. Excretion is primarily pulmonary, with freon being exhaled in the breath. Additional valid and reliable data are not available.

Current Approved Indications for Medical Use

None

Desired Action/Reason for Personal Use

Alcohol-like disinhibitory euphoria or "high"; perceptual distortion

Toxicity[6]

Acute: Airway freezing; cardiac dysrhythmias; cognitive impairment; death from suffocation; dizziness; dysesthesia of the tongue; frostbite injury to the face, mouth, esophagus, and trachea (as a direct effect of inhaling the cold freon gas); headaches; hypoxemia; local contact irritation (dryness and erythema of exposed skin); nausea; pharyngitis; psychomotor impairment; pulmonary edema; shortness of breath; slurred speech; sudden sniffing death (generally due to ventricular fibrillation)

Chronic: Anorexia; ataxia; fatigue; epistaxis; memory impairment; psychological dependence; sores or lesions in the mouth and nose; thirst (persistent); weight loss

Pregnancy & Lactation: Valid and reliable data are not available.

Abuse Potential

Physical dependence: Low (USDEA: not a scheduled drug)
Psychological dependence: Low to moderate

Withdrawal Syndrome

A freon withdrawal syndrome has not been reported. However, tolerance to the desired psychodepressant actions produced by freon reportedly occurs.

Overdosage

Freon overdosage can be fatal. The two most common causes of death are suffocation and sudden sniffing death. Death by suffocation occurs most commonly when a freon user loses consciousness with a plastic bag containing freon covering the nose and mouth. Sudden sniffing death occurs predominantly as a result of freon-induced ventricular fibrillation. In most of these latter cases, death occurs so rapidly that the freon user is dead upon arrival at the hospital. Freon overdosage requires emergency medical care, with particular attention to the cardiovascular and pulmonary systems. An intravenous beta-adrenergic blocker may be required to treat the associated tachydysrhythmias. There is no known antidote.

Notes

1. A nonmedical, commercial brand name is Freon 22® (i.e., Freon 152a [1,1-difluoroethane]; Freon 22 [monochlorodifluoromethane]).
2. Also, including the chlorofluorocarbons (CFCs).
3. Freon has been replaced in most of these applications with propane (also an inhalant gas; see the Volatile Solvents & Inhalants monograph).
4. Freon also has been obtained for the purpose of abuse from automobile air conditioner recharge units.
5. Reported abuse of freon in several southwestern states (e.g., Texas) is equally high for adolescent boys of Hispanic descent.
6. Freon generally has relatively low toxicity, except at higher concentrations (e.g., >100 ppm).

References

Avella, J., Wilson, J.C., & Lehrer, M. (2006). Fatal cardiac arrhythmia after repeated exposure to 1,1-difluoroethane (DFE). *The American Journal of Forensic Medicine and Pathology, 27*(1), 58-60.

Gotelli, M.J., Monserrat, A.J., Lo Balbo, A., et al. (2008). Freon: Accidental ingestion and gastric perforation. *Clinical Toxicology, 46*(4), 325-328.

Hahn, T., Avella, J., & Lehrer, M. (2006). A motor vehicle accident fatality involving the inhalation of 1,1-difluoroethane. *Journal of Analytical Toxicology, 30*(8), 638-642.

Koreeda, A., Yonemitsu, K., Mimasaka, S., et al. (2007). An accidental death due to Freon 22 (mono-chlorodifluoromethane) inhalation in a fishing vessel. *Forensic Science International, 168*(2-3), 208-211.

Kubota, T., & Miyata, A. (2005). Acute inhalational exposure to chlorodifluoromethane (Freon 22): A report of 43 cases. *Clinical Toxicology, 43*(4), 305-308.

Maxwell, J.C. (2001). Deaths related to the inhalation of volatile substances in Texas: 1988-1998. *American Journal of Drug and Alcohol Abuse, 27*(4), 689-697.

Police: Teens huff freon from roof air conditioner. (2002, July 23). NewsNet5. Available: http://www.newsnet5.com/crimestoppers/1573596/detail.html.

Xiong, Z., Avella, J., & Wetli, C.V. (2004). Sudden death caused by 1,1-difluoroethane inhalation. *Journal of Forensic Sciences, 49*(3), 627-629.

GAMMA-HYDROXYBUTYRATE

Names

BAN or INN Chemical Synonyms: Gamma Hydroxybutyric Acid; Sodium Oxybate

Brand/Trade: Xyrem®[1]

Chemical: 4-Hydroxybutanoic acid

Street: Battery Acid; Blue Nitro; Blue Thunder; Cherry Meth; Date Rape Drug; Easy Lay; Fantasy; G; Gamma-OH; Gamma 10; GBH; Georgia Home Boy; GHB; GH Buddy; Gook; Goop; Grave Bodily Harm; Great Hormones at Bedtime; Grievous Bodily Harm; G-Riffic; G-Riffick; Jib; Liquid E; Liquid Ecstasy; Liquid G; Liquid X; Nature's Quaalude; Organic Quaalude; Salty Water; Scoop; Sleep; Sleep-500; Soap; Somatomax; Thunder Nectar; Vita-G

Pharmacologic Classification

Psychodepressant, sedative-hypnotic: miscellaneous (endogenous cerebral inhibitory neurotransmitter)

Brief General Overview

Gamma-hydroxybutyrate (GHB) occurs naturally in the human body as both a precursor and a metabolite of GABA.[2] It was first chemically synthesized in 1960. GHB use became popular in North America during the 1980s and 1990s as a date-rape drug, when it was found to facilitate sexual assault and reduce the likelihood of a perpetrator being arrested, charged, or convicted of aggravated sexual assault because of its pharmacologic characteristics and actions. It is odorless and colorless; soluble in alcohol, and capable of causing (1) muscle relaxation, (2) profound sedation, (3) increased sexual behavior secondary to its disinhibitory effects, and (4) anterograde amnesia. During the same period of time, GHB also gained popularity among bodybuilders as a "nutritional supplement." Sales of GHB in health food stores and over the Internet flourished.

In March 2000, the use of GHB was made illegal across the United States with passage of the federal Hillory J. Farias and Samantha Reid Date-Rape Drug Prohibition Act. However, GHB and its chemical precursor, GBL (gamma-butyrolactone), continued to be widely available over the Internet until the USDEA arrested over 100 dealers in 84 cities in the United States and Canada late in 2002. Despite these efforts, GHB use remains high, and it is expected to increase with diversion of the recently approved prescription product from its legitimate clinical use as adjunctive pharmacotherapy for the symptomatic management of narcolepsy.[3]

GHB is often illicitly used in combination with other drugs and substances of abuse (see "Overdosage" section) to enhance their action or diminish their adverse effects. For example, GHB may be used with 3, 4-methylenedioxymethamphetamine (MDMA) because it reportedly attenuates the unpleasant dysphoria generally experienced during MDMA use, presumably by its action on the central dopaminergic system.[4]

Dosage Forms and Routes of Administration

GHB is available as an oral solution by its generic prescription name, sodium oxybate. Illicit powder and oral solutions also are produced in, imported into, and distributed across North America. These illicit dosage forms may be added to a container of bottled water prior to the user's attendance at a rave.[5,6] They also may be mixed into an alcoholic drink at a circuit party or dance club for self-ingestion or be secretly given to others (e.g., added to another's drink while that drink is left unattended, or mixed in a punch bowl at a social function).

The typical GHB user is a man in his early 20s of European descent. Use occurs predominantly in the social context of all-night parties, circuit parties, dance clubs, music festivals, and raves. Increasingly, sexually active adolescent boys and girls and young adult men and women deliberately use GHB to enhance sexual experiences. In this context, GHB is often used in combination with alcohol and other drugs and substances of abuse, particularly the psychodelics. Another population in which GHB use is extremely high is gay and bisexual men, regardless of race. GHB is one of the five main club drugs (i.e., cocaine, GHB, ketamine, methamphetamine, and methylenedioxymethamphetamine [MDMA, Ecstasy]) that are socially used by this population group.

Mechanism of CNS Action

The exact mechanism of GHB's psychodepressant action has not been determined.

However, the following contributory mechanisms have been confirmed: (1) GHB binds to its own endogenous receptors in the CNS, predominantly in the basal ganglia and hippocampus; (2) GHB appears to enhance the inhibitory actions that are modulated by the GABA$_B$ receptors; (3) GHB acts both presynaptically and postsynaptically to modulate the activity of other neurotransmitters in the CNS; and (4) GHB presynaptically inhibits the release of dopamine into the synaptic cleft, resulting in an accumulation of dopamine in the presynaptic neuron.

Pharmacodynamics/Pharmacokinetics

Gamma-hydroxybutyrate is rapidly but incompletely absorbed from the GI tract. Oral bioavailability is relatively low ($F = 0.25$). Peak plasma levels are obtained ~30 minutes after oral ingestion. Ingestion with a high-fat meal significantly delays and reduces absorption. The apparent volume of distribution is ~50 L, and plasma protein binding is very low (i.e., ~1%). Total body clearance is ~1.5 mL/min. Metabolism, primarily by GHB dehydrogenase and the Krebs cycle, accounts for the major elimination pathway for GHB. Less than 5% is excreted in unchanged form in the urine. The half-life of elimination is ~30 minutes. Effects may persist for 3 to 6 hours. GHB appears to follow dose-dependent (i.e., nonlinear) pharmacokinetics.

Current Approved Indications for Medical Use

Management of cataplexy associated with narcolepsy[7]; management of excessive daytime sleepiness associated with narcolepsy

Desired Action/Reason for Personal Use

Alcohol-like disinhibitory euphoria or "high" (without alcohol-like hangover effect); arousal of sexual desire (particularly among gay and bisexual men); bodybuilding aid (nutritional supplement); enhance sexual experiences (particularly among gay and bisexual men); prevention/self-management of alcohol withdrawal syndrome; prevention/self-management of opiate analgesic withdrawal syndrome; sociability (particularly among gay and bisexual men); also, purposely administered to others without their knowledge in the context of perpetration of a drug-facilitated crime (e.g., robbery; sexual assault, including date rape)[8]

Toxicity

Acute: Amnesia; bradycardia; cognitive impairment; coma (deep, unarousable); confusion; diarrhea; dizziness; drowsiness; enuresis[9]; headache; heartburn; hypotension; hypotonia; loss of consciousness; memory impairment; nausea; psychomotor impairment; respiratory depression (high dosages); sleep (deep); slurred speech; somnolence; sweating; vomiting

Chronic: Menstrual irregularities; physical dependence; psychological dependence; somnambulism (sleep walking); tinnitus

Pregnancy & Lactation: Valid and reliable data are not available.

Abuse Potential

Physical dependence: Low to moderate (USDEA Schedule I)[10]
Psychological dependence: Moderate

Withdrawal Syndrome

A specific GHB withdrawal syndrome has been reported. Signs and symptoms include agitation,[11] anxiety, autonomic excitation or instability, delirium, diaphoresis, dysphagia, hallucinations, hypertension, insomnia, muscle aches, nystagmus, psychosis, tachycardia, and tremor.[12] The GHB withdrawal syndrome may begin within 1 hour of the last use of GHB and last for up to 15 days. It may be potentially life threatening and is often quite resistant to pharmacotherapeutic management with benzodiazepines, such as diazepam (Valium®) or lorazepam (Ativan®). In cases of severe GHB withdrawal, a barbiturate may be more efficacious (see Barbiturates monograph).

Overdosage

GHB overdosage may be fatal. However, fatalities are rare and are usually associated with polydrug use. Alcohol, heroin, and methylenedioxymethamphetamine (MDMA, Ecstasy) are the other drugs most often involved in GHB overdosages.[13] Users who have overdosed present to the emergency department in an unconscious state, often in a coma. Other presenting signs and symptoms of overdosage may include agitation, blurred vision, bradycardia, confusion, delirium, headache, hypothermia, loss of bladder and bowel control, muscle jerks or twitches (i.e., myoclonic movements), muscle weakness, psychomotor impairment, respiratory impairment, seizures, sweating, and vomiting. With proper recognition and care, particularly with attention to cardiac and respiratory support, complete recovery within 6 to 8 hours, without sequelae, generally can be expected. There is no known antidote.

Notes

1. Although it is the exact same drug chemically (actually the sodium salt of GHB), when used therapeutically, GHB is preferentially referred to as "sodium oxybate" (i.e., in much the same way that THC is referred to as "dronabinol" instead of "marijuana" (see Cannabis monograph).
2. Available data suggest that GHB is probably also a neurotransmitter.
3. In 2002, the Date-Rape Drug Prohibition Act (Public Law 106-172) was amended to allow the approved therapeutic use of GHB in the form of the prescription drug Xyrem®.
4. The combined use of GHB and an amphetamine (see monograph) is referred to as "max." The combined use of GHB, ketamine (see monograph), and alcohol (see monograph) is referred to as "special k-lube."
5. A single oral liquid dose of GHB sold at raves is often referred to as a "swig."
6. When GHB is dissolved in water, it imparts a distinctly salty taste to the water.
7. GHB also has been used in Europe to treat the alcohol withdrawal syndrome. It is being reviewed for similar clinical uses in North America.
8. GHB, which is odorless and colorless, is generally used in combination with alcohol for this purpose. Intended victims lose their ability to fend off their assailant and, because of GHB-induced amnesia, become unreliable witnesses if charges are brought against the assailant.
9. Nocturnal urinary incontinence is associated with pharmacotherapeutic dosing at bedtime.
10. Xyrem®, the approved prescription form of GHB, is a Schedule III controlled substance. Currently, approved prescription use is managed under a formal, required Xyrem® Risk Management Program in order to eliminate (or at least significantly reduce) possible drug diversion.

11. May be quite severe and require appropriate physical or chemical restraint (or both) to prevent injury to self or others.
12. The chemical precursors of GHB (e.g., gamma butyrolactone [GBL] and 1,4-butanediol) also are increasingly abused and display similar signs and symptoms of withdrawal.
13. Deaths associated with GBH overdosage are generally secondary to respiratory failure.

References

Abanades, S., Farré, M., Barral, D., et al. (2007). Relative abuse liability of gamma-hydroxybutyric acid, flunitrazepam, and ethanol in club drug users. *Journal of Clinical Psychopharmacology, 27*(6), 625-638.

Abanades, S., Farré, M., Segura, M., et al. (2006). Gamma-hydroxybutyrate (GHB) in humans. Pharmacodynamics and pharmacokinetics. *Annals of the New York Academy of Sciences, 1074*, 559-576.

Abanades, S., Farré, M., Segura, M., et al. (2007). Disposition of gamma-hydroxybutyric acid in conventional and nonconventional biological fluids after single drug administration: Issues in methodology and drug monitoring. *Therapeutic Drug Monitoring, 29*(1), 64-70.

Bialer, P.A. (2002). Designer drugs in the general hospital. *Psychiatric Clinics of North America, 25*(1), 231-243.

Boyce, S.H., Padgham, K., & Miller, L.D. (2000). Gamma hydroxybutyric acid (GHB): An increasing trend in drug abuse. *European Journal of Emergency Medicine, 7*(3), 177-181.

Brenneisen, R., ElSohly, M.A., Murphy, T.P., et al. (2004). Pharmacokinetics and excretion of gamma-hydroxybutyrate (GHB) in healthy subjects. *Journal of Analytic Toxicology, 28*(8), 625-630.

Carter, L.P., Richards, B.D., Mintzer, M.Z., et al. (2006). Relative abuse liability of GHB in humans: A comparison of psychomotor, subjective, and cognitive effects of supratherapeutic doses of triazolam, pentobarbital, and GHB. *Neuropsychopharmacology, 31*(11), 2537-2551.

Castelli, M.P., Moci, I., Langlois, X., et al. (2000). Quantitative autoradiographic distribution of gamma-hydroxybutyric acid binding sites in human and monkey brain. *Brain Research. Molecular Brain Research, 78*(1-2), 91-99.

Colfax, G.N., Mansergh, G., Guzman, R., et al. (2001). Drug use and sexual risk behavior among gay and bisexual men who attend circuit parties: A venue-based comparison. *Journal of Acquired Immune Deficiency Syndromes, 28*(4), 373-379.

Couper, F.J., & Logan, B.K. (2001). GHB and driving impairment. *Journal of Forensic Sciences, 46*(4), 919-923.

Craig, K., Gomez, H.F., McManus, J.L., et al. (2000). Severe gamma-hydroxybutyrate withdrawal: A case report and literature review. *The Journal of Emergency Medicine, 18*(1), 65-70.

Doyon, S. (2001). The many faces of ecstasy. *Current Opinion in Pediatrics, 12*(2), 170-176.

Dyer, J.E., Roth, B., & Hyma, B.A. (2001). Gamma-hydroxybutyrate withdrawal syndrome. *Annals of Emergency Medicine, 37*(2), 147-153.

Fuller, D.E., & Hornfeldt, C.S. (2003). From club drug to orphan drug: Sodium oxybate (Xyrem) for the treatment of cataplexy. *Pharmacotherapy, 23*(9), 1205-1209.

Glisson, J.K., & Norton, J. (2002). Self-medication with gamma-hydroxybutyrate to reduce alcohol intake. *Southern Medical Journal, 95*(8), 926-928.

Gonzalez, A., & Nutt, D.J. (2005). Gamma hydroxy butyrate abuse and dependency. *Journal of Psychopharmacology, 19*(2), 195-204.

Halkitis, P.N., & Palamar, J.J. (2006). GHB use among gay and bisexual men. *Addictive Behaviors, 31*(11), 2135-2139.

Ingels, M., Rangan, C., Bellezzo, J., et al. (2000). Coma and respiratory depression following the ingestion of GHB and its precursors: Three cases. *The Journal of Emergency Medicine, 19*(1), 47-50.

Jenkins, D.H. (2000). Substance abuse and withdrawal in the intensive care unit. *Surgical Clinics of North America, 80*(3), 1033-1053.

Kalasinsky, K.S., Dixon, M.M., Schmunk, G.A., et al. (2001). Blood, brain, and hair GHB concentrations following fatal ingestion. *Journal of Forensic Sciences, 46*(3), 728-730.

Kintz, P., Villain, M., Pélissier, A.L., et al. (2005). Unusually high concentrations in a fatal GHB case. *Journal of Analytical Toxicology, 29*(6), 582-585.

Lemon, M.D., Strain, J.D., & Farver, D.K. (2006). Sodium oxybate for cataplexy. *The Annals of Pharmacotherapy, 40*(3), 433-440.

Mason, P.E., & Kerns, W.P. Jr. (2002). Gamma hydroxybutyric acid (GHB) intoxication. *Academic Emergency Medicine, 9*(7), 730-739.

Mattison, A.M., Ross, M.W., Wolfson, T., et al. (2001). Circuit party attendance, club drug use, and unsafe sex in gay men. *Journal of Substance Abuse, 13*(1-2), 119-126.

Mazarr-Proo, S., & Kerrigan, S. (2005). Distribution of GHB in tissues and fluids following a fatal overdose. *Journal of Analytical Toxicology, 29*(5), 398-400.

McDaniel, C.H., & Miotto, K.A. (2001). Gamma hydroxybutyrate (GHB) and gamma butyrolactone (GBL) withdrawal: Five case studies. *Journal of Psychoactive Drugs, 33*(2), 143-149.

McDonough, M., Kennedy, N., Glasper, A., et al. (2004). Clinical features and management of gamma-hydroxybutyrate (GHB) withdrawal: A review. *Drug and Alcohol Dependence, 75*(1), 3-9.

Miotto, K., Darakjian, J., Basch, J., et al. (2001). Gamma-hydroxybutyric acid: Patterns of use, effects and withdrawal. *American Journal of Addiction, 10*(3), 232-241.

Miro, O., Nogue, S., Espinosa, G., et al. (2002). Trends in illicit drug emergencies: The emerging role of gamma-hydroxybutyrate. *Journal of Toxicology. Clinical Toxicology, 40*(2), 129-135.

O'Connell, T., Kaye, L., & Plosay, J.J. 3rd (2000). Gamma-hydroxybutyrate (GHB): A newer drug of abuse. *American Family Physician, 62*(11), 2478-2483.

Okun, M.S., Boothby, L.A., Bartfield, R.B., et al. (2001). GHB: An important pharmacologic and clinical update. *Journal of Pharmacy & Pharmaceutical Sciences, 4*(2), 167-175.

Robinson, D.M., & Keating, G.M. (2007). Sodium oxybate: A review of its use in the management of narcolepsy. *CNS Drugs, 21*(4), 337-354.

Scharf, M.B. (2006). Sodium oxybate for narcolepsy. *Expert Review of Neurotherapeutics, 6*(8), 1139-1146.

Schneir, A.B., Ly, B.T., & Clark, R.F. (2001). A case of withdrawal from the GHB precursors gamma-butyrolactone and 1,4-butanediol. *Journal of Emergency Medicine, 21*(1), 31-33.

Schwartz, R.H., Milteer, R., & LeBeau, M.A. (2000). Drug-facilitated sexual assault ("date rape"). *Southern Medical Journal, 93*(6), 558-561.

Sivilotti, M.L., Burns, M.J., Aaron, C.K., et al. (2001). Pentobarbital for severe gamma-butyrolactone withdrawal. *Annals of Emergency Medicine, 38*(6), 660-665.

Smith, K.M., Larive, L.L., & Romanelli, F. (2002). Club drugs: Methylenedioxymethamphetamine, flunitrazepam, ketamine hydrochloride, and gamma-hydroxybutyrate. *American Journal of Health-System Pharmacy, 59*(11), 1067-1076.

Sodium oxybate: New drug. Fewer attacks of cataplexy in some patients. (2007). *Prescrire International, 16*(89), 98-101.

Stillwell, M.E. (2002). Drug-facilitated sexual assault involving gamma-hydroxybutyric acid. *Journal of Forensic Sciences, 47*(5), 1133-1134.

Tarabar, A.F., & Nelson, L.S. (2004). The gamma-hydroxybutyrate withdrawal syndrome. *Toxicology Reviews, 23*(1), 45-49.

Teter, C.J., & Guthrie, S.K. (2001). A comprehensive review of MDMA and GHB: Two common club drugs. *Pharmacotherapy, 21*(12), 1486-1513.

Uys, J.D., & Niesink, R.J. (2005). Pharmacological aspects of the combined use of 3,4-methyl-enedioxymethamphetamine (MDMA, ecstasy) and gamma-hydroxybutyric acid (GHB): A review of the literature. *Drug and Alcohol Review, 24*(4), 359-368.

Wedin, G.P., Hornfeldt, C.S., & Ylitalo, L.M. (2006). The clinical development of gamma-hydroxybutyrate (GHB). *Current Drug Safety, 1*(1), 99-106.

Weir, E. (2000). Raves: A review of the culture, the drugs and the prevention of harm. *CMAJ: Canadian Medical Association Journal, 162*(13), 1843-1848.

Winickoff, J.P., Houck, C.S., Rothman, E.L., et al. (2000). Verve and Jolt: Deadly new Internet drugs. *Pediatrics, 106*(4), 829-830.

World Health Organization (2001). WHO expert committee on drug dependence. Thirty-second report. *World Health Organization Technical Report Series, 903*, i-iv, 1-26.

Xyrem approved for muscle problems in narcolepsy. (2002). *FDA Consumer Magazine, 36*(5), 7.

GASOLINE

Names

BAN or INN Generic Synonyms: None

Brand/Trade: None

Chemical: Petrol[1]

Street: Gas; Motor Spirit; Petro; Petrol

Pharmacologic Classification

Psychodepressant, volatile solvents & inhalants: volatile solvent, petroleum distillate (aliphatic hydrocarbon)

Brief General Overview

Despite numerous efforts by North American government agencies and the media over the past three decades, gasoline remains one of the most popular of the volatile solvents used for its psychodepressant actions. Undoubtedly, its ubiquitous availability contributes to its popularity. Users are typically younger adolescents, both boys and girls, of European, Mexican (Hispanic), or Native American descent. The use of gasoline by youth of African and Asian descent is, by comparison, relatively uncommon. Other factors that tend to correlate positively with gasoline use include family dysfunction, juvenile delinquency, lower socioeconomic status, and poor academic performance.

Dosage Forms and Routes of Administration

Gasoline is readily available across North America wherever motorized vehicles are used (i.e., in every city, hamlet, reservation, town, and village). Abusers typically soak a rag in gasoline and inhale the gasoline fumes while holding the soaked rag over the nose and mouth. This method of use is commonly referred to as "huffing." Another method of use is to put the gasoline-soaked rag into a heavy paper or plastic bag, hold the bag securely over the nose and mouth, and inhale deeply. This method of use is commonly referred to as "bagging."[2] Abuse of gasoline typically occurs in the company of friends while at home, on the street, or at school (i.e., on school playgrounds or parking lots).

Mechanism of CNS Action

The exact mechanism of psychodepressant action associated with the inhalation of gasoline fumes has not been determined. However, it is believed that specific binding sites in the CNS are not involved and that the actions are somewhat similar to those of alcohol (see monograph).

Pharmacodynamics/Pharmacokinetics

Gasoline is poorly absorbed after oral ingestion. However, its concentrated vapors are relatively well absorbed from the lungs following pulmonary inhalation. Additional valid and reliable data are not available.

Current Approved Indications for Medical Use

None

Desired Action/Reason for Personal Use

Alcohol-like disinhibitory euphoria or "high"

Toxicity

Acute: Ataxia; cognitive impairment; contact dermatitis; coughing; dizziness; dyspnea; erythema of exposed skin surfaces; headache; lethargy; nausea; pneumonitis; pulmonary irritation; sneezing

Chronic: Aspiration pneumonia; cognitive impairment; memory impairment; neurological impairment, permanent[3]; neurological impairment, transient (e.g., abnormal neurological testing in regard to brisk deep reflexes, finger-to-nose movement, rapid alternating hand movements, postural tremor, and tandem gait); organic lead encephalopathy[4]; peripheral neuropathy; psychological dependence

Pregnancy & Lactation: Valid and reliable data are not available. However, a large retrospective study of women working at a petrochemical company showed a significant increase in risk for spontaneous abortion after regular exposure to gasoline. In a single case report of gasoline ingestion by a woman during week 38 of pregnancy, acute distress in both mother and fetus was noted, but both were normal 2 weeks later after an emergency cesarean section. Additional valid and reliable data are needed on the effects of maternal gasoline use on pregnancy and lactation.

Abuse Potential

Physical dependence: None (USDEA: not a scheduled drug)
Psychological dependence: Low to moderate

Withdrawal Syndrome

Although a gasoline withdrawal syndrome has not been reported for North American youth (or other users), a gasoline inhalation withdrawal syndrome has been reported as occurring in regular, long-term daily adolescent users in other countries. Signs and symptoms include anhedonia, craving for gasoline, dry mouth, insomnia, irritability, increased lacrimation, and psychomotor retardation. Additional valid and reliable data are required to confirm the occurrence of this syndrome, further characterize its signs and symptoms, and formulate optimal effective treatment.

Overdosage

Exposure to gasoline fumes is usually not life threatening, but it can result in coma, respiratory arrest, and death. Aspiration pneumonia and pneumonitis are much more commonly seen after gasoline overdosage. Other sequelae, primarily related to anoxia, require emergency medical management and support. There is no known antidote.

Notes

1. Gasoline is a complex mixture of hydrocarbons that also typically contains trace amounts of other chemicals such as benzene and hexane. The exact composition of a particular sample depends on both the source of the crude oil from which it is produced and the method of refinement.
2. Fumes also can be directly inhaled from the gasoline storage container (e.g., gasoline can or tank). Some young adolescents pour the gasoline into a large plastic garbage bag, twist the open end to partially close the bag, place the partially closed bag over their nose and mouth, and directly inhale the gasoline fumes.
3. Permanent neurological impairment (i.e., symmetric sensorimotor polyneuropathy) associated with gasoline use is most likely caused by various gasoline additives (e.g., manganese in the form of methylcyclopentadienyl manganese tricarbonyl [MMT], an engine "anti-knock" additive) that are meant to increase engine performance or clean engines but were never intended for human inhalation.
4. Encephalopathy is extremely rare since the addition of lead (i.e., tetraethyl lead) to gasoline was largely discontinued in the late 1960s.

References

Burns, T.M., Shneker, B.F., & Juel, V.C. (2001). Gasoline sniffing multifocal neuropathy. *Pediatric Neurology, 25*(5), 419-421.

Cairney, S., Maruff, P., Burns, C., et al. (2002). The neurobehavioral consequences of petrol (gasoline) sniffing. *Neuroscience and Biobehavioral Reviews, 26*(1), 81-89.

GLUE

Names

BAN or INN Generic Synonyms: None

Brand/Trade: None

Chemical: Various[1]

Street: Gluey

Pharmacologic Classification

Psychodepressant, volatile solvents & inhalants: volatile solvent

Brief General Overview

Glue, which generally refers to any liquid or paste adhesive product, is commonly used for its psychodepressant actions, primarily by children and young adolescents 8 to 12 years of age, because it is readily accessible to them[2] and produces a relatively brief (i.e., typically 5- to 20-minute) period of euphoria or "high." The most frequently reported locations for the use of glue and other solvents and inhalants are a user's own home or a friend's home, party settings, playgrounds, schools and school grounds, and the street. Approximately one-third of users engage in the behavior while alone, but most users prefer glue sniffing in the company of small groups of friends. Some children may continue to use glue during later adolescence, but most replace the use of glue with other drugs and substances of abuse (e.g., alcohol, marijuana) that become more readily available to them.

Dosage Forms and Routes of Administration

Glue is commercially available and legally distributed in a variety of liquid and paste formulations (e.g., bicycle tire repair glue, contact cement, household glue, model airplane or car cement, rubber cement).[3] Glue sniffers typically sniff vapors directly from a glue container or put the glue into a paper or plastic bag, place the bag over their nose and mouth, and inhale (i.e., huffing). Glue sniffing is a common occurrence in North America and worldwide, particularly among children and adolescents 8 to 12 years of age. Poverty, a history of childhood abuse, and poor scholastic performance all correlate highly with risk for glue and other solvent and inhalant use. Two-thirds of glue-using children are boys, although the proportion of girls has been steadily increasing over the past two decades. In North America, children and adolescents of European descent and Native American descent have the highest rates of glue use, with rates for girls now equal to boys in some surveys.

Mechanism of CNS Action

Valid and reliable data are not generally available because glue is not intended for human pulmonary inhalation. However, data on toluene[4] indicate that its actions in the CNS are similar to those of alcohol. Toluene appears to inhibit glutamatergic neurotransmission. It also appears to have some dopaminergic actions. Additional valid and reliable data are needed.

Pharmacodynamics/Pharmacokinetics

Valid and reliable data are not available.

Current Approved Indications for Medical Use

None, other than surgical wound closure with specially prepared glues

Desired Action/Reason for Personal Use

Alcohol-like disinhibitory euphoria or "high"; dissociation (i.e., escape from reality); perceptual distortions (illusions)

Toxicity

Acute: Ataxia; blurred vision; cognitive impairment; coughing; dizziness; drowsiness; epistaxis; eye irritation; headache; lethargy; nausea; slurred speech; sneezing; vomiting; weakness

Chronic: Anorexia; aspiration pneumonia; deafness (specifically associated with the toluene component); memory impairment; mental depression; metabolic acidosis (specifically associated with the toluene component); myopathy (specifically associated with the toluene component); neurological damage; psychological dependence; psychosis; rash (local) around the nose and mouth (with some glues); renal tubular damage (specifically associated with the toluene component); respiratory tract irritation and local damage; rhabdomyolysis

Pregnancy & Lactation: Valid and reliable data are not available in regard to the maternal use of glue and its effects on pregnancy and lactation. However, toluene embryopathy, including cognitive and learning disorders (e.g., attention-deficit/hyperactivity disorder), developmental delay, microcephaly, minor craniofacial and limb anomalies, and variable growth deficiency, has been reported. Definitive interpretation of data is confounded by possible concurrent use of other drugs and substances of abuse, notably alcohol and tobacco, by pregnant young adolescent girls (and women) who use glue. Additional valid and reliable data are needed.

Abuse Potential

Physical dependence: None to low (USDEA: not a scheduled drug)
Psychological dependence: Moderate

Withdrawal Syndrome

A glue withdrawal syndrome has not been reported.

Overdosage

Death has been commonly associated with glue sniffing. The major mechanisms of these fatalities include (1) choking from aspiration of vomitus, (2) fatal accidents (e.g., motor vehicle and bicycle or pedestrian accidents resulting from glue intoxication), and (3) suffocation as a result of the plastic bag used to sniff the glue occluding the respiratory passages. Signs and symptoms of overdosage involving glue are variable and depend upon both the type of glue used and its specific formulation. Bronchospasm, cardiac dysrhythmias, coma, and respiratory insufficiency or arrest may occur. Therefore, glue overdosage requires emergency medical support and monitoring of body systems. There is no known antidote.

Notes

1. A wide variety of types of glue are available, including cyanoacrylate (i.e., "super glue"), epoxy (i.e., two-part resin/hardener glue), paper glue (i.e., paste or white glue), polyvinyl acetate (i.e., plastic adhesive), and urea-formaldehyde glue (i.e., casamite). All types contain a wide variety of additives. Some types, such as glass cement alloy, contain heavy metals, including bismuth, lead, and tin.
2. Glue is legal to purchase and possess, relatively inexpensive, packaged in small containers that are easy to steal and conceal, and readily available (e.g., in school and home settings).
3. None of these products are intended for human pulmonary inhalation. Thus, they may contain a variety of toxic ingredients (e.g., acetone, aluminum, toluene), usually in unlabeled and undisclosed amounts.
4. Toluene (methylbenzene) is an aromatic solvent. It is both a principal ingredient in many glues and a chemical capable of being used for its own psychodepressant actions. (See also the Volatile Solvents & Inhalants monograph.)

References

Adlaf, E.M., Paglia, A., Ivis, F.J., et al. (2000). Nonmedical drug use among adolescent students: Highlights from the 1999 Ontario Student Drug Use Survey. *CMAJ: Canadian Medical Association Journal, 162*(12), 1677-1680.

Akay, C., Kalman, S., Dündaröz, R., et al. (2008). Serum aluminum levels in glue-sniffer adolescent and in glue containers. *Basic & Clinical Pharmacology & Toxicology, 102*(5), 433-436.

Alper, A.T., Akyol, A., Hasdemir, H., et al. Glue (toluene) abuse: Increased QT dispersion and relation with unexplained syncope. *Inhalation Toxicology, 20*(1), 37-41.

Buszewicz, G., & Madro, R. (2004). Stability of toluene and reduction of acetone to 2-propanol in homogenates of the human liver, brain and lungs. *Forensic Science International, 141*(1), 63-68.

Field-Smith, M.E., Bland, J.M., Taylor, J.C., et al. (2002, July 15). *Trends in death associated with abuse of volatile substances 1971-2000.* Report number 15. London: Department of Public Health Sciences, St. George's Hospital Medical School.

Kao, K.C., Tsai, Y.H., Lin, M.C., et al. (2000). Hypokalemic muscular paralysis causing acute respiratory failure due to rhabdomyolysis with renal tubular acidosis in a chronic glue sniffer. *Journal of Toxicology. Clinical Toxicology, 38*(6), 679-681.

Tang, H.L., Chu, K.H., Cheuk, A., et al. (2005). Renal tubular acidosis and severe hypophosphataemia due to toluene inhalation. *Hong Kong Medical Journal, 11*(1), 50-53.

Vural, M., & Ogel, K. (2006). Dilated cardiomyopathy associated with toluene abuse. *Cardiology, 105*(3), 158-161.

HARMALA ALKALOIDS

Names

BAN or INN Generic Synonyms: Harmaline; Harmine

Brand/Trade: None

Chemical: See "Brief General Overview"

Street: *Yage*; *Yajè*

Pharmacologic Classification

Psychodelic, LSD-like psychodelic: indole (natural alkaloid)

Brief General Overview

The harmala alkaloids include harmaline, harmine, 6-methoxyharmalan, norharmane, and tetrahydroharmine. They occur naturally in plant species, particularly in the bark of the South American vine *Banisteriopsis caapi* and the seeds of the Near Eastern desert shrub *Peganum harmala*.[1] Although the use of harmala alkaloids is legal, their use is extremely uncommon in North America, probably because (1) the culture of use is not indigenous to North America, (2) each use is accompanied by severe vomiting and purging (diarrhea), and (3) a number of other psychodelic drugs are readily available that are not associated with such adverse effects as severe vomiting and diarrhea. Still, over the past 5 years, the use of harmala alkaloids has increased significantly in the large urban centers of North America, South America, and Europe. In addition, in a manner similar to the use of peyote by members of the Native American Church (see Mescaline monograph), two religions of Brazilian origin (i.e., *Santo Daime* and *Uñiao do Vegetal*) have sought the right to use *ayahuasca* as a sacrament in their syncretic churches in the United States under the Religious Freedom Act.

The ceremonial use of *ayahuasca* by indigenous Amazonian tribes is increasing as is its integration into *mestizo* folk medicine in the northwest Amazon. "*Ayahuasca* tourism" in the Amazon is likewise increasing as Europeans and North Americans seek *ayahuasca's* psychodelic actions through their own personal use. While suggestions for its use in the treatment of alcoholism and other substance use disorders have been made, clinical investigative support for its potential efficacy in this regard is currently lacking.

Dosage Forms and Routes of Administration

The harmala alkaloids are commonly consumed together with N,N-dimethyltryptamine (DMT; see N,N-Dimethyltryptamine monograph) in a South American (Amazonian) ceremonial tea called *ayahuasca*.[2]

Mechanism of CNS Action

The harmala alkaloids are selective, reversible inhibitors of monoamine oxidase A (MAOA). When harmala alkaloids are orally ingested together with DMT, the reversible inhibition of MAOA, which appears to occur predominantly in the GI tract and liver, significantly reduces the first-pass hepatic metabolism of DMT. The harmala alkaloids also appear to weakly inhibit serotonin reuptake. These two actions increase serotonergic activity and enable DMT to elicit its psychodelic actions after oral ingestion (see N,N-Dimethyltryptamine [DMT] monograph).

Pharmacodynamics/Pharmacokinetics

Harmala alkaloids are readily absorbed after oral ingestion, with peak blood concentration occurring in ~1.5 hours. Maximal mental (e.g., "high") and physical (e.g., increased blood pressure) effects occur at this time. Additional valid and reliable data are not available.

Current Approved Indications for Medical Use

None[3]

Desired Action/Reason for Personal Use

Dreamlike experience with vividly colored images; hallucinations (auditory and vivid visual); magico-religious and ceremonial use among members of indigenous Amazonian tribes and Brazilian religions

Toxicity

Acute: Agitation; ataxia; confusion; diarrhea (stimulant purging effect); dizziness; hallucinations (auditory and visual); nausea; numbness of the limbs; psychosis; sweating; tremor; vomiting

Chronic: Psychological dependence

Pregnancy & Lactation: Valid and reliable data are not available.

Abuse Potential

Physical dependence: None to low (USDEA: not a scheduled drug)
Psychological dependence: Low to moderate

Withdrawal Syndrome

A harmala alkaloids withdrawal syndrome has not been reported.

Overdosage

The harmala alkaloids appear to have a relatively high therapeutic index. No deaths directly related to their use have been confirmed. There is no known antidote. Additional valid and reliable data are needed.

Notes

1. *Peganum harmala* is commonly known as "Syrian vine" and is found and used from Iran to Pakistan. Seeds from which an infusion can be made are available over the Internet. The harmala alkaloids also are found in *Passiflora incarnata*.
2. *Ayahuasca*, the use of which is akin to a religious sacrament to many South American Indians, particularly in Brazil, Ecuador, and Peru, also is known as *caapi, hoasca, natema, pinde*, or *yajè* (*yage*). Its use dates back to pre-Columbian times. It is generally prepared by infusing the shredded stalk of the malpighiaceous plant *Banisteriopsis caapi* together with DMT-containing plants such as *Anadenanthera peregrina*, *Virola calophylla*, or *Psychotria viridis*. In Bolivia and Peru, its use has been associated with healing, shamanism, and other social rituals. Psychodelic effects after oral ingestion generally peak between 1.5 and 2 hours (i.e., at the time of maximal blood concentration of DMT) and can last for up to 4 hours.
3. Although not approved for medical use in North America, the harmala alkaloids are used as antineoplastic drugs in some other countries (e.g., Iran) and for shamanistic healing ceremonies by certain South American Indians. See also the discussion of religious use in the Brief General Overview.

References

Callaway, J.C., Brito, G.S., & Neves, E.S. (2005). Phytochemical analyses of Banisteriopsis caapi and Psychotria viridis. *Journal of Psychoactive Drugs, 37*(2), 145-150.

Frison, G., Favretto, D., Zancanaro, F., et al. (2008). A case of β-carboline alkaloid intoxication following ingestion of Peganum harmala seed extract. *Forensic Science International, 179*(2-3), e37-e43.

Gable, R.S. (2007). Risk assessment of ritual use of oral dimethyltryptamine (DMT) and harmala alkaloids. *Addiction, 102*(1), 24-34.

Halpern, J.H. (2004). Hallucinogens and dissociative agents naturally growing in the United States. *Pharmacology & Therapeutics, 102*(2), 131-138.

Ott, J. (2001). Pharmepena-Psychonautics: Human intranasal, sublingual and oral pharmacology of 5-methoxy-N,N-dimethyl-tryptamine. *Journal of Psychoactive Drugs, 33*(4), 403-407.

Riba, J., Anderer, P., Jané, F., et al. (2004). Effects of the South American psychoactive beverage ayahuasca on regional brain electrical activity in humans: A functional neuroimaging study using low-resolution electromagnetic tomography. *Neuropsychobiology, 50*(1), 89-101.

Riba, J., Rodriguez-Fornells, A., Urbano, G., et al. (2001). Subjective effects and tolerability of the South American psychoactive beverage Ayahuasca in healthy volunteers. *Psychopharmacology, 154*(1), 85-95.

Riba, J., Valle, M., Urbano, G., et al. (2003). Human pharmacology of ayahuasca: Subjective and cardiovascular effects, monoamine metabolite excretion, and pharmacokinetics. *The Journal of Pharmacology and Experimental Therapeutics, 306*(1), 73-83.

Saleem, A., Engstrom, M., Wurster, S., et al. (2002). Interaction of folk medicinal plant extracts with human α2-adrenoceptor subtypes. *Naturforsch, 57*(3-4), 332-338.

Santos, R.G., Landeira-Fernandez, J., Strassman, R.J., et al. (2007). Effects of ayahuasca on psychometric measures of anxiety, panic-like and hopelessness in Santo Daime members. *Journal of Ethnopharmacology, 112*(3), 507-513.

Sklerov, J., Levine, B., Moore, K.A., et al. (2005). A fatal intoxication following the ingestion of 5-methoxy-N,N-dimethyltryptamine in an ayahuasca preparation. *Journal of Analytical Toxicology, 29*(8), 838-841.

Sobhani, A.M., Ebrahimi, S.A., & Mahmoudian, M. (2002). An in vitro evaluation of human DNA topoisomerase I inhibition by Peganum harmala L. seeds extract and its β-carboline alkaloids. *Journal of Pharmacy & Pharmaceutical Sciences, 5*(1), 19-23.

Tupper, K.W. (2008). The globalization of ayahuasca: Harm reduction or benefit maximization? *International Journal on Drug Policy, 19*(4), 297-303.

HASHISH (See Cannabis)

HEROIN

Names

BAN or INN Generic Synonyms: Diacetylmorphine; Diamorphine

Brand/Trade: None

Chemical: (5α,6α)-7,8-Didehydro-4,5-epoxy-17-methylmorphinan-3,6-diol diacetate

Street: 747; 2000; A-Bomb; AIP; Al Capone; Alquitran; Amelia; Antifreeze; Aries; A-Sidani; Aunt Hazel; Batman; Beast; Big Bad Boy; Big Bag; Big Boy; Big H; Big Harry; Bin Laden; Black Dragon; Black Eagle; Black Girl; Black Pearl; Black Powder; Black Stuff; Black Tar; Blue; Blue Bag; Bobby Brown; *Bonita*; Boy; Bozo; Brad Nowell; Brain Damage; *Brea*; Brick Gum; *Broja*; Brown; Brown Bag; Brown Crystal; Brown Rhine; Brownstone; Brown Sugar; Brown Tape; Bull Dog; Bundle; Butu; *Caballo*; *Caca*; *Calbo*; Capital H; Captain Jack; *Carga*; *Carne*; *Chapopote*; Charley; Chatarra; Cheeba; Cheese; 57 Chevy; Chiba; Chicken; *Chicle*; China Cat; China White; Chinese Red; Chinese Rocks; *Chieva*; Chip; *Chiva*; Choco-fan; *Cocofan*; Cotics; Cotton Candy; Crap; Crop; Crown Crap; *Cura*; Cut-Deck; Dead on Arrival; Dead President; Desert Storm; Diesel; Dirt; D.O.A.; Dog Food; Doggie; Dolphin; Doogie; Doojee; Dooley; Doosey; Dope; Downtown; Dragon; Dreck; Dr. Feelgood; Dugie; Duji; Dujre; Dyno; Dyno-Pure; Eighth; *Estuffa*; Ferry Dust; Flea Powder; Foil; Foo Foo Stuff; Furra; Galloping Horse; Gallup; Gamot; *Gato*; George; George Smack; Ghost; Girl; Glacines; Golden Girl; Golpe; *Goma*; Good and Plenty; Good H; Good Horse; H; Hache; Hairy; Hard Candy; Harry; Hayron; Hazel; H-Bomb; H Caps; Helen; Henry; Hera; Hero; Hero of the Underworld; *Heroina*; Heron; Herone; Hessle; Him; *Hombre*; Homicide; Horse; Horsebite; Hot Dope; HRN; Isda; Jack Bauer; Jazz; Jee Gee; Jerry Springer; Jive Doo Jee; *Joharito*; Jojee; Joy; Joy Flakes; Joy Powder; Junco; Junk; Kabayo; Kaka Water; Kermit the Frog; *La Buena*; Lady H; Layne Staley; *Manteca*; Matsakow; Mexican Black Tar; Mexican

Brown; Mexican Horse; Mexican Mud; Morotgara; Mr. Brownstone; Mud; Murder; Murder One; Muzzle; Nanoo; Nice and Easy; Nickel Deck; Noise; Number Eight; Nurse; Ogoy; Old Navy; Old Steve; Orange Line; Pangonadalot; Papers; Peg; Perfect High; *Perica*; *Perico*; Poison; Poppy; Predator; Pure; Pure Hell; Rain; Rambo; Raw; Raw Fusion; Raw Hide; Red Chicken; Red Eagle; Red Rock; Reindeer Dust; Rob Flaherty; Sack; Salt; Scag; Scat; Scate; Scott; Second to None; Sheeba; Shit; Shiva; Shmack; Shmeck/Schmeek; Silk; Skag; Skid; Skunk; Slam; Slime; Smack; Spider; Spider Blue; Stuff; Suicide; Sweet Dreams; Tang; Tar; *Tecata*; Thanie; The Beast; The Witch; Thunder; *Tigre*; *Tigre Blanco*; *Tigre del Norte*; Tits; TNT; Tommy Hilfiger; Tongs; Tootsie Roll; Top Drool; Train; Twin Towers; *Vidrio*; West Side; White Angel; White Bitch; White Boy; White Dragon; White Girl; White Horse; White Junk; White Nurse; White Pony; White Stuff; White Tiger; Witch Hazel; WTC; Yellow Bag; Yen-Shee; *Zoquette*

Pharmacologic Classification

Psychodepressant, opiate analgesic: pure agonist (semisynthetic)

Brief General Overview

Heroin was first synthesized and introduced into clinical practice over 125 years ago as a "nonaddictive" treatment for "the great army of suffering"—the soldiers who had become physically dependent on morphine during the American Civil War (1861–1865). Heroin is produced by chemical modification of morphine (see monograph), which is formed naturally in the resin of the opium poppy *Papaver somniferum*. The opium poppy can be cultivated worldwide in temperate climates but is indigenous to Burma, Laos, and Thailand.[1] In addition to these three countries, much of the world's illicit supply of opium (and heroin) is cultivated in Afghanistan, Colombia, Mexico, and Pakistan. In fact, Afghanistan is currently the largest producer of opium in the world. (See also the Opiate Analgesics monograph.)

Dosage Forms and Routes of Administration

Heroin is produced for illicit use in North America in clandestine chemical laboratories, primarily in Colombia, France, and Italy.[2] It is primarily intravenously injected.[3] However, since the late 1980s, with the growing risk of HIV transmission by shared contaminated needles and the increased availability of a significantly purer form of heroin (i.e., the concentration of illicit heroin increased from 5% to over 90%),[4] the preferred method of use has been steadily shifting to intranasal sniffing (snorting) and smoking ("chasing the dragon").[4] The use of Black Tar heroin from Mexico, which is actually a poorly refined gummy resin form of heroin that is quite similar to opium, also became prevalent during this time. Black in color, it is typically sold in quantities the size of a large tablet. It is estimated that at least 17% of the San Francisco Hispanic community has tried this form of heroin. It is preferred by some users because, unlike the powdered form of heroin, it is difficult to "cut."[5] It also is about one-tenth of the usual street cost of powdered heroin, a factor that has made it attractive to school-age adolescents. Black Tar heroin is difficult to filter and, thus, its intravenous injection is significantly more likely than powdered heroin to cause infections at injection sites and phlebitis. It is sometimes injected subcutaneously, a pattern of use that has been related to infection with botulism.

Historically, the typical North American heroin user was a man 20 to 40 years of age of European descent. He generally injected heroin intravenously and had a history of antisocial behavior characterized by the use of other drugs and substances of abuse, and he often had a criminal record and history of incarceration. Reflecting the increasing availability of heroin and changing methods of heroin use, the demographics of the heroin user have changed significantly. Heroin users are now female and male, younger and older, richer and poorer, "chippers" and "hardcore" users, representing all ethnic groups. Since the 1980s, an important factor in use patterns has been the changing drug culture, including the association of heroin use with cocaine use (heroin is often used to "come down" from a "coke high") and the "crack house" culture (see Cocaine monograph for patterns of combination use). Another major factor has been the involvement of global organized crime syndicates and outlaw motorcycle gangs, along with their association with widespread North American youth gangs, in the illicit distribution and sale of heroin.

By the beginning of the 21st century, women, from every major ethnic background, accounted for more than one-third of heroin users in North America. Women of African, Asian, Hispanic, and Native American descent are found in significant numbers among the new heroin users. The new users are characteristically poorly educated, unemployed—other than employment in the drug or sex trade—and otherwise socially disadvantaged and living in the inner cities. In New York City, users of Hispanic descent are currently the predominant users of heroin.[6]

Mechanism of CNS Action

Five major groups of opiate receptors have been identified: delta, epsilon, kappa, mu, and sigma. Opiate analgesic activity occurs at the mu, kappa, and sigma receptors (see Opiate Analgesics monograph). As a pure opiate analgesic agonist, heroin acts primarily at the mu receptors, which are found in the highest concentrations in the hypothalamus, limbic system, midbrain, spinal cord, and thalamus. In addition to analgesia, opiate agonists suppress the cough reflex, alter mood (e.g., produce euphoria or dysphoria), cause mental clouding, and stimulate respiratory depression. The nausea and vomiting associated with heroin use probably are caused by stimulation of the chemoreceptor trigger zone.

Pharmacodynamics/Pharmacokinetics

After intravenous injection, heroin is rapidly peripherally deacetylated to 6-acetylmorphine, which is further deacetylated to morphine (see monograph),[7] which in turn undergoes metabolism to morphine-3-glucuronide and morphine 6-O-glucuronide. The elimination half-life of heroin after intravenous injection is ~2 minutes (range, 1.3 to 2.2 minutes). When orally ingested, heroin is rapidly deacetylated in the liver and GI tract and undergoes virtually complete presystemic conversion, or first-pass hepatic metabolism, to morphine (i.e., when ingested, heroin is completely converted into morphine and thus offers no advantage over morphine).[8,9] Although pulmonary inhalation of heroin by smoking results in rapid, dose-related effects (both objective and subjective), bioavailability is ~50%. Moderate hepatic impairment does not appear to significantly affect the pharmacokinetics of heroin. However, moderate renal impairment may affect the elimination of its morphine metabolite.

Current Approved Indications for Medical Use[10]

None

Desired Action/Reason for Personal Use

Euphoria; feeling of tranquility; prevention/self-management of the opiate analgesic withdrawal syndrome; rapid, generalized sensation of warmth ("rush," which physiologically is associated with histamine release and a consequent increase in peripheral blood flow); sleepy, trancelike state (i.e., "on the nod") during which visions or vivid daydreams ("pipe dreams") may occur

Toxicity

Acute: Anorexia; asthma, acute exacerbation[11]; bradycardia; cognitive impairment; constipation; drowsiness; dry mouth; edema; headaches; heavy feeling of the extremities; hives; miosis; nausea; psychomotor impairment; pruritus (may be severe); respiratory depression or arrest; sedation; sex drive, diminished; sweating, excessive; vomiting; weakness

Chronic: Complications associated with improper intravenous injection technique (e.g., abscesses, bacteremia, gangrene and amputation, septicemia, skin breakdown, thrombophlebitis, thrombosis, and ulceration; these complications are particularly common in homeless or mentally ill intravenous heroin users)[12]; impaired lung function and dyspnea related to chronic heroin smoking (i.e., "chasing the dragon")[13]; infections, including hepatitis and HIV (a consequence of both contaminated needles or syringes and drug-related unprotected sexual intercourse); peripheral neuropathy; physical dependence; psychological dependence

Pregnancy & Lactation: FDA Pregnancy Category "not established." Safety of heroin use by adolescent girls and women who are pregnant has not been established. Heroin crosses the placenta. However, it does not appear to be associated with the development of congenital malformations. Neonates born to mothers who regularly used heroin during their pregnancies, especially near term, display the neonatal opiate analgesic withdrawal syndrome. In addition, these neonates have a significantly greater risk for postnatal growth deficiency as well as for sudden infant death syndrome (SIDS). However, the causative factor may not be heroin (i.e., it may be related to the mother's lifestyle as a heroin user and her socioeconomic status). Adolescent girls and women who are pregnant should not use heroin.

Safety of heroin use by adolescent girls and women who are breast-feeding has not been established. Heroin is excreted in breast milk. Neonates and infants may display expected pharmacologic actions (e.g., drowsiness, lethargy). They also may become physically dependent. In addition, neonatal physical dependency developed in utero may be prolonged in breast-fed neonates. Adolescent girls and women who are breast-feeding should not use heroin.

Abuse Potential

Physical dependence: High (USDEA Schedule I; use is prohibited)[14]
Psychological dependence: High

Withdrawal Syndrome

Abrupt discontinuation of regular, long-term heroin use may result in a heroin withdrawal syndrome. The syndrome also may occur in heroin users if a mixed opiate agonist/antagonist (e.g., pentazocine [Talwin®]) or the opiate analgesic antagonist (e.g., naloxone [Narcan®]) is used.

Signs and symptoms of the heroin withdrawal syndrome resemble those associated with withdrawal from other opiate analgesic agonists and include abdominal pain, anorexia, body aches, chills, diarrhea, difficulty sleeping, esotropia (rare), insomnia, leg movements (involuntary ["kicking the habit"]), muscle pain, nervousness, piloerection (gooseflesh), restlessness, rhinitis, shivering, sneezing, stomach cramps, sweating (excessive), tachycardia, tremors, unexplained fever, vomiting, weakness, and yawning. These signs and symptoms usually peak within 24 to 48 hours after the last heroin dose and subside after about 1 week. The heroin withdrawal syndrome is not usually life threatening, but gradual discontinuation of regular, long-term use will prevent or minimize these signs and symptoms.

Overdosage

Overdosage fatalities have been associated with every method of heroin use but are most often associated with intravenous use. Generally the signs and symptoms of heroin overdosage are an exacerbation of its psychodepressant and other actions and include limb paralysis (temporary), peripheral neuropathy, rhabdomyolysis-induced renal failure, seizures (occasionally), and vomiting. Pulmonary edema often is a major contributor to mortality. Heroin overdosage requires emergency medical support, with attention to increasing heroin elimination. The opiate antagonist naloxone (Narcan®) is usually effective in reversing associated respiratory depression.[15] The duration of action of heroin may exceed that of naloxone, so repeated doses of naloxone may be required during the course of the emergency medical management of heroin overdosage. Overdosage also may be complicated by multiple toxicities and synergistic effects of other drugs, because most heroin users are poly-drug and substance users who commonly use alcohol, cocaine, and other drugs and substances of abuse concurrently with heroin.

Notes

1. These opium-producing countries were commonly referred to during the last half of the 20th century as the Golden Triangle.
2. The heroin found at street level in North America is usually "cut" or "stepped on" (i.e., diluted with an adulterant in order to increase profit). Commonly used adulterants include lactose, powdered milk, quinine, starch, strychnine, and sugar.
3. Prior to injection, the heroin powder is dissolved in a spoon or metal bottle cap. It is heated (often with a match or cigarette lighter) to facilitate dissolution. Some heroin users have discovered that adding a small amount of organic acid (i.e., two or three drops of lemon or lime juice) may facilitate dissolution—and may also eliminate the need for heating. This heroin has come to be referred to "on the street" as "lemon heroin" or "lime heroin." Before injection, the dissolved heroin is usually filtered (i.e., drawn into the syringe through a filter removed from a cigarette) to remove any undissolved drug or other particulate matter.
4. Pulmonary inhalation of heroin, "chasing the dragon," also has been extended to other drugs and substances of abuse. Basically, the user places the dried powder form of the drug or substance on a small piece of aluminum foil. The aluminum foil is then heated from underneath, generally with a match or cigarette lighter, and as it heats up the drug changes from a solid to a volatile state. The

wafting smoke columns of drug are then followed (i.e., "chasing the dragon") and inhaled through a tube—often a rolled-up piece of paper currency. Subcutaneous self-injection of heroin, "skin popping," also has been a common method of use over the past 50 years. However, it, too, has been largely replaced by intranasal snorting. Skin poppers usually have a lower level of dependence on heroin, and use is less frequent (i.e., once daily to once weekly).

5. High purity heroin is usually "cut" before illicit distribution and sale at the "street" level. The average concentration of heroin available for injection is about 27%, compared with about 7% during the 1980s. Street-level Colombian heroin typically ranges from 25% to 80% pure, while Mexican Black Tar heroin typically ranges from 14% to 60% pure, with the highest purity found in U.S.–Mexican border cities (e.g., El Paso, Texas). In response to growing demand, more opium poppies are being grown in Mexico: in 2008, more than 7000 hectares producing over 50 tons of Mexican Black Tar heroin.

6. In 2005 a new pattern of heroin use began to be reported among Hispanic-American adolescents in Texas—the use of "Cheese." Cheese is the street name for a mixture of heroin, acetaminophen (Tylenol®), and diphenhydramine (see monograph). The mixture resembles grated parmesan cheese—thus its name—and it is intranasally sniffed (snorted). The heroin concentration in the mixture is relatively low (i.e., generally 2% to 8%).

7. Both 6-acetylmorphine and morphine are active metabolites of heroin. Some data suggest that deacetylation (hydrolysis) of 6-acetylmorphine to morphine is significantly impaired by the presence of high blood alcohol concentrations. This is postulated to contribute to the higher rate of heroin overdosage deaths when alcohol intoxication is simultaneously present.

8. For this reason, heroin offers no advantage over methadone in opiate-dependence maintenance programs.

9. Heroin is not detectable in plasma after oral or rectal administration because of its short elimination half-life.

10. An effective opiate analgesic, heroin was widely available for use in a variety of patent medicines and tonics in North America until early in the 20th century. At that time, because of its abuse potential and the availability of therapeutic alternatives, federal regulations were enacted to prohibit its domestic production and importation. During the mid-1980s, Canadian drug laws were modified to allow regulated medical use of heroin for the treatment of severe, intractable pain. However, legitimate medical use has remained at very low levels (i.e., far below forecasts). Although heroin is still used in the United Kingdom as part of prescribed maintenance programs for opiate-dependent people, this use has been largely replaced by the therapeutic use of methadone (see monograph) and, more recently, buprenorphine (see monograph). However, interest in and research on heroin-assisted treatment programs continues in several European countries and Canada.

11. Intranasal snorting of heroin can cause acute, potentially life-threatening exacerbation of asthma.

12. Complications increase as the user progresses to other vein sites (i.e., from antecubital fossa or forearm sites to hand, foot, or leg sites and ultimately to neck and groin sites) as the initial sites are damaged (i.e., "lost") and can no longer be used for intravenous injection.

13. Pulmonary dysfunction is exacerbated by the high rate of tobacco smoking noted by regular long-term heroin users.

14. Heroin, under its generic name of diacetylmorphine, is legally available in Canada by prescription for the management of severe pain.

15. Caution is required when naloxone is administered to heroin users who may be physically dependent, because it may precipitate the heroin withdrawal syndrome.

References

Brugal, M.T., Barrio, G., De, L.F., et al. (2002). Factors associated with non-fatal heroin overdose: Assessing the effect of frequency and route of heroin administration. *Addiction, 97*(3), 319-327.

Buster, M., Rook, L., van Brussel, G.H., et al. (2002). Chasing the dragon, related to the impaired lung function among heroin users. *Drug and Alcohol Dependence, 68*(2), 221-228.

Cullen, W., Bury, G., & Langton, D. (2000). Experience of heroin overdose among drug users attending general practice. *The British Journal of General Practice, 50*(456), 546-549.

Darke, S., & Ross, J. (2000). Fatal heroin overdoses resulting from non-injecting routes of administration. NSW, Australia, 1992-1996. *Addiction, 95*(4), 569-573.

Darke, S., Ross, J., & Kaye, S. (2001). Physical injecting sites among injecting drug users in Sydney, Australia. *Drug and Alcohol Dependence, 62*(1), 77-82.

Dettmeyer, R., Schmidt, P., Musshoff, F., et al. (2000). Pulmonary edema in fatal heroin overdose: Immunohistological investigations with IgE, collagen IV and laminin—No increase of defects of alveolar-capillary membranes. *Forensic Sciences International, 110*(2), 87-96.

Finnie, A., & Nicolson, P. (2002). Injecting drug use: Implications for skin and wound management. *British Journal of Nursing, 11*(6 Suppl), S17-S28.

Firth, A.Y. (2001). Heroin withdrawal as a possible cause of acute concomitant esotropia in adults. *Eye, 15*(Part 2), 189-192.

Fischer, B., Rehm, J., Kirst, M., et al. (2002). Heroin-assisted treatment as a response to the public health problem of opiate dependence. *European Journal of Public Health, 12*(3), 228-234.

Frank, B. (2000). An overview of heroin trends in New York City: Past, present and future. *Mount Sinai Journal of Medicine, 67*(5-6), 340-346.

Gonzalez, G., Oliveto, A., & Kosten, T.R. (2002). Treatment of heroin (diamorphine) addiction: Current approaches and future prospects. *Drugs, 62*(9), 1331-1343.

Gyarmathy, V.A., Neaigus, A., Miller, M., et al. (2002). Risk correlates of prevalent HIV, hepatitis B virus, and hepatitis C virus infections among noninjecting heroin users. *Journal of Acquired Immune Deficiency Syndrome, 30*(4), 448-456.

Gyr, E., Brenneisen, R., Bourquin, D., et al. (2000). Pharmacodynamics and pharmacokinetics of intravenously, orally and rectally administered diacetylmorphine in opioid dependents, a two-patient pilot study within a heroin-assisted treatment program. *International Journal of Clinical Pharmacology and Therapeutics, 38*(10), 486-491.

Hendriks, V.M., van den Brink, W., Blanken, P., et al. (2001). Heroin self-administration by means of 'chasing the dragon': Pharmacodynamics and bioavailability of inhaled heroin. *European Neuropsychopharmacology, 11*(3), 241-252.

Hopfer, C.J., Mikulich, S.K., & Crowley, T.J. (2000). Heroin use among adolescents in treatment for substance use disorders. *Journal of the American Academy of Child & Adolescent Psychiatry, 39*(10), 1316-1323.

Hosztafi, S. (2001). [Heroin. II. Preparation, hydrolysis, stability, pharmacokinetics] [Hungarian]. *Acta Pharmaceutica Hungarica, 71*(3), 373-383.

Klous, M.G., Van den Brink, W., Van Ree, J.M., et al. (2005). Development of pharmaceutical heroin preparations for medical co-prescriptions to opioid dependent patients. *Drug and Alcohol Dependence, 80*(3), 283-295.

Krantz, A.J., Hershow, R.C., Prachand, N., et al. (2003). Heroin insufflation as a trigger for patients with life-threatening asthma. *Chest, 123*(2), 510-517.

Metrebian, N., Carnwath, T., Stimson, G.V., et al. (2002). Survey of doctors prescribing diamorphine (heroin) to opiate-dependent drug users in the United Kingdom. *Addiction, 97*(9), 1155-1161.

Miller, C.L., Spittal, P.M., LaLiberte, N., et al. (2002). Females experiencing sexual and drug vulnerabilities are at elevated risk for HIV infection among youth who use injection drugs. *Journal of Acquired Immune Deficiency Syndrome, 30*(3), 335-341.

Minozzi, S., Amato, L., Vecchi, S., et al. (2008). Maintenance agonist treatments for opiate dependent pregnant women. *Cochrane Database of Systematic Reviews, 16*(2), CD006318.

Page, J.B., & Fraile, J.S. (1999). Lemon juice as a solvent for heroin in Spain. *Substance Use & Misuse, 34*(8), 1193-1197.

Rentsch, K.M., Kullak-Ublick, G.A., Reichel, C., et al. (2001). Arterial and venous pharmacokinetics of intravenous heroin in subjects who are addicted to narcotics. *Clinical Pharmacology and Therapeutics, 70*(3), 237-246.

Rice, E.K., Isbel, N.M., Becker, G.J., et al. (2000). Heroin overdose and myoglobinuric acute renal failure. *Clinical Nephrology, 54*(6), 449-454.

Rook, E.J., Huitema, A.D., van den Brink, W., et al. (2006). Pharmacokinetics and pharmacodynamic variability of heroin and its metabolites: Review of the literature. *Current Clinical Pharmacology, 1*(1), 109-118.

Rook, E.J., Huitema, A.D., van den Brink, W., et al. (2006). Population pharmacokinetics of heroin and its major metabolites. *Clinical Pharmacokinetics, 45*(4), 401-417.

Rook, E.J., van Ree, J.M., van den Brink, W., et al. (2006). Pharmacokinetics and pharmacodynamics of high doses of pharmaceutically prepared heroin, by intravenous or by inhalation route in opioid-dependent patients. *Basic & Clinical Pharmacology & Toxicology, 98(1)*, 86-96.

Roy, E., Haley, N., Leclerc, P., et al. (2002). Drug injection among street youth: The first time. *Addiction,* 97(8), 1003-1009.

Sanchez, J., Comerford, M., Chitwood, D.D., et al. (2002). High risk sexual behaviours among heroin sniffers who have no history of injection drug use: Implications for HIV risk reduction. *AIDS Care,* 14(3), 391-398.

Schoener, E.P., Hopper, J.A., & Pierre, J.D. (2002). Injection drug use in North America. *Infectious Disease Clinics of North America, 16(3)*, 535-551.

Smith, M.L., Shimomura, E.T., Summers, J., et al. (2001). Urinary excretion profiles for total morphine, free morphine, and 6-acetylmorphine following smoked and intravenous heroin. *Journal of Analytical Toxicology, 25(7)*, 504-514.

Tarabar, A.F., & Nelson, L.S. (2003). The resurgence and abuse of heroin by children in the United States. *Current Opinion in Pediatrics, 15(2)*, 210-215.

Warner-Smith, M., Darke, S., & Day, C. (2002). Morbidity associated with non-fatal heroin overdose. *Addiction, 97(8)*, 963-967.

Warner-Smith, M., Darke, S., Lynskey, M., et al. (2001). Heroin overdose: Causes and consequences. *Addiction, 96(8)*, 1113-1125.

HYDROCODONE

Names

BAN or INN Generic Synonyms: Dihydrocodeine

Brand/Trade: Hycodan®[1]

Chemical: 4,5-α-Epoxy-3-methoxy-17-methylmorphinan-6-one

Street: Diffs; Duncan Flockharts; Hyke; Tuss; Vikes

Pharmacologic Classification

Psychodepressant, opiate analgesic: pure agonist, semisynthetic (antitussive)

Brief General Overview

Hydrocodone was first synthesized nearly 100 years ago. It is structurally related to codeine. Although its efficacy and pharmacologic actions closely resemble those of morphine, its potency is only about two-thirds that of morphine. During the 1990s, the personal use of opiate analgesics for their psychodepressant actions came back into vogue in North America. The use of hydrocodone skyrocketed, with production increasing over 400%, prescription use increasing over 300%, and hydrocodone-related emergency department visits increasing 500%. Hydrocodone is the most frequently prescribed opiate analgesic in the United States.

Dosage Forms and Routes of Administration

Hydrocodone is produced by several licit pharmaceutical manufacturers in North America. It is available in oral elixir, syrup, and tablet formulations[2] and is usually orally ingested. However, some hydrocodone users crush or pulverize the oral tablet into a fine powder that they intranasally sniff (snort). Hydrocodone is not clandestinely produced. All the hydrocodone that is obtained for personal use has been diverted from licit pharmaceutical manufacturers (e.g., by forged or altered prescriptions; nursing home and pharmacy break and entries). North American women of European descent between 20 and 40 years of age are the most common hydrocodone users. Many hydrocodone users, women and men alike of all races, are being medically managed for chronic pain. Increasingly over the past 5 years, hydrocodone use has been reported among high school students.

Mechanism of CNS Action

Hydrocodone elicits its analgesic, psychodepressant, and respiratory depressant actions primarily by binding to the endorphin (opiate) receptors in the CNS. However, its exact mechanism of action has not been determined (see Opiate Analgesics monograph).

Pharmacodynamics/Pharmacokinetics

Hydrocodone is adequately absorbed after oral ingestion. Peak blood concentrations generally are achieved within 1.5 hours. The duration of action is 4 to 8 hours. Hydrocodone is extensively metabolized in the liver. The mean elimination half-life is ~4 hours.

Current Approved Indications for Medical Use

Cough suppression (particularly for the management of exhausting, nonproductive cough); pain, moderate

Desired Action/Reason for Personal Use

Euphoria; "rush"[3]; prevention/self-management of the hydrocodone, or other opiate analgesic, withdrawal syndrome

Toxicity[4]

Acute: Blurred vision; cognitive impairment; constipation; dizziness; drowsiness; lethargy; nausea; psychomotor impairment; respiratory depression; sedation; vomiting

Chronic: Fungal rhinosinusitis, invasive (with intranasal snorting); hearing loss, sensorineural; nasal mucosal irritation and damage (with intranasal snorting)[5]; physical dependence; psychological dependence

Pregnancy & Lactation: FDA Pregnancy Category C (see Appendix B). Safety of hydrocodone use by adolescent girls and women who are pregnant has not been established. Hydrocodone crosses the placenta. Neonates whose mothers regularly used hydrocodone during pregnancy display signs and symptoms of the opiate analgesic withdrawal syndrome. Adolescent girls and women who are pregnant should not use hydrocodone.

Safety of hydrocodone use by adolescent girls and women who are breast-feeding has not been established. Additional valid and reliable data are needed.

Abuse Potential

Physical dependence: High (USDEA Schedule II; high potential for abuse)[6]
Psychological dependence: Moderate to high

Withdrawal Syndrome

A hydrocodone withdrawal syndrome has been reported. Abrupt discontinuation of hydrocodone after regular, long-term use results in signs and symptoms of the opiate analgesic withdrawal syndrome (see Opiate Analgesics monograph).

Overdosage

Signs and symptoms of hydrocodone overdosage are an exacerbation of its psycho-depressant and other actions and include apnea; bradycardia; cardiac arrest; cold, clammy skin; extreme somnolence progressing to stupor or coma; respiratory depression; and skeletal muscle flaccidity. Hydrocodone overdosage may be fatal and requires emergency medical support of body systems, with attention to increasing hydrocodone elimination and re-establishment of adequate respiratory function. The opiate analgesic antagonist naloxone (Narcan®) usually is effective for the medical management of associated respiratory depression.[7] The duration of action of hydrocodone may exceed that of naloxone, so repeated doses of naloxone may be required during the course of emergency medical management of hydrocodone overdosage.

Notes

1. Hydrocodone is most commonly available in combination products that usually contain acetaminophen. Examples are Lortab® and Vicodin®.
2. The oral elixir and syrup formulations are generally used for cough suppression. The oral tablets are usually used for the medical management of acute pain (moderate to moderately severe).
3. Rapid, generalized sensation of warmth that is physiologically associated with histamine release and a consequent increase in peripheral blood flow.
4. Abuse of combination products increases toxicity (e.g., products containing acetaminophen present an additional risk for liver toxicity).
5. Nasal septal perforation and erosion of the lateral nasal walls, nasopharynx, and soft palate have been reported.
6. Combination products containing hydrocodone and nonopiate medicinal ingredients are classified as USDEA Schedule III (moderate potential for abuse).
7. Caution is required when naloxone is administered to hydrocodone users who are physically dependent, because it may precipitate signs and symptoms of the opiate analgesic withdrawal syndrome in these users.

References

Baker, D.D., & Jenkins, A.J. (2008). A comparison of methadone, oxycodone, and hydrocodone related deaths in Northeast Ohio. *Journal of Analytical Toxicology, 32*(2), 165-171.

Friedman, R.A., House, J.W., Luxford, W.M., et al. (2000). Profound hearing loss associated with hydrocodone/acetaminophen abuse. *The American Journal of Otology, 21*(2), 188-191.

Havens, J.R., Walker, R., & Leukefeld, C.G. (2008). Prescription opioid use in the rural Appalachia: A community-based study. *Journal of Opioid Management, 4*(2), 63-71.

Katz, N., Fernandez, K., Chang, A., et al. (2008). Internet-based survey of nonmedical prescription opioid use in the United States. *The Clinical Journal of Pain, 24*(6), 528-535.

Yewell, J., Haydon, R., Archer, S., et al. (2002). Complications of intranasal prescription narcotic abuse. *The Annals of Otology, Rhinology, and Laryngology, 111*(2), 174-177.

HYDROMORPHONE

Names

BAN or INN Generic Synonyms: Dihydromorphinone

Brand/Trade: Dilaudid®; Hydromorph Contin®; Hydromroph IR®; HydroStat®; OROS® Hydromorphone

Chemical: 4,5-α-Epoxy-3-hydroxy-17-methylmorphinan-6-one

Street: Big D; Delantz; Delats; Delaud; Delida; Dillies; Ds; DS; Dust; Footballs; Hillbilly Heroin; Juice; Little D; Lords

Pharmacologic Classification

Psychodepressant, opiate analgesic: pure agonist (semisynthetic)

Brief General Overview

Hydromorphone is synthetically produced by the chemical modification of morphine. It is approximately 10 times more potent than morphine when both drugs are administered intravenously, but it shares essentially the same efficacy and clinical profile. (Also see the Morphine monograph.)

Dosage Forms and Routes of Administration

Hydromorphone is produced by several licit pharmaceutical manufacturers in North America. It is available in several dosage formulations, including injectables for intramuscular, intravenous, and subcutaneous use; rectal suppositories; and oral tablets, including controlled-release formulations. Hydromorphone is personally used for its psychodepressant actions and is sometimes used as a substitute for heroin. Users often obtain the hydromorphone oral tablets, which they dissolve and intravenously inject. Hydromorphone is not clandestinely produced. All the hydromorphone that is personally used has been diverted from licit pharmaceutical manufacturers (e.g., by forged or altered prescriptions; nursing home and pharmacy break and entries).

Mechanism of CNS Action

Although the exact mechanism of action has not been clearly established, hydromorphone appears to elicit its analgesic, psychodepressant (e.g., drowsiness, changes in mood, and mental clouding), and respiratory depressant actions primarily by binding to the endorphin (opiate) receptors in the CNS. Hydromorphone preferentially binds to the mu receptors. It also has been demonstrated to significantly increase cerebral blood flow in the limbic system (e.g., amygdala, anterior cingulate cortex, and thalamus). However, this action has not been clearly related to its mechanism of CNS action. Also see the Opiate Analgesics monograph.

Pharmacodynamics/Pharmacokinetics

Hydromorphone is rapidly absorbed after oral ingestion and produces analgesia within 30 minutes. Oral bioavailability is ~30%. Intranasal bioavailability is ~50%. After intravenous injection, hydromorphone produces analgesia within 5 minutes. Hydromorphone is extensively metabolized in the liver to a glucuronide conjugate that is excreted in the urine. The mean elimination half-life is ~3 hours and the mean total body clearance is 1.7 L/minute.

Dose-dumping (i.e., the premature and exaggerated release of drug from its delivery system) has been associated with the concomitant use of alcohol and the oral extended-release formulations of hydromorphone (e.g., Palladone®, which was voluntarily withdrawn from the market in 2005). This interaction has not been reported with other controlled-release formulations (e.g., OROS® Hydromorphone). In addition, the ingestion of food does not significantly affect the bioavailability of some hydromorphone controlled-release products (i.e., OROS® Hydromorphone).

Current Approved Indications for Medical Use

Cough suppression; pain, moderate to severe

Desired Action/Reason for Personal Use

Euphoria (mild); prevention/self-management of the opiate analgesic withdrawal syndrome; relaxation

Toxicity

Acute[1]: Apnea; cognitive impairment; constipation; dizziness; drowsiness; dry mouth; flushing; hypotension, postural; lethargy; lightheadedness; miosis; nausea; pain at injection site; pruritus; reduced interest in sex; respiratory depression; sedation; sweating; vomiting

Chronic: Constipation; menstrual irregularity; physical dependence; psychological dependence

Pregnancy & Lactation: FDA Pregnancy Category C (see Appendix B). Safety of hydromorphone use by adolescent girls and women who are pregnant has not been established. Neonates whose mothers regularly used hydromorphone during pregnancy display signs and symptoms of the opiate analgesic withdrawal syndrome (see Opiate Analgesics monograph). Adolescent girls and women who are pregnant should not use hydromorphone.

Safety of hydromorphone use by adolescent girls and women who are breast-feeding has not been established. It is not known whether hydromorphone is excreted in breast milk. Additional valid and reliable data are needed.

Abuse Potential

Physical dependence: High (USDEA Schedule II; high potential for abuse)
Psychological dependence: Moderate to high

Withdrawal Syndrome

Several weeks of regular hydromorphone use may result in physical and psychological dependence. Abrupt discontinuation will result in the hydromorphone withdrawal syndrome, which is generally similar to but less severe than the withdrawal syndrome associated with heroin or morphine. Signs and symptoms of the hydromorphone withdrawal syndrome include abdominal pain, anorexia, anxiety, diarrhea, gooseflesh, insomnia, muscle pain, muscle spasms, tachycardia, tremor, watery eyes, and yawning. Most of the signs and symptoms resolve within 1 week after the discontinuation of hydromorphone use.

Overdosage

Signs and symptoms of hydromorphone overdosage include respiratory depression (decreased rate and tidal volume, Cheyne-Stokes respiration, cyanosis), extreme somnolence progressing to stupor or coma, skeletal muscle flaccidity, cold and clammy skin, and, sometimes, bradycardia and hypotension. Severe overdosage, particularly that associated with intravenous injection, may result in apnea, circulatory collapse, cardiac arrest, and death.

Hydromorphone overdosage requires emergency medical support of body systems, with attention to increasing hydromorphone elimination, particularly when the overdosage has involved the oral dosage forms. The opiate antagonist naloxone (Narcan®) is the specific antidote for respiratory depression.[2] The duration of action of hydromorphone may exceed that of naloxone, so repeated doses of naloxone may be required during the course of emergency medical management of hydromorphone overdosage.

Notes

1. Rapid intravenous injection significantly increases the risk for both hypotension and respiratory depression.
2. Caution is required when naloxone is administered to hydromorphone users who are physically dependent, because it may precipitate the hydromorphone withdrawal syndrome in these users.

References

Hill, J.L., & Azcny, J.P. (2000). Comparing the subjective, psychomotor, and physiological effects of intravenous hydromorphone and morphine in healthy volunteers. *Psychopharmacology, 152*(1), 31-39.

Hong, D., Flood, P., & Diaz, G. (2008). The side effects of morphine and hydromorphone patient-controlled analgesia. *Anesthesia and Analgesia, 107*(4), 1384-1389.

Quigley, C. (2002). Hydromorphone for acute and chronic pain. *Cochrane Database of Systematic Reviews* (1), CD003447.

Sarhill, N., Walsh, D., & Nelson, K.A. (2001). Hydromorphone: Pharmacology and clinical applications in cancer patients. *Supportive Care in Cancer, 9*(2), 84-96.

Sathyan, G., Sivakumar, K., & Thipphawong, J. (2008). Pharmacokinetic profile of a 24-hour controlled-release OROS formulation of hydromorphone in the presence of alcohol. *Current Medical Research and Opinion, 24*(1), 297-305.

Sathyan, G., Xu, E., Thipphawong, J., et al. (2007). Pharmacokinetic profile of a 24-hour controlled-release OROS formulation of hydromorphone in the presence and absence of food. *BioMed Central(BMC) Clinical Pharmacology, 7,* 2.

7-HYDROXYMITRAGYNINE (See *Kratom*)

IBOGAINE

Names

BAN or INN Generic Synonyms: None

Brand/Trade: None

Chemical: 12-Methoxyibogamine

Street: Bocca; Boga; *Eboga*; *Eboge*; Eboka; Iboga; *Lebuga*; *Leoga*; Libuga

Pharmacologic Classification

Psychostimulant (lower dosages) and Psychodelic (higher dosages), miscellaneous: iboga alkaloid (natural)

Brief General Overview

Ibogaine is extracted from the roots of the equatorial African rain forest shrub *Tabernanthe iboga*.[1] It is used for its psychostimulant actions and, at higher dosages, for inducing hallucinations as a component of tribal religious ceremonies and rites (e.g., within the Bwiti religion in West Central Africa).

Dosage Forms and Routes of Administration

Ibogaine can be chemically synthesized, but the synthetic form is rarely available. The most common source is the natural alkaloid directly obtained from the root of *Tabernanthe iboga*. The root bark, preferably from a fresh plant, is rasped off, dried, and ground into a powder. The powder is orally ingested, usually after mixing with water. Although widely used in traditional religious ceremonies and rites by certain tribes in equatorial Africa, in North America ibogaine is used only occasionally by immigrants from these regions. Rarely, ibogaine is used by "drug experimenters" for its psychostimulant and psychodelic actions. These groups of users are usually men 18 to 30 years of age of European descent who either have traveled to parts of Africa where "iboga root" is used and available for purchase or have some background in college-level organic chemistry that enables them to synthesize the ibogaine.

Mechanism of CNS Action

The exact mechanisms of ibogaine's psychostimulant and psychodelic actions have not been determined. However, it appears that its psychostimulant actions are related to its binding to N-methyl-D-aspartate (NMDA) receptors in the CNS. In addition, ibogaine has been demonstrated to cause functional blockade of both human muscle-type and ganglionic nicotinic acetylcholine (nACh) receptors.

Ibogaine's hallucinogenic actions putatively are related to its interactions with serotonin receptors, specifically 5-HT2A and 5-HT2C. This action may involve the noncompetitive inhibition of serotonin transporter (see the "Pharmacodynamics/Pharmacokinetics" section).

Pharmacodynamics/Pharmacokinetics

Ibogaine is metabolized predominantly in the liver by microsomal enzyme cytochrome P450 2D6 to several metabolites. 0-demethylation of ibogaine results in the production of the active metabolite, 12-hydroxyibogamine (i.e., noribogaine). Noribogaine has a high affinity for the 5-HT transporter and elevates extracellular concentrations of 5-HT (i.e., serotonin). Additional valid and reliable data are not available.

Current Approved Indications for Medical Use

None[2]

Desired Action/Reason for Personal Use

Alertness, vigilance, or wakefulness; appetite or hunger suppression; decrease fatigue; diminish craving for cocaine or heroin; enhance ceremonial dancing and drumming abilities[3]; euphoria (mild); hallucinations (primarily visual, with vivid colors and bright lights); self-management of the opiate analgesic withdrawal syndrome; sexual arousal or desire (increased); visions[4]

Toxicity

Acute: Appetite suppression; cardiac dysrhythmias; distortion of sense of time; hypotension; loss of consciousness; nausea; psychomotor stimulation; vomiting

Chronic: Valid and reliable data are not available.

Pregnancy & Lactation: Valid and reliable data are not available.

Abuse Potential

Physical dependence: None to low (USDEA Schedule I; use is prohibited)
Psychological dependence: Low

Withdrawal Syndrome

An ibogaine withdrawal syndrome has not been reported.

Overdosage

Oral ingestion of high dosages of ibogaine has resulted in seizures, respiratory paralysis, and death. Ibogaine overdosage may require emergency medical management of body systems, with particular attention to controlling seizures and maintaining respiratory function. There is no known antidote.

Notes

1. Ibogaine is the principal active alkaloid found in the root of *Tabernanthe iboga*. It is isomeric with tabernanthine (i.e., it has the same molecular formula but its chemical structure is a mirror image).
2. Ibogaine has been researched and touted for pharmacotherapeutic use to attenuate drug craving and resultant drug-seeking behavior, particularly in regard to problematic patterns of alcohol, cocaine, nicotine, and opiate analgesic use. To date, however, satisfactory scientific evidence to support this claim is lacking.
3. Generally, in conjunction with the rites of African iboga cults, such as in Gabonian initiation ceremonies in which a "near death" experience is purposely induced by the tribal priest/healer.
4. At relatively high dosages, hallucinogenic visions are induced. Members of African iboga cults believe the visions facilitate communication with deceased ancestors.

References

Alper, K.R., Lotsof, H.S., & Kaplan, C.D. (2008). The ibogaine medical subculture. *Journal of Ethnopharmacology, 115*(1), 9-24.

He, D.Y., & Ron, D. (2006). Autoregulation of glial cell line-derived neurotrophic factor expression: Implications for the long-lasting actions of the anti-addiction drug, ibogaine. *Journal of the Federation of American Societies for Experimental Biology, 20*(13), 2420-2422.

Helsley, S., Rabin, R.A., & Winter, J.C. (2001). Drug discrimination studies with ibogaine. *Alkaloids and Chemical Biology, 56*, 63-77.

Hittner, J.B., & Quello, S.B. (2004). Combating substance abuse with ibogaine: Pre- and posttreatment recommendations and an example of successive model fitting analyses. *Journal of Pyschoactive Drugs, 36*(2), 191-199.

Jacobs, M.T., Zhang, Y.W., Campbell, S.D., et al. (2007). Ibogaine, a noncompetitive inhibitor of serotonin transport, acts by stabilizing the cytoplasm-facing state of the transporter. *Journal of Biological Chemistry, 282*(40), 29441-29447.

Maas, U., & Strubelt, S. (2006). Fatalities after taking ibogaine in addiction treatment could be related to sudden cardiac death caused by autonomic dysfunction. *Medical Hypotheses, 67*(4), 960-964.

Mash, D.C., Kovera, C.A., Pablo, J., et al. (2000). Ibogaine: Complex pharmacokinetics, concerns for safety, and preliminary efficacy measures. *Annals of the New York Academy of Sciences, 914*, 394-401.

Onaivi, E.S., Ali, S.F., Chirwa, S.S., et al. (2002). Ibogaine signals addiction genes and methamphetamine alteration of long-term potentiation. *Annals of the New York Academy of Sciences, 965*, 28-46.

Szumlinski, K.K., Haskew, R.E., Balogun, M.Y., et al. (2001). Iboga compounds reverse the behavioural disinhibiting and corticosterone effects of acute methamphetamine: Implications for their antiaddictive properties. *Pharmacology, Biochemistry, and Behavior, 69*(3-4), 485-491.

Szumlinski, K.K., Maisonneuve, I.M., & Glick, S.D. (2001). Iboga interactions with psychomotor stimulants: Panacea in the paradox? *Toxicon, 39*(1), 75-86.

INHALANTS (See Volatile solvents & inhalants)

ISOBUTANE (See Volatile solvents & inhalants)

ISOMEPROBAMATE (See Meprobamate)

KAVA

Names

BAN or INN Generic Synonyms: None

Brand/Trade: None

Chemical: See "Mechanism of CNS Action"

Street: *Ava; 'Awa; Gea; Gi;* Grog; Intoxicating Long Pepper; Intoxicating Pepper; Kao; *Kava-Kava;* Kawa-Kawa; Kawa Pepper; Kew; Malohu; Maluk; Meruk; Milik; *Pepe Kava;* Sakau; Tonga; Wurzelstock; *Yagona; Yangona; Yaqona; Yongona*

Pharmacologic Classification

Psychodepressant, sedative-hypnotic: miscellaneous (naturally occurring kava pyrones)

Brief General Overview

Kava is obtained from the roots (rhizomes) of the shrublike perennial plant *Piper methysticum,* a member of the black pepper family. *Piper methysticum* appears to grow best in tropical climates near sea level and is indigenous to the South Pacific islands, including Fiji, Hawaii, New Guinea, Samoa, Tahiti, the Solomons, and Tonga. Its ceremonial and other social use by various Polynesian tribes dates back thousands of years.

Dosage Forms and Routes of Administration

Kava is now grown by many farmers, particularly in Polynesia, as a cash crop. *Kava*-containing herbal products, generally in the form of oral capsules, are widely available across North America. In addition, the root of *Piper methysticum* can be purchased from several Internet sites for priority delivery anywhere in North America.[1] Traditionally, the root is dried, pounded into a powder, and then mixed into a beverage. The primary mode of use of *kava,* both historically and currently, has been as a nonfermented beverage that causes relatively mild and tranquil intoxication.[2] Reportedly, this beverage does not cause the cognitive and memory impairment that is generally associated with the use of similarly acting psychodepressants, such as alcohol (see monograph) and the benzodiazepines (see monograph). However, concomitant *kava* use can potentiate alcohol-induced impairment.

Mechanism of CNS Action

The CNS actions of *kava* are related to several *kava* pyrones (kava lactones), including 5,6-demethoxyyangonin (5,6-desmethoxyyangonin), 7,8-dihydrokawain (7,8-dihydrokavain), 4,8-dihydromethysticin, dihydroyangonin, kawain (kavain), methysticin, and yangonin. The exact mechanism of *kava's* psychodepressant action has not been determined. However, it has been determined that *kava* inhibits the cyclooxygenase enzyme and MAO-B. In addition, binding inhibition has been demonstrated at dopamine (D2), GABA, histamine (H1 and H2), and opiate (mu and delta) receptor sites. Areas of action within the CNS appear to primarily involve the amygdala complex, limbic system structures, and the reticular formation.

Pharmacodynamics/Pharmacokinetics

Valid and reliable data are not available.

Current Approved Indications for Medical Use[3]

None

Desired Action/Reason for Personal Use

Anxiety/stress reduction; euphoria; magico-religious ceremonial use by tribal priests of various South Pacific island cultures; relaxation[4]; sleep promotion; sociability

Toxicity

Acute: Anorexia; blurred vision; dizziness; fatigue; headache; GI irritation; mydriasis; nausea; numbing/tingling of the mouth (due to *kava's* local anesthetic effects); psychomotor impairment

Chronic: Dry, scaly skin rash (ichthyosiform kava dermopathy) known in Fijian as *Kanikani*; hepatic dysfunction[5]; mental depression; neurological impairment; parkinsonism (extrapyramidal reactions), in genetically susceptible users[6]; pulmonary hypertension; shortness of breath

Pregnancy & Lactation: Safety of *kava* use by adolescent girls and women who are pregnant has not been established. However, *kava* may decrease uterine muscle strength. Therefore, adolescent girls and women who are pregnant, particularly near term or during labor, should not use *kava*. Additional valid and reliable data are needed.

Kava appears to be excreted in breast milk. However, no adverse effects have been reported in breast-fed neonates or infants. Additional valid and reliable data are needed.

Abuse Potential

Physical dependence: None to low (USDEA: not a scheduled drug)
Psychological dependence: Low

Withdrawal Syndrome

A *kava* withdrawal syndrome has not been reported.

Overdosage

Valid and reliable data are not available.

Notes

1. The root can be purchased whole, pounded, as shavings, or in powdered form.
2. This method of use has sometimes been referred to as the "Fiji" method. An alternative method of use, sometimes referred to as the "Tonga" method, involves chewing the kava root (rhizome), spitting

the chewed root into a bowl, filtering the concoction, and then drinking the filtered liquid in a single gulp to avoid the bitter, pungent taste.

3. *Kava* has a long use in traditional folk medicine. It has been used for a variety of conditions and diseases, including addiction, anxiety, arthritis, asthma, birth control, indigestion, joint pain, kidney stones, leprosy, menopausal symptoms, migraine headaches, pain, premenstrual syndrome, seizures, stroke, syphilis, toothache, tuberculosis, vaginitis, and weight reduction.

4. In conjunction with tribal social use among friends and relatives, usually males. The social use of *kava* is similar to that of *khat* (see *Catha edulis* monograph). In a somewhat related context of use, several "*kava* bars" and lounges have been established in the United States specifically to sell *kava* drinks.

5. Has reportedly resulted in liver failure (relatively rare). The hepatoxicity associated with *kava* use may be due to a direct hepatotoxic effect of *kava*, possibly as a result of inhibition of cyclooxygenase activity, inhibition of cytochrome P450, mitochondrial toxicity, reduction in liver glutathione content, or a combination of these. Other reports have suggested contaminants in the *kava* formulations as a result of different extraction processes (e.g., acetonic or alcoholic). Additional valid and reliable data are needed.

6. *Kava* also has been found to reduce the efficacy of levodopa when used to treat parkinsonism (i.e., concomitant *kava* use results in increased "off" periods).

References

Bilia, A.R., Gallon, S., & Vincieri, F.F. (2002). Kava-kava and anxiety: Growing knowledge about the efficacy and safety. *Life Sciences, 70*(22), 2581-2597.

Centers for Disease Control and Prevention (CDC). Hepatic toxicity possibly associated with kava-containing products United States, Germany, and Switzerland, 1999-2002. *MMWR Morbidity and Mortality Weekly Report, 51*(47), 1065-1067.

Clouatre, D.L. (2004). Kava kava: Examining new reports of toxicity. *Toxicology Letters, 150*(1), 85-96.

Denham, A., McIntyre, M., & Whitehouse, J. (2002). Kava—the unfolding story: Report on a work-in-progress. *Journal of Alternative and Complementary Medicine, 8*(3), 237-263.

Dinh, L.D., Simmen, U., Bueter, K.B., et al. (2001). Interaction of various Piper methysticum cultivars with CNS receptors in vitro. *Planta Medica, 67*(4), 306-311.

Ernst, E. (2002). The risk-benefit profile of commonly used herbal therapies: Ginkgo, St. John's wort, ginseng, echinacea, saw palmetto, and kava. *Annals of Internal Medicine, 136*(1), 42-53.

Fu, P.P., Xia, Q., Guo, L., et al. (2008). Toxicity of kava kava. *Journal of Environmental Science and Health –Part C: Environmental Carcinogenesis & Ecotoxicology Reviews, 26*(1), 89-112.

Gounder, R. (2006). Kava consumption and its health effects. *Pacific Health Dialog, 13*(2), 131-135.

Humberston, C.L., Akhtar, J., & Krenzelok, E.P. (2003). Acute hepatitis induced by kava kava. *Journal of Toxicology-Clinical Toxicology, 41*(2), 109-113.

Izzo, A.A., & Ernst, E. (2001). Interactions between herbal medicines and prescribed drugs: A systematic review. *Drugs, 61*(15), 2163-2175.

Kava, R. (2001). The adverse effects of kava. *Pacific Health Dialog, 8*(1), 115-118.

Kraft, M., Spahn, T.W., Menzel, J., et al. (2001). [Fulminant liver failure after administration of the herbal antidepressant kava-kava] [German]. *Deutsche Medizinische Wochenschrift, 126*(36), 970-972.

Lüde, S., Török, M., Dieterie, S., et al. (2008). Hepatocellular toxicity of kava leaf and root extracts. *Phytomedicine, 15*(1-2), 120-131.

Meseguer, E., Taboada, R., Sanchez, V., et al. (2002). Life-threatening parkinsonism induced by kava-kava. *Movement Disorders, 17*(1), 195-196.

O'Sullivan, H.M., & Lum, K. (2001). Herbal medicine on the rise: The case of 'awa. *Pacific Health Dialog, 8*(2), 380-387.

Pittler, M.H., & Ernst, E. (2000). Efficacy of kava extract for treating anxiety: Systematic review and meta-analysis. *Journal of Clinical Psychopharmacology, 20*(1), 84-89.

Stevinson, C., Huntley, A.M., & Ernst, E. (2002). A systematic review of the safety of kava extract in the treatment of anxiety. *Drug Safety, 25*(4), 251-261.

Stickel, F., Baumüller, H.M., Seitz, K., et al. (2003). Hepatitis induced by Kava (Piper methysticum rhizoma). *Journal of Hepatology, 39*(1), 62-67.

Wheatley, D. (2001). Kava and valerian in the treatment of stress-induced insomnia. *Phytotherapy Research, 15*(6), 549-551.

Whitton, P.A., Lau, A., Salisbury, A., et al. (2003). Kava lactones and the kava-kava controversy. *Phytochemistry, 64*(3), 673-679.

Wu, D., Yu, L., Nair, M.G., et al. (2002). Cyclooxygenase enzyme inhibitory compounds with antioxidant activities from Piper methysticum (kava kava) roots. *Phytomedicine, 9*(1), 41-47.

KETAMINE

Names

BAN or INN Generic Synonyms: None

Brand/Trade: Ketajet®; Ketalar®; Ketaset®

Chemical: 2-(2-Chlorophenyl)-2-(methylamino)-cyclohexanone

Street: Blind Squid; Breakfast Cereal; Bump; Cat; Cat Tranquilizer; Cat Valium; Green; Horse Tranquilizer; Jet; Jet Fuel; K; Kay Jay; Keezy; Keller; Keller's Day; Kenny; Ket; Ket Kat; KFC; Kit-Kat; Kitty; KKK; Klarko K Kat; Klarky Kat; K-Train; Kustard; K Wire; New Ecstasy; Old Man; Property of Sir John; Psychedelic Heroin; Purple; Regretamine; Special "K"; Special La Coke; Super Acid; Super C; Super K; Triple K; Vetamine; Vitamin K; Vit K; Wonky

Pharmacologic Classification

Psychodelic, miscellaneous: cataleptic (dissociative) general anesthetic

Brief General Overview

Ketamine was originally developed during the early 1960s as an "eyes open," or dissociative, anesthetic that would not excessively suppress respiratory function (similar in many ways to phencyclidine [PCP; see monograph]). It was widely used on the battlefields of the Vietnam War. Today it is used primarily in veterinary medicine as an anesthetic, but it is also used in humans, particularly for short surgical procedures or as an adjunct to other general anesthetics. Ketamine is personally used for its psychodelic actions. However, over the last decade it also has been used in the context of date rape and other crimes.

Ketamine is manufactured by licit pharmaceutical companies, primarily outside of North America (i.e., Belgium, China, Colombia, Germany, and India). It is legally imported for both human (10%) and animal (90%) use. Ketamine is illegally obtained for illicit use, often through burglary of veterinary clinics. Although a significant amount of ketamine is smuggled into North America, Mexico has become the primary source of illicit ketamine in the United States over the past 5 years.

Ketamine is reportedly used by high school students at all grade levels. However, it is primarily used at dance clubs and raves by young men, usually of middle-class European descent, in their late 20s.[1] Other users are gay and bisexual men of all ages. Ketamine use is extremely high among members of the gay and bisexual community, regardless of race. These men commonly intranasally snort ketamine as one of their five main party or club drugs (i.e., cocaine, gamma-hydroxybutyrate [GBH], ketamine, methamphetamine, and methylenedioxymethamphetamine [MDMA]; see monographs). These party drugs are used to facilitate social disinhibition, arouse sexual desire, and enhance sexual experiences among members of the gay and bisexual community.

Dosage Forms and Routes of Administration

Ketamine is generally available as an aqueous solution for intramuscular injection or as a dry powder. Although users can intramuscularly inject the ketamine solution, a more popular method of use involves evaporating the liquid from the injectable formulation until all that remains is the dry residue of the drug. The residue is then ground into a crystalline powder and intranasally sniffed (snorted).[2] Ketamine also can be smoked. Smoking involves dipping a marijuana or tobacco cigarette into the ketamine solution and then smoking the cigarette. If preferred, the ketamine powder from the residue can be sprinkled on marijuana buds or tobacco leaves prior to rolling a "joint" or cigarette.

Mechanism of CNS Action

Ketamine and other dissociative anesthetics allow sensory impulses to reach the brain but cause them to be interpreted in a distorted manner. As the dosage increases, analgesia progresses to anesthesia and then coma. The eyes remain open. Ketamine appears to elicit its anesthetic action by selectively depressing the thalamoneocortical system prior to obtunding the reticular activating and limbic systems (i.e., it selectively interrupts association pathways in the CNS prior to producing somesthetic sensory blockade). The analgesic action of ketamine, which is noted at subanesthetic dosages, appears to be related to its antagonism (i.e., blocking) of the N-methyl-D-aspartate (NMDA) receptors. This action in turn prevents the excitatory amino acids aspartate and glutamate from eliciting their actions in various CNS locations, including the cerebral cortex.

Pharmacodynamics/Pharmacokinetics

Ketamine blood concentrations and actions appear to be poorly correlated, and the pharmacokinetics of ketamine displays significant intersubject variability. Available data suggest that much of the variability is due to enantiomer-specific differences; variability depends on whether the S(+), R(-), or racemic form (±) is used. In addition, variability reportedly decreases with advancing age in children.

Onset of action is dependent on the route of administration: 1 to 5 minutes, intramuscular injection; 5 to 15 minutes, intranasal snorting; and 5 to 30 minutes, oral ingestion. Some ketamine is excreted unchanged in the urine together with its major metabolite, norketamine. Total body clearance of ketamine usually ranges from 1 to 1.5 L/minute. Effects tend to last ~1 hour. However, some users have reported residual effects lasting for up to 24 hours. Additional valid and reliable data are not available.

Current Approved Indications for Medical Use

Anesthesia (generally, for brief procedural sedation in the emergency department)

Desired Action/Reason for Personal Use[3]

Arouse sexual desires (particularly, among gay and bisexual men); dreamy, semi-conscious state of intoxication; enhance sexual experiences (particularly, among gay and bisexual men); euphoria; hallucinations; social disinhibition (particularly, among gay and bisexual men); vivid dreaming; also, ketamine is purposely given to others, without their knowledge, in the context of the perpetration of drug-facilitated crime (e.g., robbery; sexual assault, including date rape)

Toxicity

Acute: Amnesia, anterograde; anesthesia paralysis (loss of voluntary motion or inability to move the body); anxiety; ataxia; blood pressure, increased; blurred vision; cognitive impairment; confusion, severe; delirium; disorientation; dissociation, severe; dizziness; dysphoria; flashbacks; heart rate, increased; memory encoding impairment; memory loss; nausea; salivation, excessive; slurred speech; vomiting

Chronic: Egocentric thinking; paranoia; psychological dependence; tolerance

Pregnancy & Lactation: FDA Pregnancy Category C (see Appendix B). Safety of ketamine use by adolescent girls and women who are pregnant has not been established. However, it has been reported that when ketamine is used as an anesthetic during labor, moderate depression of neurobehavioral tests administered to exposed neonates may last for up to 2 days following delivery. Additional valid and reliable data are needed.

Safety of ketamine use by adolescent girls and women who are breast-feeding has not been established. Valid and reliable data are needed.

Abuse Potential

Physical dependence: None to low (USDEA Schedule III; moderate potential for abuse)
Psychological dependence: Low to moderate

Withdrawal Syndrome

A ketamine withdrawal syndrome has not been substantiated. However, tolerance to ketamine can develop with continued regular use. In addition, a significant incidence of "recovery agitation" following brief procedural sedation in the emergency department has been reported; it is responsive to medical management with a benzodiazepine sedative-hypnotic (e.g., diazepam [Valium®]; see monograph).

Overdosage

Ketamine has a relatively high therapeutic index. Overdosage deaths have been reported, but they are relatively rare. With appropriate recognition and medical management, recovery from most ketamine overdosages is usually complete. Respiratory depression can occur and should be treated with supportive ventilation. If required, mechanical ventilation should be used. Ketamine can induce vomiting, particularly if foods or beverages were consumed prior to use. Semiconscious and unconscious patients should be protected against aspiration of vomitus. There is no known antidote.

Notes

1. Homeless young men, 15 to 30 years of age who are predominantly of European descent are another major group of ketamine users. These users, who preferentially inject ketamine intramuscularly—often together in a small group of acquaintances—are found in every major urban center across the United States. The communal tradition of these groups of young men is to share a common needle, syringe, and multidose vial of ketamine, each member taking his turn at an intramuscular injection (similar in many regards to a group of homeless men sharing a bottle of alcohol while standing together in a small circle in an alleyway).
2. Prior to snorting, users often cut the ketamine powder into lines—similar to cocaine use. The lines of ketamine are known as "bumps."
3. The experience produced by ketamine is often described by users as being comparable, in many regards, to a "near death experience;" or as "being in the k-hole"—"being removed from reality," where there is "an intense mind-body dissociation"; or as being "set adrift,"—an "out of body experience in an introspective dreamlike world," with highly realistic, intense, and immersive visual images.

References

Chazan, S., Ekstein, M.P., Marouani, N., et al. (2008). Ketamine for acute and subacute pain in opioid-tolerant patients. *Journal of Opioid Management, 4*(3), 173-180.

Dallimore, D., Herd, D.W., Short, T., et al. (2008). Dosing ketamine for pediatric procedural sedation in the emergency department. *Pediatric Emergency Care, 24*(8), 529-533.

Halkitis, P.N., & Palamar, J.J. (2008). Multivariate modeling of club drug use initiation among gay and bisexual men. *Substance Use & Misuse, 43*(7), 871-879.

Herd, D., & Anderson, B.J. (2007). Ketamine disposition in children presenting for procedural sedation and analgesia in a children's emergency department. *Paediatric Anaesthsia, 17*(7), 622-629.

Ihmsen, H., Geisslinger, G., & Schuttler, J. (2001). Stereoselective pharmacokinetics of ketamine: R(-)-ketamine inhibits the elimination of S(+)-ketamine. *Clinical Pharmacology and Therapeutics, 70*(5), 431-438.

Jansen, K.L., & Darracot-Cankovic, R. (2001). The nonmedical use of ketamine, part two: A review of problem use and dependence. *Journal of Psychoactive Drugs, 33*(2), 151-158.

Lankenau, S., Clatts, M., Welle, D., et al. (2005). Street careers: Homelessness, drug use, and hustling among young men who have sex with men. *International Journal of Drug Policy, 16*, 10-18.

Lankenau, S.E., & Clatts, M. (2004). Drug injection practices among high-risk youth: The first shot of ketamine. *Journal of Urban Health, 81*(2), 232-248.

Lankenau, S.E., Sanders, B., Bloom, J.J., et al. (2002). Ketamine injection among high-risk youth: Preliminary findings from New York City. *Journal of Drug Issues, 32*(3), 893-905.

Lofwall, M.R., Griffiths, R.R., & Mintzer, M.Z. (2006). Cognitive and subjective acute dose effects of intramuscular ketamine in healthy adults. *Experimental and Clinical Psychopharmacology, 14*(4), 439-449.

Moore, K.A., Sklerov, J., Levine, B., et al. (2001). Urine concentrations of ketamine and norketamine following illegal consumption. *Journal of Analytical Toxicology, 25*(7), 583-588.

Newton, A., & Fitton, L. (2008). Intravenous ketamine for adult procedural sedation in the emergency department: A prospective cohort study. *Emergency Medicine Journal, 25*(8), 498-501.

Pal, H.R., Berry, N., Kumar, R., et al. (2002). Ketamine dependence. *Anaesthesia and Intensive Care, 30*(3), 382-384.

Persson, J., Hasselstrom, J., Maurset, A., et al. (2002). Pharmacokinetics and non-analgesic effects of S- and R-ketamines in healthy volunteers with normal and reduced metabolic capacity. *European Journal of Clinical Pharmacology, 57*(12), 869-875.

Sinner, B., & Graf, B.M. (2008). Ketamine. *Handbook of Experimental Pharmacology, 182*, 313-333.

Stewart, C.E. (2001). Ketamine as a street drug. *Emergency Medical Services, 30*(11), 30, 32, 34.

Wolff, K., & Winstock, A.R. (2006). Ketamine: From medicine to misuse. *CNS Drugs, 20*(3), 199-218.

KHAT (See *Catha edulis*)

KRATOM

Names

BAN or INN Generic Synonyms: None

Brand/Trade: None[1]

Chemical: See "Mechanism of Action"

Street: *Air Ketum*[2]; *Biak*; *Gra-Tom*; *Ithang*; *Kakuam*; *Ketum*; *Krathom*; *Thom*

Pharmacologic Classification[3]

Psychodepressant (higher dosages) and psychostimulant (lower dosages)

Brief General Overview

Kratom is the leaf from a large tropical tree that is native to the rainforests of Southeast Asia, where it grows to over 40 feet in height (family: Rubiaeae[4]; genus: *Mitragyna*; species: *speciosa*). It is used in its native regions for both its medicinal and its psychoactive actions. Red- and white-veined (petiole) leaf varieties are available, with the white-veined leaf reportedly possessing stronger effects.[5] Generally, *kratom* is traditionally used by peasant laborers to increase their work production. *Kratom* use is legal in North America, and its use has been steadily increasing over the past decade.

Dosage Forms and Routes of Administration

In Southeast Asia, fresh *kratom* leaves are generally chewed by men, often continuously, for their psychostimulant actions. This pattern of use is similar to that of *coca* leaves and *betel cutch*, which are chewed for buccal absorption of their psychostimulant juices (see Cocaine and *Betel Cutch* monographs). The stringy central vein of the leaf is often removed to facilitate chewing. An alternative method of use involves orally ingesting the dried, powdered leaves mixed with apple sauce or fruit juice. *Kratom* is rarely smoked. When smoked, it is mixed with marijuana or tobacco leaves and rolled into joints or cigarettes, respectively.

In North America and Europe, *kratom* leaves are generally made into a "tea" by infusion or steeping, and the resultant brew is orally ingested.[6] The *kratom* can also be extracted into water, the water then evaporated, and the resultant concentrated tarry, gummy resin hand-rolled into a "pill" that is then coated with flour for oral ingestion. Virtually all of the *kratom* used in North America is purchased on-line over the Internet. It is available in a variety of forms for oral ingestion, including loose leaves for making a tea;, a powder, usually in oral capsule form; and a gummy resin pill. Some users in North America grow their own *kratom*, generally in large greenhouses or hothouses.[7]

Mechanism of CNS Action

At lower concentrations, *kratom* acts as a psychostimulant, whereas at higher concentrations it acts as a psychodepressant. The exact mechanism of these actions has not been determined. *Kratom* contains over 25 different alkaloids, and it is thought that 7-hydroxymitragynine and mitragynine are the most active of these alkaloid constituents.[8,9] Although structurally related to the tryptamines, these alkaloids appear to elicit their CNS actions primarily by functioning as agonists mainly at the mu and kappa opiate analgesic receptors. In addition, they display alpha-adrenergic receptor activity.

Pharmacodynamics/Pharmacokinetics

Kratom is buccally absorbed upon chewing the leaves. Psychoactive actions are generally short-lived (i.e., <2 hours). However, some effects may persist for up to 6 hours depending on dosage or amount used.[10] The ingestion of food with *kratom* significantly reduces its psychoactive actions, probably by means of decreased bioavailability. Additional valid and reliable data are not available.

Current Approved Indications for Medical Use[11]

None

Desired Action/Reason for Personal Use

Psychostimulant use (dose-dependent, achieved at lower kratom concentrations): alertness and vigilance or wakefulness; decrease fatigue and drowsiness; elevate mood (mild)
Psychodepressant use (dose-dependent, achieved at higher *kratom* concentrations): alcohol-like disinhibitory euphoria or "high" (relatively mild); prevent/manage the opiate analgesic withdrawal syndrome; self-medicate/manage chronic pain

Toxicity

Acute: Anorexia, constipation, dry mouth; nausea[12]; tremors; urinary frequency; vomiting[13]

Chronic: Dark facial pigmentation, particularly on the cheeks; physical dependence; psychological dependence; psychosis (rare); weight loss

Pregnancy & Lactation: Valid and reliable data are not available.

Abuse Potential[14]

Physical dependence: Low to moderate (USDEA: not a scheduled drug)
Psychological dependence: Moderate

Withdrawal Syndrome

A *kratom* withdrawal syndrome has been reported upon abrupt discontinuation of regular, long-term, high dosage use. It appears to be, in most regards, quite similar to the opiate analgesic withdrawal syndrome (see Opiate Analgesics monograph). Signs and symptoms of the *kratom* withdrawal syndrome include "bone pain," crying, diarrhea, irritability, muscle aches and twitching, and running nose.

Overdosage

Valid and reliable data are not available.

Notes

1. Several brands of *kratom*, such as "Dragonfly" and "Purple Sticky," are available for purchase and delivery over the Internet.
2. In Malaysia, *kratom* tea is commonly sold at roadside stands. This form of *kratom* is referred to as *"air ketum,"* which translates to *"kratom* water."
3. This mixed classification is due to the multiple psychoactive constituents of *kratom* and its apparent dose-related CNS actions (see "Mechanism of CNS Action").
4. Same family as the coffee plant (see Caffeine monograph).
5. The white-veined leaf also is referred to as green-veined.
6. The tea is made from an infusion of the *kratom* leaves, fresh or dried, and often mixed with black or herbal teas. One part 80 proof (i.e., 40%) alcohol is commonly added to three parts *kratom* tea solution in order to preserve the tea for consumption at a later date (i.e., longer than the maximal recommended 3 to 5 days under refrigeration).
7. However, it is widely believed, predominantly on the basis of popular folklore, that the *kratom* obtained from greenhouses is significantly less potent than that obtained from native sources in Southeast Asia. To deal with both the issue of potency and the issue of getting the plant cuttings to properly root, several *kratom* clone strains have been developed.
8. *Kratom* also contains other alkaloids, such as epicatechin, a potent antioxidant that contributes to its other suggested actions, including lowering blood pressure (anti-hypertensive action) and supporting the immune system (i.e., immunostimulant action).
9. Other identified active constituents of *kratom* include ajmalicine, corynantheidine, corynoxeine, corynoxine A, corynoxine B, (-)-epicatechin, 9-hydroxycorynantheidine, 7-hydroxymitragynine, isomitraphylline, isopteropodine, mitragynine, mitraphylline, paynantheine, rhynchophylline, speciociliatine, speciofoline, speciogynine, speciophylline, stipulatine, and tetrahydroalstonine.
10. Psychostimulant actions are predominantly experienced at lower *kratom* dosages and psycho-depressant actions, at higher dosages.
11. In its native Southeast Asia, *kratom* is ethnomedically used (i.e., in the practice of folk medicine) to treat cough, diarrhea, pain, and opium addiction.
12. Associated with drinking *kratom* tea, which is extremely bitter. Reportedly, the nausea can be minimized by consuming the tea with honey or sugar (see "Pharmacodynamics/Pharmacokinetics").
13. Generally associated with the repugnant taste of the concentrated tea form of *kratom*. However, vomiting also has been reported after smoking *kratom*.
14. *Kratom* has been widely used throughout its native Southeast Asia. However, its sale and use have been restricted or banned by several countries, including Australia, Malaysia, Myanmar (i.e., Burma), and Thailand.

References

Babu, K.M., McCurdy, C.R., & Boyer, E.W. (2008). Opioid receptors and legal highs: Salvia divinorum and Kratom. *Clinical Toxicology, 46*(2), 146-152.

Boyer, E.W., Babu, K.M., Adkins, J.E., et al. (2008). Self-treatment of opioid withdrawal using kratom (Mitragynia speciosa korth). *Addiction, 103*(6), 1048-1050.

LORAZEPAM

Names

BAN or INN Generic Synonyms: None

Brand/Trade: Ativan®; Lorazepam Intensol®; Novo-Lorazem®; Nu-Loraz®

Chemical: 7-Chloro-5-(o-chlorophenyl)-1,3-dihydro-3-hydroxy-2H-1,4-benzodiazepin-2-one

Street: Zzz

Pharmacologic Classification

Psychodepressant, sedative-hypnotic: benzodiazepine

Brief General Overview

Lorazepam was widely abused as a prescription drug, particularly during the 1980s and 1990s. Professionals of both genders (e.g., businessmen and businesswomen, teachers) have been the largest group of abusers in North America. However, more women than men abuse this drug.

The typical lorazepam abuser is a woman 35 to 55 years of age or a man or woman 60 to 80 years of age. Generally, these men and women began using lorazepam when it was prescribed for them for the medical management of an approved and valid indication. However, they continued to use lorazepam for longer than recommended (i.e., usually for more than 3 months of continuous daily use)—long enough for the development of physical and psychological dependence. For these users, the prescribing physician and dispensing pharmacist are the drug suppliers. When access becomes restricted (i.e., they are unable to obtain lorazepam through a legal prescription by their physician or to get their prescription refilled by their pharmacist), they increasingly use Internet web sites to obtain lorazepam, which is shipped directly to them at their home address by various postal and courier delivery services.

Dosage Forms and Routes of Administration

Lorazepam is legitimately produced by pharmaceutical manufacturers in North America and is available in several dosage formulations, including injectables for intravenous use, solutions for oral use, and tablets for oral or sublingual use. People who abuse lorazepam primarily use the oral route, although use of the sublingual route is increasing.

Mechanism of CNS Action

Lorazepam has anticonvulsant, anxiolytic, and sedative actions. The exact mechanism of these actions has not been determined. However, the anxiolytic action appears to be mediated by, or work in concert with, the inhibitory neurotransmitter GABA, apparently by binding to benzodiazepine receptors within the GABA complex. (See also the Benzodiazepines monograph.)

Pharmacodynamics/Pharmacokinetics

Lorazepam is well absorbed after oral ingestion, with a mean bioavailability of 93%. Peak blood concentrations of lorazepam are achieved within 2 hours after oral ingestion and 60 minutes after sublingual placement. Onset of action is dependent on the route of administration: 1 to 5 minutes, intravenously; 15 to 30 minutes, intramuscularly; and 1 to 6 hours, orally. Lorazepam is 85% bound to plasma proteins. Its mean apparent volume of distribution is 1.3 L/kg. It is rapidly conjugated to an inactive glucuronide. Less than 1% of lorazepam is excreted in unchanged form in the urine. The mean elimination half-life is ~14 hours and the mean total body clearance is ~80 mL/minute.

Current Approved Indications for Medical Use

Anxiety disorders, short-term use (less than 30 consecutive days)

Desired Action/Reason for Personal Use

Alcohol-like disinhibitory euphoria; prevention/self-management of the lorazepam withdrawal syndrome; tension reduction

Toxicity

Acute[1]**:** Amnesia, anterograde (dose-related); cognitive impairment; confusion; dizziness; drowsiness; fatigue; impaired vigilance; mental depression; psychomotor impairment; sedation; unsteadiness; weakness

Chronic: Physical dependence; psychological dependence

Pregnancy & Lactation: FDA Pregnancy Category D (see Appendix B). Safety of lorazepam use by adolescent girls and women who are pregnant has not been established (see Benzodiazepines monograph). Additional valid and reliable data are needed.

Safety of lorazepam use by adolescent girls and women who are breast-feeding has not been established. However, lorazepam has been detected in breast milk. Additional valid and reliable data are needed.

Abuse Potential

Physical dependence: Moderate (USDEA Schedule IV; low potential for abuse)
Psychological dependence: Moderate to high

Withdrawal Syndrome

Lorazepam use (particularly regular, long-term, high-dosage use) has been associated with physical and psychological dependence. Abrupt discontinuation of regular, long-term, high dosage use may result in the benzodiazepine withdrawal syndrome (see Benzodiazepines monograph).

Overdosage

Signs and symptoms of lorazepam overdosage include ataxia, coma, confusion, delirium, drowsiness, hypotonia, and somnolence. Fatal overdosage solely involving lorazepam is rare. Lorazepam overdosage requires emergency medical support of body systems, with attention to increasing lorazepam elimination. The benzodiazepine antagonist flumazenil (Anexate®, Romazicon®) may be required[2] (see Benzodiazepines monograph).

Notes

1. Inadvertent injection of lorazepam into an artery may result in arteriospasm and resultant gangrene that may require amputation of the digits or limb distal to the injection site.
2. Caution is required, because flumazenil antagonism may precipitate the benzodiazepine withdrawal syndrome in people who are physically dependent on lorazepam.

References

Blin, O., Simon, N., Jouve, E., et al. (2001). Pharmacokinetic and pharmacodynamic analysis of sedative and amnesic effects of lorazepam in healthy volunteers. *Clinical Neuropharmacology, 24*(2), 71-81.

Fernandez-Torre, J.L. (2001). De novo absence status of late onset following withdrawal of lorazepam: A case report. *Seizure, 10*(6), 433-437.

Pandharipande, P., Shintani, A., Peterson, J., et al. (2006). Lorazepam is an independent risk factor for transitioning to delirium in intensive care unit patients. *Anesthesiology, 104*(1), 21-26.

Pompéia, S., Pradella-Hallinan, M., Manzano, G.M., et al. (2008). Effects of lorazepam on visual perceptual abilities. *Human Psychopharmacology, 23*(3), 183-192.

LYSERGIC ACID AMIDE

Names

BAN or INN Generic Synonyms: Ergine; d-Lysergamide

Brand/Trade: None

Chemical: (8β)-9,10-Didehydro-6-methyl-ergoline-8-carboxamide

Street: *Badoh Negro*; Blue Stars; Flying Saucers; Heavenly Blue; LA-lll; LAA; LSA; Morning Glory; *Ololiuqui*; Pearly Gates; Summer Skies; Wedding Bells

Pharmacologic Classification

Psychodelic, LSD-like psychodelic: natural indole, ergot (i.e., ergoline alkaloid)

Brief General Overview

Lysergic acid amide (LSA), present in the seeds of the morning glory *Ipomoea violacea*,[1] was used by ancient Aztecs and continues to be used by shamans in some southern Mexican Indian tribes in religious ceremonies to facilitate prophecy and spiritual cure of disease. It is structurally and pharmacologically similar to lysergic acid diethylamide (LSD; see monograph), but is significantly less potent (i.e., LSD is 10 to 100 times as potent as LSA on a microgram per microgram basis). LSA also is found in some other plants, notably the Hawaiian baby woodrose.[2]

The Hawaiian baby woodrose, *Argyreia nervosa*, is not a rose, but rather a woody climbing vine or liana. LSA is found in a much higher concentration in the seeds of the Hawaiian baby woodrose than in morning glory seeds (i.e., the Hawaiian baby woodrose seeds are about 25 times more concentrated).

Dosage Forms and Routes of Administration

Although LSA can be synthesized, it is almost always obtained from the seeds of either morning glory or Hawaiian baby woodrose. Typically, the seeds are ground into a flour that is then soaked in water and strained through cheesecloth. The filtered liquid, which contains the LSA, is orally ingested.[3]

Mechanism of CNS Action

Valid and reliable data are not available.

Pharmacodynamics/Pharmacokinetics

Valid and reliable data are not available.

Current Approved Indications for Medical Use

None

Desired Action/Reason for Personal Use

Dreamlike conscious state; hallucinations, illusions, synesthesia; mystical religious experiences

Toxicity

Acute: Abdominal cramps; anorexia; anxiety; blood pressure, increased; fever; hangover[4]; heart rate, increased; memory impairment, particularly short-term memory; mydriasis; nausea; psychomotor impairment; uterine contractions; vomiting

Chronic: Valid and reliable data are not available.

Pregnancy & Lactation: The safety of LSA use by adolescent girls and women who are pregnant has not been established. However, because of the documented uterotonic action of ergometrine, one of the amides found in morning glory seeds, LSA should not be used by adolescent girls and women who are pregnant. Additional valid and reliable data are needed.

The safety of LSA use by adolescent girls and women who are breast-feeding has not been established. It is unknown if LSA is excreted in significant amounts in breast milk. Additional valid and reliable data are needed.

Abuse Potential

Physical dependence: None (USDEA Schedule III; low potential for abuse)
Psychological dependence: Low

Withdrawal Syndrome

A specific LSA withdrawal syndrome has not been reported.

Overdosage

Valid and reliable data are not available. However, morning glory seeds are commonly treated with insecticides, fungicides, and other chemicals that may contribute to any toxicity associated with LSA overdosage. On rare occasions, death has been reported. Therefore, LSA overdosage requires emergency medical support of body systems, with attention to increasing LSA elimination. There is no known antidote. (See also LSD monograph, "Overdosage.")

Notes

1. Morning glory seeds contain other active amides, including ergometrine, elymoclavine, and chanoclavine.
2. LSA also is found in *Acremonium coenophialum*, *Claviceps paspali*, *Claviceps purpurea*, *Stipa robusta* (sleepy grass), and *Turbina corymbosa*.
3. Users who have a little chemistry background often use various nonpolar (e.g., naphtha; Zippo® lighter fluid) and polar (e.g., alcohol, methanol) solvents in "cookbook" extraction procedures to produce a relatively pure white powder containing LSA. This powder is sometimes dissolved and injected intravenously to obtain a more immediate and intense action.
4. Headaches occur occasionally in some users, who also may have the following concomitant signs and symptoms: blurred vision, constipation, dizziness, nausea, and physical inertia.

References

Argyreia nervosa: Hawaiian baby woodrose (pp. 1-2). (2002). Available: http://leda.lycaeum.org/?ID=2658.

Ipomoea violacea: Morning glory (p. 1). (2002). Available: http://leda.lycaeum.org/?ID=263.

LSA extraction (pp. 1-3). (2002). Available: http://leda.lycaeum.org/Documents/LSA_Extraction.13393.shtml.

LYSERGIC ACID DIETHYLAMIDE

Names

BAN or INN Chemical Synonyms: Lysergide; *Lyserg-SaeureDiaethylamid*[1] (German)

Brand/Trade: None

Chemical: 9,10-Didehydro-N,N-diethyl-6-methylergoline-8β-carboxamide

Street: 25; A; Acid; Acid-25; Alice; Alphabet; Animal; Barrels; Battery Acid; Beavis & Butthead; Bells; Big D; Birdhead; Black Acid; Black Star; Black Sunshine; Black Tabs; Blotter; Blotter Acid; Blotter Cube; Blue Acid; Blue Barrels; Blue Chairs; Blue Cheers; Blue Dot; Blue Heaven; Blue Microdot; Blue Mist; Blue Moons; Blue Vials; Boomers; Brown Bombers; Brown Dots; California Sunshine; Cheers; Chocolate Chips; Cid; Cid Drip; Coffee; Colors; Conductor; Contact Lens; Crystal Tea; Cube; Cupcakes; Deeda; Diamonds;

Disney Productions; Domes; Doses; Dot; Dots; Double Dome; DSL; Electric Kool Aid; Elvis; Eye Candy; Felix; Felix the Cat; Fields; Flash; Flat Blues; Flats; Frogs; Ghost; Glories; Goofy's; Grape Parfait; Green Double Domes; Green Single Dome; Green Wedge; Grey Shields; Hats; Hawaiian Sunshine; Hawk; Haze; Head Light; Heavenly Blue; Illusions; Instant Zen; L; LAA; LAD; Lakeshore Drive; *Lason Sa Daga*; Lavender; Lens; Let Sunshine Do; Lime Acid; Logor; Loony Toons; LSD; Lucy in the Sky with Diamonds; Magic Tickets; Mickey's; Microdots; Mighty Quinn; Mind Blow; Mind Detergent; Mind-Tripper; Monterey Purple; Moons; Optical Illusions; Orange Barrels; Orange Cubes; Orange Haze; Orange Micro; Orange Sunshine; Orange Wedges; Owsley; Owsley's Acid; Pane; Paper Acid; Peace; Peaks; Pearly Gates; Pellets; Pink Blotters; Pink Panther; Pink Robots; Pink Wedges; Pink Witches; Potato; Pure Love; Purple Barrels; Purple Flats; Purple Haze; Purple Mikes; Purple Ozoline; Rainbow; Rain Drops; Recycle; Red Lips; Rips; Royal Blues; Russian Sickles; Sacrament; Sandoz; Smears; Square Dancing Tickets; Squirrels; Strawberries; Strawberry Fields; Sugar Cube; Sugar Lumps; Sunshine; Tabs; Tail Lights; The Ghost; The Hawk; Ticket; Timothy Leary Ticket; Trips; Twenty-Five; Uncle Sid; Uncle Sidney; Vodka Acid; Wedding Bells; Wedges; White Lightning; White Owsley's; Window Glass; Window Pane; Woodstock; Yellow Dimples; Yellow Sunshines; Yin Yang; Zen

Pharmacologic Classification

Psychodelic, LSD-like psychodelic: natural indole, ergot (i.e., ergoline alkaloid)

Brief General Overview

Lysergic acid diethylamide (LSD) was first synthesized in 1938. Its chemical precursors are the ergot alkaloids ergonovine and ergotamine. However, LSD did not receive much attention or interest in use until the 1960s, when it became the embodiment of the hippie generation—the "Turn on, tune in, drop out" antiestablishment drug. Popularity and use of LSD declined significantly during the 1970s but resurged with the explosion of psychodelic drug use associated with attendance at dance clubs and raves during the 1990s. Typical users are adolescents and young adults. Most users appear to "mature out" and voluntarily discontinue LSD use without external assistance. LSD is still one of the most potent psychodelics known and is regarded by many as the prototype for this class of drugs and substances of abuse.

Dosage Forms and Routes of Administration

Virtually all of the tens of millions of doses, or "hits," of LSD used each year in North America come from chemical synthesis in illicit clandestine laboratories in Canada and the United States.[2] Although LSD can be, and has been, administered by virtually every route, including gelatin squares, or "window panes," which are inserted into the conjunctival sac for ophthalmic absorption, over 99% of all doses are orally ingested. Drops[3] of LSD have been added to various vehicles for distribution and sale. Among the most common are blotter paper; gel wraps, which resemble small blue-colored bubble wrap packing material; "Pez®", "Smarties®", and "Sweet Tarts®" candies; and sugar cubes. LSD also is available as a powder or crystal that is often incorporated into capsules or tablets for oral ingestion. The U.S. Department of Justice has identified over 200 illicit brands of LSD tablets and over 350 different illicit brands of LSD blotter paper, which generally have their own stamp design (e.g., a common or popular cartoon character or other symbol).[4] Doses of LSD are often orally ingested, particularly by adolescents, with a gulp of alcohol (i.e., a beer "chaser") to "wash the dose down."[5]

Mechanism of CNS Action

The exact mechanism of LSD's psychodelic action has not been determined. However, it is known that LSD interacts with the neurotransmitter receptors for both serotonin (i.e., 5-HT1A; 5-HT1C; 5-HT2) and dopamine (i.e., D1; D2), resulting in agonistic actions.

Pharmacodynamics/Pharmacokinetics

After LSD is ingested, the onset of action is within about 30 to 60 minutes. Physical effects include blurred vision, diaphoresis, incoordination, mydriasis, palpitations, and tachycardia. Psychological effects include euphoria, tension, visual illusions, perceptual changes (e.g., micropsia, macropsia), difficulty locating the source of a sound, fear of fragmentation or disintegration of self, prolongation of visual afterimages, synesthesias (i.e., "hearing colors," "seeing sounds"), distortion of body image, mood swings from happiness to sadness, vivid thoughts and memories, and the perception of time passing extremely slowly (i.e., temporal disintegration). The intensity of these effects is directly related to the amount of LSD used. Its effects peak over 1 to 6 hours and usually dissipate by 8 to 12 hours. The elimination half-life has been estimated to be 2 to 5 hours, but questionable analytical techniques were used for this estimate. Additional valid and reliable data are unavailable.

Current Approved Indications for Medical Use

None

Desired Action/Reason for Personal Use

Distorted time perception; euphoria; hallucinations (primarily visual); heightened awareness of sensory input; sense of clarity of intelligence (i.e., "mind-expanding"); synesthesia

Toxicity

Acute: Anorexia; anxiety; body temperature, increased; chills; cognitive impairment; confusion; headache; hyperglycemia; hypertension; insomnia; muscle weakness; mydriasis; panic; psychomotor impairment; psychosis (rare), usually of brief duration; respirations, deep and rapid; sweating, increased; tachycardia; tremor; vomiting

Chronic: Flashbacks (particularly, with the use of larger dosages)[6]; triggering or exacerbation of latent mental disorders, particularly schizophrenia

Pregnancy & Lactation: LSD does not appear to be a human teratogen. Although LSD use by women during pregnancy has not been directly related to teratogenic effects, human chromosomal breakage induced by high concentrations of LSD has been demonstrated in vitro. The clinical significance of this finding remains unknown. However, LSD use during pregnancy has reportedly been associated with an increased rate of spontaneous abortion. In addition, LSD is an ergot alkaloid derivative and, as such, can cause uterine contractions. Adolescent girls and women who are pregnant should not use LSD.

Safety of LSD use by adolescent girls and women who are breast-feeding has not been established. It is unknown if LSD is excreted in breast milk. Additional valid and reliable data are needed.

Abuse Potential

Physical dependence: None (USDEA Schedule I; use is prohibited)
Psychological dependence: Low

Withdrawal Syndrome

An LSD withdrawal syndrome has not been reported. However, tolerance to the behavioral or psychological effects of LSD may be seen after 3 to 4 days of daily use. The extent of tolerance to LSD can be significant—in the same order of magnitude as that observed with phencyclidine (PCP; see monograph), and alcohol (see monograph) or other sedative-hypnotics. Less tolerance develops to the cardiovascular effects of LSD. Reversed tolerance, or increased sensitivity, has been reported by some users but is considered rare. In addition, cross-tolerance has been reported to occur among LSD, mescaline, and psilocybin, suggesting a common molecular mechanism of action. When LSD has not been used for 3 to 4 days, sensitivity to its effects increases rapidly, returning to pre-use levels.

Overdosage

LSD has a relatively high therapeutic index, and no deaths have been directly related to LSD use alone. However, LSD may rarely cause death from associated accidents (e.g., attempting to fly from a rooftop) or acts of violence. Overdosage of LSD most often results in "bad trips." Signs and symptoms of "bad trips," which usually persist for up to 12 hours after ingestion of LSD, include anxiety (intense), combativeness, confusion, fear of "disintegration of self," labile mood, and panic. Users who are experiencing a "bad trip" can usually be "talked-down" or given a benzodiazepine (e.g., diazepam [Valium®]) to relieve associated anxiety. In severe and otherwise unresponsive cases, an antipsychotic phenothiazine drug (e.g., chlorpromazine [Thorazine®]) may be required to manage the signs and symptoms of LSD overdosage. There is no known antidote.

Notes

1. The German name is the source of the most common term used for lysergic acid diethylamide, LSD.
2. Although the recipe for synthesis of LSD is available on the Internet, the actual chemical synthesis and production of LSD is not a straightforward "cookbook" task. It requires an experienced organic chemist and appropriate laboratory facilities and supplies. Most of these chemists have illicitly operated in northern California, with a few laboratories in the Midwest producing LSD more recently.
3. In pure liquid form, LSD is colorless, odorless, and virtually tasteless, although reportedly it has a slightly bitter taste.

4. Some popular illicit LSD blotter paper designs include Albert Hoffman (the chemist who first synthesized LSD in 1938), Alice in Wonderland, Bart Simpson, Beavis and Butthead, Bill and Opus, Campbell's® Tomato Soup, Cheshire Cat, Daffy Duck, Felix the Cat, Ganesh, and Popeye the Sailor Man.
5. LSD is often consumed at raves in combination with MDMA, or Ecstasy (see 3,4-Methylenedioxymethamphetamine monograph). The combination is commonly known as "X and L" or "flip-flops." This pattern of use is referred to as "candy flipping."
6. Generally, LSD-related flashbacks are reported less frequently today than during the 1960s and 1970s, probably because significantly lower dosages of LSD are used today.

Reference

Wu, L.T., Schlenger, W.E., & Galvin, D.M. (2006). Concurrent use of methamphetamine, MDMA, LSD, ketamine, GHB, and flunitrazepam among American youths. *Drug and Alcohol Dependence, 84*(1), 102-113.

MARIJUANA (See Cannabis)

MAZINDOL

Names

BAN or INN Generic Synonyms: None

Brand/Trade: Sanorex®

Chemical: 5-(p-Chlorophenyl)-2,5-dihydro-3H-imidazo[2,1-α]isoindol-5-ol

Street: None

Pharmacologic Classification

Psychostimulant, miscellaneous: amphetamine congener

Brief General Overview

Mazindol is an anorexiant that is prescribed for short-term management of exogenous obesity. People who exceed the recommended dosage, or continue to use mazindol for longer than 6 weeks, are at risk for developing severe psychological dependence. Mazindol is chemically and pharmacologically related to the amphetamines, which have high abuse potential. People who become psychologically dependent may increase their mazindol dosage to many times the usual medically recommended dosage.

Dosage Forms and Routes of Administration

Mazindol is licitly produced by pharmaceutical manufacturers in North America. It is available in oral tablet form and is orally ingested.

Mechanism of CNS Action

Mazindol is an imidazoisoindole anorexiant that shares many pharmacologic actions with the amphetamines and their congeners. Tolerance to the anorexiant (anorectant, anorectic) actions reportedly occurs with all drugs in this class. The exact mechanism of mazindol's anorexiant action for the management of exogenous obesity has not been fully determined. It appears to involve appetite suppression and other as yet unspecified CNS actions. It has been demonstrated that mazindol binds to striatal dopamine transporters and functions as an indirect dopamine agonist.

Pharmacodynamics/Pharmacokinetics

Mazindol is well absorbed after oral ingestion. Its onset of action is within 30 to 60 minutes. Peak blood concentrations are generally achieved within 1 to 2 hours. Mazindol has a high tissue affinity. Thus, the blood contains the lowest relative concentration 2 hours after ingestion. It has a duration of action of 8 to 15 hours and is slowly excreted in the urine and feces. The excretion rate can be increased with continued use. Additional valid and reliable data are not available.

Current Approved Indications for Medical Use

Exogenous obesity (short-term symptomatic management)

Desired Action/Reason for Personal Use

Alertness; appetite/hunger suppression and associated weight loss or maintenance; decrease fatigue; energy

Toxicity

Acute: Anxiety; blurred vision; constipation; dry mouth; dizziness; dysuria; headache; insomnia; mydriasis; nausea; nervousness; peripheral neuropathy; sweating (excessive)

Chronic: Physical dependence; psychological dependence

Pregnancy & Lactation: FDA Pregnancy Category "not established." Safety of mazindol use by adolescent girls and women who are pregnant has not been established. Additional valid and reliable data are needed.

Safety of mazindol use by adolescent girls and women who are breast-feeding has not been established. Additional valid and reliable data are needed.

Abuse Potential

Physical dependence: Moderate (USDEA Schedule IV; low potential for abuse)
Psychological dependence: Moderate to high

Withdrawal Syndrome

Abrupt discontinuation of regular, long-term mazindol use reportedly has been associated with an amphetamine-like withdrawal syndrome. The signs and symptoms of this syndrome include extreme fatigue and mental depression. Regular, long-term mazindol use should be gradually discontinued.

Overdosage

Mazindol overdosage rarely has been reported. Signs and symptoms include agitation, hyperactivity, irritability, and tachycardia. Mazindol overdosage requires emergency medical support of body systems, with attention to increasing mazindol elimination. There is no known antidote.

References

Bray, G.A. (2000). A concise review on the therapeutics of obesity. *Nutrition, 16*(10), 953-960.

Kosten, T.R., George, T.P., & Kosten, T.A. (2002). The potential of dopamine agonists in drug addictions. *Expert Opinion on Investigational Drugs, 11*(4), 491-499.

Norris, S.L., Zhang, X., Avenell, A., et al. (2005). Pharmacotherapy for weight loss in adults with type 2 diabetes mellitus. *Cochrane Database of Systematic Reviews, 25*(1), CD004096.

MEPERIDINE

Names

BAN or INN Generic Synonyms: Pethidine

Brand/Trade: Demerol®

Chemical: l-Methyl-4-phenylisoipecotic acid ethyl ester; ethyl 1-methyl-4-phenyliso-nipecotate

Street: Bam; Demis; Dems; Mep; Meps; Morals; Synthetic Heroin

Pharmacologic Classification

Psychodepressant, opiate analgesic: pure agonist (synthetic)

Brief General Overview

Meperidine was introduced into clinical practice in the 1930s. A commonly used opiate analgesic in hospitals and health care settings in North America, it was originally developed as an anticholinergic. Most of the people who become physically dependent on the opiate analgesics generally prefer heroin (see monograph) or morphine (see monograph) to meperidine.[1] However, health care professionals who become physically dependent on opiate analgesics usually begin their opiate analgesic use with meperidine (probably because of its availability in hospitals and other health care settings). These users commonly continue to use meperidine as their opiate analgesic of choice.[2] They also are at high risk for relapse following treatment for meperidine dependence if they have a dual diagnosis and family history of substance use disorders.

Dosage Forms and Routes of Administration

Meperidine is legally produced by pharmaceutical manufacturers in North America.[3] It is available in oral (i.e., syrup, tablet) and injectable (i.e., intravenous, intramuscular, subcutaneous) formulations. Meperidine is significantly less effective after oral ingestion; compared with injection, a higher oral dose is needed to achieve desired effects. Meperidine's availability and the option of several routes of administration appear to make it attractive for abuse by health care professionals.[4]

Mechanism of CNS Action

Meperidine appears to elicit its psychotropic actions, including analgesic and respiratory depressant actions, primarily by binding to endorphin receptors, particularly mu receptors, in the CNS. However, the exact mechanism has not been determined (see Opiate Analgesics monograph).

Pharmacodynamics/Pharmacokinetics

Meperidine has several therapeutic actions qualitatively similar to those of morphine, one of which is analgesia. When injected in doses of 80 to 100 mg, meperidine is approximately equivalent in analgesic action to 10 mg of morphine. The onset of action is slightly more rapid than that for morphine, although the duration of action is slightly shorter. Meperidine is significantly less effective after oral ingestion than after injection because it undergoes extensive first-pass hepatic metabolism ($F = 0.52$).[5] Thus, in order to achieve comparable pharmacologic actions, an oral dose of meperidine that is approximately twice the injectable dose is required, although the exact ratio of oral to injectable analgesia has not been determined. Peak analgesia generally occurs within 1 hour after oral ingestion or intramuscular, intravenous, or subcutaneous injection. Analgesia may last for up to 2 to 4 hours.

Meperidine is weakly (about 60%) bound to plasma proteins and has a mean apparent volume of distribution of ~4.5 L/kg. It is extensively metabolized, primarily in the liver, with about 5% eliminated in unchanged form in the urine. Total body clearance is ~850 mL/minute. The mean elimination half-life is ~3 hours. Normeperidine, an active metabolite of meperidine, is associated with CNS excitation[6] and may accumulate in users who have kidney dysfunction. Meperidine is a weak acid, so alkalinization of the urine decreases its excretion and acidification of the urine increases its excretion.[7] These changes in urinary pH may significantly affect the total body clearance and the elimination half-life of meperidine and its metabolite.

Current Approved Indications for Medical Use[8]

Acute pain (moderate to severe); cancer pain (moderate to severe)

Desired Action/Reason for Personal Use

Euphoria (mild); prevention/self-management of the meperidine or other opiate analgesic withdrawal syndrome; self-management of pain

Toxicity

Acute: Bradycardia; cardiovascular depression; cognitive impairment (particularly during the first few days of meperidine use); constipation; disorientation; dizziness; dry mouth; flushing; headache; lightheadedness; miosis; nausea; normeperidine neurotoxicity[9]; postural hypotension (orthostatic); pruritus (severe); respiratory depression; sedation; seizures (particularly users with preexisting seizure disorders); sweating; syncope; visual changes; vomiting

Chronic: Abscesses at injection site (with injectable use); physical dependence; psychological dependence; scarring of skin (with injectable use)

Pregnancy & Lactation: FDA Pregnancy Category B (see Appendix B). Safety of meperidine use by adolescent girls and women who are pregnant has not been established. However, meperidine does cross the placental barrier, and neonatal physical dependence and withdrawal are associated with maternal meperidine use during pregnancy or near term. In addition, neonates exposed in utero to meperidine tend to have increased nonnutritive sucking (i.e., a lower sucking frequency and a less stable sucking rhythm) in comparison with nonexposed neonates. This lower sucking frequency also appears to occur when meperidine is used as an analgesic during labor, particularly if the dose is administered less than 5 hours before delivery. Adolescent girls and women who are pregnant should not use meperidine.

Safety of meperidine use by adolescent girls and women who are breast-feeding has not been established. Meperidine is excreted in breast milk. The use of repeated doses of meperidine can result in significant concentrations in breast milk of both meperidine and its active metabolite, normeperidine. These concentrations may place breast-fed infants at risk for expected pharmacologic actions (e.g., drowsiness) and physical dependence.[10] Adolescent girls and women who are breast-feeding should not use meperidine.

Abuse Potential

Physical dependence: High (USDEA Schedule II; high potential for abuse)
Psychological dependence: High

Withdrawal Syndrome

Long-term, regular use of meperidine is associated with physical and psychological dependence. Abrupt discontinuation of long-term regular use may result in the meperidine withdrawal syndrome. The signs and symptoms include abdominal pain, anorexia, body aches, chills, diarrhea, difficulty sleeping, fever (unexplained), nervousness, piloerection (gooseflesh), restlessness, rhinitis, shivering, sneezing, stomach cramps, sweating (excessive), tachycardia, tremors, weakness, and yawning. The meperidine withdrawal syndrome may have its onset as soon as 3 hours after the last use of meperidine. The signs and symptoms of withdrawal generally peak within 8 to 12 hours and gradually resolve over a period of up to 5 days.

Overdosage

Signs and symptoms of meperidine overdosage include bradycardia (sometimes),

Cheyne-Stokes respiration, cold and clammy skin, cyanosis, hypotension, respiratory depression (with a decrease in rate and tidal volume), skeletal muscle flaccidity, and somnolence (extreme, progressing to stupor or coma). In severe overdosage, particularly that involving the intravenous injection of meperidine, apnea, circulatory collapse, cardiac arrest, and death may occur.[11] Meperidine overdosage requires emergency medical support of body systems, with attention to maintaining or re-establishing adequate respiratory function and increasing meperidine elimination (when the overdosage involved oral ingestion).

The opiate antagonist naloxone (Narcan®) is a specific antidote for treating the respiratory depression associated with overdosage of meperidine. However, use of the opiate antagonist in people who are physically dependent on meperidine precipitates an acute meperidine withdrawal syndrome. The severity of the withdrawal syndrome depends on the degree of physical dependence, the amount of meperidine involved in the overdosage, the time elapsed before seeking medical treatment, and the dose of the antagonist injected. An initial lower dosage of the opiate analgesic antagonist (10% to 20% of the usual recommended initial dosage) is generally recommended for these patients.

Notes

1. Meperidine is associated with significantly less euphoria than either heroin (see monograph) or morphine (see monograph).
2. Among physicians in the United States, anesthesiologists have the highest reported rate of abuse of opiate analgesics, particularly meperidine.
3. It is also illegally synthesized in clandestine laboratories. When its chemical analogue, 1-methyl-4-phenyl-4-propionoxypiperidine (MPPP), is produced it often contains a neurotoxic byproduct (1-methyl-4-phenyl-1,2,3,6-tetrahydropyridine [MPTP]). MPTP has been demonstrated to cause drug-induced parkinsonism (often irreversible) by means of destroying the same neurons in the substantia nigra that are damaged by Parkinson's disease.
4. Meperidine users often take nonprescription antacids (e.g., Mylanta®, Rolaids®, Tums®) to enhance and prolong the desired actions of meperidine, because it is a weak acid and alkalinization of the urine decreases its renal excretion (see "Pharmacodynamics/Pharmacokinetics" section).
5. First-pass hepatic metabolism has been reported to be significantly decreased (by up to 50%) and oral bioavailability correspondingly increased in the presence of significant hepatic disease or dysfunction (e.g., cirrhosis).
6. The mean elimination half-life of normeperidine is ~18 hours.
7. For example, acidification of the urine can significantly increase the percentage of meperidine eliminated in unchanged form to up to 25%.
8. Meperidine is not considered to be an analgesic of first choice because of the availability of other more efficacious opiate analgesics (e.g., morphine) that are also less toxic, particularly in patients with renal impairment.
9. Normeperidine, the active metabolite of meperidine, is neurotoxic. Use of meperidine for longer than 3 consecutive days, particularly at higher dosages or in the presence of renal impairment, significantly increases the risk for developing related toxicity, including anxiety, hallucinations, nervousness, seizures (potentially fatal), tremors, and twitching. Agitation, exaggerated startle response, excitement, hallucinations (generally transient), mydriasis, and psychosis (rare) may also occur.
10. Cases have been reported in which the neonate required resuscitation.
11. In addition, accumulation of the active metabolite, normeperidine, may produce convulsions, hyperactive reflexes, mydriasis, and tremors.

References

Capogna, G. (2001). Effect of epidural analgesia on the fetal heart rate. *European Journal of Obstetrics, Gynecology, and Reproductive Biology, 98*(2), 160-164.

Domino, K.B., Hornbein, T.F., Polissar, N.L., et al. (2005). Risk factors for relapse in health care professionals with substance use disorders. *JAMA: The Journal of the American Medical Association, 293*(12), 1453-1460.

Hafstrom, M., & Kjellmer, I. (2000). Non-nutritive sucking by infants exposed to pethidine in utero. *Acta Paediatrica, 89*(10), 1196-1200.

Hubbard, G.P., & Wolfe, K.R. (2003). Meperidine misuse in a patient with sphincter of Oddi dysfunction. *The Annals of Pharmacotherapy, 37*(4), 534-537.

Joranson, D.E., Ryan, K.M., Gilson, A.M., et al. (2000). Trends in medical use and abuse of opioid analgesics. *JAMA: The Journal of the American Medical Association, 283*(13), 1710-1714.

Latta, K.S., Ginsberg, B., & Barkin, R.L. (2002). Meperidine: A critical review. *American Journal of Therapeutics, 9*(1), 53-68.

Ransjo-Arvidson, A.B., Matthiesen, A.S., Lilja, G., et al. (2001). Maternal analgesia during labor disturbs newborn behavior: Effects on breastfeeding, temperature, and crying. *Birth, 28*(1), 5-12.

Riordan, J., Gross, A., Angeron, J., et al. (2000). The effect of labor pain relief medication on neonatal suckling and breastfeeding duration. *Journal of Human Lactation, 16*(1), 7-12.

Seifert, C.F., & Kennedy, S. (2004). Meperidine is alive and well in the new millennium: Evaluation of meperidine usage patterns and frequency of adverse drug reactions. *Pharmacotherapy, 24*(6), 776-783.

Shipton, E. (2006). Should New Zealand continue signing up to the Pethidine Protocol? *The New Zealand Medical Journal, 119*(1230), U1875.

Simopoulos, T.T., Smith, H.S., Peeters-Asdourian, C., et al. (2002). Use of meperidine in patient-controlled analgesia and the development of a normeperidine toxic reaction. *Archives of Surgery, 137*(1), 84-88.

Strassels, S.A., (2008). Cognitive effects of opioids. *Current Pain and Headache Reports, 12*(1), 32-36.

MEPROBAMATE[1]

Names

BAN or INN Generic Synonyms: 1,3-Propanediol, 2-methyl-2-propyl-, dicarbamate

Brand/Trade: Equanil®; Meprospan®; Miltown®; Novo-Mepro®

Chemical: 2-Methyl-2-propyl-1,3-propanedioldicarbamate

Street: Housewife's Delight; Tranks; Tranx

Pharmacologic Classification

Psychodepressant, sedative-hypnotic: miscellaneous (carbamate derivative)

Brief General Overview

Meprobamate was introduced into clinical use as an anxiolytic in the mid-1950s and was the first of the so-called minor tranquilizers. It was initially promoted as a safe, "nonaddicting" alternative to the barbiturates. These claims proved to be false, and its clinical use diminished significantly with the development and increased use of the benzodiazepines over the last half of the 20th century.

Dosage Forms and Routes of Administration

Meprobamate is licitly produced by pharmaceutical manufacturers in North America. It is available in a number of oral capsule and tablet formulations, which are usually orally ingested. Popular as a street drug in the 1960s and 1970s, meprobamate is now abused primarily by middle-aged women and the elderly. (Also see Note 1.)

Mechanism of CNS Action

Although the exact mechanism of action for meprobamate has not yet been determined, it appears to act at multiple sites in the CNS, including the thalamus and the limbic system. These actions appear to be mediated through interaction with the $GABA_A$ receptor complex.

Pharmacodynamics/Pharmacokinetics

Meprobamate is well absorbed after oral ingestion. Its onset of action is within 1 hour. Peak blood concentrations are achieved within 1 to 3 hours. Meprobamate is only slightly bound to plasma proteins (~20%) but appears to be uniformly distributed throughout the body tissues. It is extensively metabolized in the liver to several inactive metabolites. Approximately 10% of meprobamate is excreted in unchanged form in the urine. The mean elimination half-life is 10 hours (range, 6 to 16 hours).

Current Approved Indications for Medical Use[2]

Anxiety disorders (adjunctive, short-term symptomatic management)

Desired Action/Reason for Personal Use

Euphoria; prevention/self-management of the meprobamate withdrawal syndrome

Toxicity

Acute: Ataxia; cognitive impairment; disorientation; dizziness; drowsiness; headache; psychomotor impairment; slurred speech; syncope; vertigo; weakness

Chronic: Hypersensitivity reactions (generally occurring between the first and fifth doses of meprobamate); physical dependence; psychological dependence; neutropenia; porphyria (exacerbation of)

Pregnancy & Lactation: FDA Pregnancy Category D (see Appendix B). Meprobamate crosses the placenta. Use during the first trimester of pregnancy has been associated with increased risk for congenital malformations. Adolescent girls and women who are pregnant should not use meprobamate.

Meprobamate is excreted in breast milk at concentrations two to four times that in maternal blood. The higher concentration in breast milk may result in expected pharmacologic actions in neonates and infants (e.g., drowsiness, lethargy), who also may become physically dependent. Adolescent girls and women who are breast-feeding should not use meprobamate.

Abuse Potential

Physical dependence: Moderate (USDEA Schedule IV; low potential for abuse)[3]
Psychological dependence: Moderate

Withdrawal Syndrome

Abrupt discontinuation of regular, long-term use of meprobamate may precipitate the meprobamate withdrawal syndrome. The signs and symptoms of meprobamate withdrawal occur within 12 to 48 hours after its last use. Signs and symptoms include anxiety, ataxia, confusion, hallucinations (auditory and visual), insomnia, muscle twitching, tremors, vomiting, and, rarely, seizures. Seizures are more likely to occur in people who have histories of CNS injury/dysfunction, or those who have preexisting or latent seizure disorders.

Overdosage

Signs and symptoms of meprobamate overdosage include ataxia, coma, drowsiness, lethargy, stupor, and vasomotor and respiratory collapse. Meprobamate overdosage has been frequently associated with the concurrent use of alcohol or other psychotropic drugs. It also has been associated with suicide attempts, some of which have been successful. Meprobamate overdosage, alone or in combination with other psychotropic drugs, may be fatal and, thus, requires emergency medical support of body systems, with attention to increasing meprobamate elimination. There is no known antidote.

Notes

1. Carisoprodol (Soma®; Vanadom®) (N-isopropyl-2-methyl-2-propyl-1,3-propanedioldicabamate) is a skeletal muscle relaxant. Its active metabolite is meprobamate. Carisoprodol also is chemically known as isomeprobamate. Although a recognized drug and substance of abuse, it is neither widely prescribed nor abused in the United States. However, its use has been increasing over the past 5 years among adolescent boys living in states along the U.S.-Mexican border. In addition to sharing all of the actions and effects of meprobamate, carisoprodol may cause some adverse drug reactions (i.e., hand tremor, horizontal gaze nystagmus, involuntary movements, and tachycardia) that may be unique to the parent compound.
2. Given the availability of more efficacious and less toxic alternative drugs (e.g., the benzodiazepines), neither meprobamate nor carisoprodol should be considered to be drugs of first choice in the pharmacotherapy of anxiety disorders.
3. Carisoprodol is not a USDEA scheduled drug.

References

Bailey, D.N., & Briggs, J.R. (2002). Carisprodol: An unrecognized drug of abuse. *American Journal of Clinical Pathology, 117*(3), 396-400.

Bramness, J.G., Skurtveit, S., & Mørland, J. (2004). Impairment due to intake of carisoprodol. *Drug and Alcohol Dependence, 74*(3), 311-318.

Briggs, G.G., Ambrose, P.J., Nageotte, M.P., et al. (2008). High-dose carisoprodol during pregnancy and lactation. *The Annals of Pharmacotherapy, 42*(6), 898-901.

Forrester, M.B. (2006). Carisoprodol abuse in Texas, 1998-2003. *Journal of Medical Toxicology, 2*(1), 8-13.

Høiseth, G., Bramness, J.G., Christophersen, A.S., et al. (2007). Carisoprodol intoxications: A retrospective study of forensic autopsy material from 1992-2003. *International Journal of Legal Medicine, 121*(5), 403-409.

Logan, B.K., Case, G.A., & Gordon, A.M. (2000). Carisoprodol, meprobamate, and driving impairment. *Journal of Forensic Science, 45*(3), 619-623.

Nordeng, H., Zahlsen, K., & Spigset, O. (2001). Transfer of carisoprodol to breast milk. *Therapeutic Drug Monitoring, 23*(3), 298-300.

Reeves, R.R., Beddingfield, J.J., & Mack, J.E. (2004). Carisoprodol withdrawal syndrome. *Pharmacotherapy, 24*(12), 1804-1806.

Reeves, R.R., Hammer, J.S., & Pendarvis, R.O. (2007). Is the frequency of carisoprodol withdrawal syndrome increasing? *Pharmacotherapy, 27*(10), 1462-1466.

MESCALINE

Names

BAN or INN Generic Synonyms: 3,4,5-Trimethoxybenzeneethanamine

Brand/Trade: None

Chemical: 3,4,5-Trimethoxyphenethylamine

Street: Big Chief; Britton; Buttons; Cactus; Cactus Buttons; *Chalbete*; Devil's Root; Dry Whiskey; Dusty; Green Whiskey; Half Moon; *Hikori*; Hikuli; *Ho*; Hyatari; Indian Dope; M; Mesc; Mescal; Mescalina; *Mescalito*; Mese; Mezc; Moon; Nubs; Peyote; *Peyotyl*; Pixie Sticks; *Raiz Diabolica*; *Seni*; The Substance; Topi; Tops; White Mule

Pharmacologic Classification

Psychodelic, amphetamine-like psychodelic: phenethylamine (natural alkaloid)

Brief General Overview

Mescaline is found in several cactus species, principally in the peyote cactus (*Lophophora williamsii*).[1] The peyote cactus is indigenous to areas of northern Mexico and the southwestern United States The psychodelic effects of mescaline are quite similar to those produced by lysergic acid diethylamide (LSD; see monograph) or psilocybin mushrooms (see monograph). The use of mescaline reportedly increased significantly in North America during the 1990s, particularly among youth of European descent.[2]

The use of peyote is considered a sacrament by members of the Native American Church of North America and the Peyote Way Church of God.[3] Historians believe peyote has been used by indigenous peoples[4] in what is now Mexico for several thousands of years. Today, Native American adolescent boys quite often report having used peyote in a nonceremonial context, but usually only once or twice.

Dosage Forms and Routes of Administration

Although mescaline can be produced by chemical synthesis,[5] it is virtually always obtained from its natural source, the peyote cactus *Lophophora williamsii*. Mescaline is prepared by drying, chopping, and grinding the buttons of the cactus, which contain not only mescaline but also several other active alkaloids. Traditionally, the cactus is dried and eaten in a ritual to induce visions.[6] Sometimes it is consumed as a medicinal tea.

Mechanism of CNS Action

Valid and reliable data are not available.

Pharmacodynamics/Pharmacokinetics

The onset of action after oral ingestion is approximately 45 to 60 minutes. Psychodelic effects peak ~4 hours after oral ingestion and gradually diminish over a period of 8 hours. Additional valid and reliable data are not available.

Current Approved Indications for Medical Use

None

Desired Action/Reason for Personal Use

Alteration in sense of time and space; magico-religious/ceremonial experience[7]; hallucinations (primarily visual, including brilliantly colored kaleidoscopic visions); heightened sensory experiences; illusions; synesthesia

Toxicity

Acute: Anorexia; anxiety; bitter taste (extreme); cognitive impairment; confusion; de-realization; disorientation; hunger (particularly for sweets), following use; hypertension; hyperthermia; insomnia; memory impairment; mydriasis; nausea (may be severe); panic reactions; personality changes; sour taste (of peyote cactus "buttons"); tachycardia; tremors; vomiting; weakness

Chronic: Psychosis (particularly among susceptible users)

Pregnancy & Lactation: Although the teratogenic potential of mescaline has been suggested by some animal studies, valid and reliable human data are not available.

Abuse Potential

Physical dependence: Low (USDEA Schedule I; use is prohibited)[8]
Psychological dependence: Moderate

Withdrawal Syndrome

A mescaline withdrawal syndrome has not been reported.

Overdosage

Mescaline has a high therapeutic index, and no reported fatalities have been directly attributed to its use. Medical support may be required. There is no known antidote.

Notes

1. Mescaline is *not* derived from either the mescal bean, which is extremely poisonous, or the mescal plant. Peyote, the common name, is thought to be a corruption of the Aztec *peyotl*. It also is known by various names by the North American Indian tribes who use it. For example, to the Tarahumare of Mexico, it is known as *hikori*; to the Mescalero, *ho*; to the Kiowa, *seni*; and to the Delawares, *biisung* (medicine).
2. The actual extent of use is difficult to estimate because most of what is sold "on the street" as synthetic mescaline is either methylenedioxymethamphetamine (MDMA, Ecstasy; see monograph) or phencyclidine (PCP; see monograph).
3. Current federal laws banning mescaline possession and use contain exemptions for the use of peyote in bona fide religious ceremonies of the Native American Church.
4. Including the Aztec, Chichimeca, Huichols, Tarahumaras, and Toltec peoples.
5. Mescaline was first isolated from peyote in 1887 and first synthesized in 1919.
6. To reduce the occurrence of associated nausea and vomiting, preparatory fasting is often part of the ritual of use.
7. North American Indians have used peyote cactus containing mescaline at least since the 1600s. During the late 1800s, Mescalero Apaches in the western United States adopted the peyote ritual from Mexican tribes. Peyote continues to be used in religious ceremonies of the Native American Church, established in 1918. Peyote is eaten ritualistically to the accompaniment of songs, drumbeat, and rattle-shaking with an attitude of prayer and religious reverie. The ceremony, which continues for 12 to 18 hours, begins at night when the "spirit-forces" (e.g., moon, stars and planets, the winds, the earth, fire, and water) are present.

    The peyote is consumed in three forms: the green plant, which is especially desirable though the most disagreeable in taste; the dry "button," which is the most common form; and a tea, which is given to the sick and to women. Each devotee eats as much as he can during the course of the night, regardless of associated nausea. It is stressed that peyote must be eaten with abandon, for if the desired state of purity is attained, no "bad effects" will be experienced. It is interesting to note that several studies have failed to find significant mental or physical adverse sequelae associated with the regular use of peyote by Native Americans within this religious context.
8. See Note 3 regarding religious exemption for peyote use.

References

Adlaf, E.M., Paglia, A., Ivis, F.J., et al. (2000). Nonmedical drug use among adolescent students: Highlights from the 1999 Ontario Student Drug Use Survey. *CMAJ. Canadian Medical Association Journal, 162*(12), 1677-1680.

Fickenscher, A., Novins, D.K., & Manson, S.M. (2006). Illicit peyote use among American Indian adolescents in substance abuse treatment: A preliminary investigation. *Substance Use & Misuse, 41*(8), 1139-1154.

Garrity, J.F. (2000). Jesus, peyote, and the holy people: Alcohol abuse and the ethos of power in Navaho healing. *Medical Anthropology Quarterly, 14*(4), 521-542.

Gilmore, H.T. (2001). Peyote use during pregnancy. *South Dakota Journal of Medicine, 54*(1), 27-29.

Halpern, J.H., Sherwood, A.R., & Hudson, J.I., et al. (2005). Psychological and cognitive effects of long-term peyote use among Native Americans. *Biological Psychiatry, 58*(8), 624-631.

METHADONE

Names

BAN or INN Generic Synonyms: None

Brand/Trade: Dolophine®; Metadol®; Methadose®; Methadose® Oral Concentrate

Chemical: 6-(Dimethylamino)-4,4-diphenyl-3-heptanone

Street: Adolph; Amidone; Biscuits; Bisquits; Chalk; Dollies; Dolls; Dollys; Dolo; Done; Doses; Fixer; Fizzies; German Boy; Juice; *Medicina;* Medicine; Meth[1]; Meth-A-Done; Nazi; Phy; Pixie; Synthetic Heroin; Wafer

Pharmacologic Classification

Psychodepressant, opiate analgesic: pure agonist (synthetic)

Brief General Overview

Methadone was developed in Germany during World War II (1939–1945) because of the shortage of morphine. Subsequently, however, it was not widely used for its analgesic actions, nor was it widely abused except when other opiate analgesics (e.g., heroin) were unavailable, because of its less intense euphoria and significantly more severe withdrawal syndrome.

Over the past 50 years, methadone has become the mainstay of opiate analgesic maintenance pharmacotherapy because of its good oral bioavailability, long duration of action (24 hours), relatively low manufacturing cost, very mild euphoria, and effectiveness in preventing the opiate analgesic withdrawal syndrome in regular, long-term users of opiate analgesics (e.g., heroin, meperidine, morphine) who are trying to discontinue their use[2] (Table 5, page 208). Methadone is abused, however, by some opiate analgesic maintenance program enrollees (generally estimated as less than 5%), particularly younger enrollees. It also is used by many more people who are addicted to opiate analgesics, particularly when their opiate analgesic of choice (e.g., heroin) is unavailable because of a lack of supply or because they lack the money or other means to obtain it.

Dosage Forms and Routes of Administration

Methadone is legally produced by pharmaceutical manufacturers in North America. It is available in a variety of injectable (i.e., intramuscular, subcutaneous) and oral (i.e., concentrate, dispersible diskette, solution, syrup, tablet) dosage formulations.

Mechanism of CNS Action

Methadone has several actions quantitatively similar to those of morphine. The most prominent actions involve the CNS and body organs composed of smooth muscle (e.g., intestine, lungs). However, the major actions of concern to people who abuse methadone and those in opiate maintenance programs are its analgesic and psychodepressant actions. Methadone elicits its analgesic and psychodepressant actions primarily by

TABLE 5

Advantages and Disadvantages of Methadone Opiate Analgesic Maintenance Programs

Advantages	Disadvantages
Produces minimal euphoria	Maintains opiate analgesic dependence
Prevents the opiate analgesic withdrawal syndrome in opiate analgesic (e.g., heroin)-dependent people	Produces a more severe withdrawal syndrome when discontinued than that associated with heroin or other opiate analgesics
Orally effective; thus, eliminates risks associated with intravenous injection of heroin or other opiate analgesics (e.g., HIV infection)	Produces cognitive impairment and other adverse effects related to the pharmacologic action of methadone
Reduces craving for heroin	Does not prevent the craving for, or use of, other nonopiate analgesic drugs and substances of abuse (e.g., alcohol, benzodiazepines, cannabis, cocaine)
Inexpensive compared with maintaining use of heroin or other opiate analgesics	Opiate analgesic dependency programs remain financially costly to run in relation to medical, pharmacy, and other costs
Legal; thus, reduces illegal activity (e.g., prostitution, burglary) associated with maintaining opiate analgesic (i.e., heroin) use	Methadone doses may be diverted and sold "on the street," usually for other drugs and substances of abuse
Encourages maintenance or resumption of normal activities of daily living (e.g., employment, child care)	Generally, users are kept dependent on others to provide daily maintenance dose (may also interfere with travel and other activities)

Source: Adapted from Pagliaro, L.A., & Pagliaro, A.M. (2004). *Pagliaros' comprehensive guide to drugs and substances of abuse*. Washington, DC: American Pharmacists Association.

binding to endorphin receptors in the CNS. However, the exact mechanism of action has not been determined (see Opiate Analgesics monograph).

Pharmacodynamics/Pharmacokinetics

Methadone is well absorbed (~90%) after oral ingestion. However, oral ingestion is associated with delayed onset of action, lowering of peak blood concentration, and increased duration of analgesic action. Methadone's duration of action is 3 to 5 hours after intramuscular or subcutaneous injection. After oral ingestion, it is 6 to 8 hours. However, it is approximately one-half as potent when orally ingested as when injected, presumably because of significant first-pass hepatic metabolism. Prolonged duration of action makes methadone an effective drug for the management of opiate analgesic dependency or addiction. Methadone is approximately 90% bound to plasma proteins and has a mean apparent volume of distribution of ~4 L/kg. Total body clearance is ~90 mL/minute, and the mean elimination half-life is 36 hours. Methadone is primarily metabolized by the cytochrome P450 hepatic microsomal enzymes (particularly isoenzymes 3A4, 3A5, and 2B6) to 2-ethylidene-1,5-dimethyl-3,3-diphenylpyrrolidine. Genetic polymorphism causes significant interindividual variability in methadone blood concentrations resulting from a particular dosage.

Current Approved Indications for Medical Use

Pain, moderate to severe (acute); opiate analgesic detoxification; opiate analgesic maintenance therapy (i.e., long-term prevention of opiate analgesic withdrawal)

Desired Action/Reason for Personal Use

Euphoria; prevention/self-management of the opiate analgesic withdrawal syndrome; relaxation

Toxicity

Acute: Anorexia; bradycardia; cognitive impairment; constipation; dizziness; drowsiness; dry mouth; flushing of the skin; headache; hypotension; lightheadedness; miosis; nausea; pruritus; sexual desire (decreased); visual acuity (reduced); urinary retention; vomiting; weakness

Chronic: Cognitive impairment; constipation; menstrual irregularities; night vision, impaired; physical dependence; psychological dependence; sexual desire, decreased; *torsades de pointes* (rare)[3]; urinary retention

Pregnancy & Lactation: FDA Pregnancy Category C (see Appendix B). Safety of methadone use by adolescent girls and women who are pregnant has not been established. Methadone crosses the placenta. Regular, long-term use during pregnancy results in the neonatal opiate withdrawal syndrome. Adolescent girls and women who are pregnant should not use methadone.

Methadone is excreted in breast milk in concentrations up to 85% of those in the maternal blood. Expected pharmacologic actions (e.g., drowsiness, lethargy, respiratory depression) may be observed in neonates and infants, who also may become physically dependent. Adolescent girls and women who are breast-feeding should not use methadone.

Abuse Potential

Physical dependence: High (USDEA Schedule II; high potential for abuse)
Psychological dependence: Moderate

Withdrawal Syndrome

Methadone users, including those enrolled in opiate analgesic dependency maintenance programs, should carry a card to alert medical personnel in the event of an emergency. These individuals may experience the opiate analgesic withdrawal syndrome if they receive the opiate analgesic agonist/antagonist pentazocine (Talwin®) or the pure opiate analgesic antagonist naloxone (Narcan®). The methadone withdrawal syndrome, although qualitatively similar to that of morphine and other opiate analgesics, differs in several ways. Its onset is slower, its course is more prolonged, and the signs and symptoms are more intense or severe. People who want to decrease their dosage of methadone or completely discontinue its use require medically supervised opiate analgesic detoxification.

Overdosage

Signs and symptoms of methadone overdosage, which begin within seconds after intravenous injection or within minutes after oral ingestion, intranasal sniffing (snorting), or rectal insertion, include coma, cool and clammy skin, miosis, respiratory depression, skeletal muscle flaccidity, and somnolence. In cases of severe overdosage, these signs and symptoms can progress to apnea, bradycardia, hypotension, and death.

Methadone overdosage requires emergency medical support, with attention to increasing methadone elimination. The opiate antagonist naloxone (Narcan®) is an essential component of the emergency medical management of overdosage of methadone.[4] Repeated doses of naloxone are usually required, because methadone's duration of action is prolonged (36 to 48 hours) and that of naloxone is short (1 to 3 hours).

Notes

1. Street names for many of the drugs and substances of abuse can sometimes refer to several different drugs or substances. For example, "Meth" also refers to the psychostimulant methamphetamine.

2. Methadone opiate analgesic maintenance programs require participants to be enrolled in an opiate addiction maintenance program. Methadone pharmacotherapy is individualized according to the degree of the participant's opiate analgesic physical dependence or addiction and other factors. For example, generally, the individualized dosage of methadone is orally ingested once daily under close supervision. However, some participants may require additional doses to prevent the onset of the opiate analgesic withdrawal syndrome. As another example, intramuscular injection may be required for those participants who are unable to ingest the oral dosage formulation. Regardless of these and other factors, the individualized dosage should always be sufficient to prevent the onset of the opiate analgesic withdrawal syndrome.

3. Reportedly occurs predominantly in people who have a predisposing risk factor for cardiac dysrhythmias and who use higher dosages of methadone.

4. Particular caution is indicated because the use of naloxone may precipitate the methadone withdrawal syndrome in people who are physically dependent on methadone.

References

Ballard, J.L. (2002). Treatment of neonatal abstinence syndrome with breast milk containing methadone. *Journal of Perinatal and Neonatal Nursing, 15*(4), 76-85.

Chhabra, S., & Bull, J. (2008). Methadone. *American Journal of Hospice Palliative Care, 25*(2), 146-150.

De Fazio, S., Gallelli, L., De Siena, A., et al. (2008). Role of CYP3A5 in abnormal clearance of methadone. *The Annals of Pharmacotherapy, 42*(6), 893-897.

Fiellin, D.A., O'Connor, P.G., Chawarski, M., et al. (2001). Methadone maintenance in primary care: A randomized controlled trial. *JAMA, 286*(14), 1724-1731.

Hulse, G.K., & O'Neill, G. (2001). Methadone and the pregnant user: A matter of careful clinical consideration. *Australian, New Zealand Journal of Obstetrics and Gynecology, 41*(3), 329-332.

King, V.L., Stoller, K.B., Hayes, M., et al. (2002). A multicenter randomized evaluation of methadone medical maintenance. *Drug and Alcohol Dependence, 65*(2), 137-148.

Krambeer, L.L., von McKnelly, W. Jr., Gabrielli, W.F., et al. (2001). Methadone therapy for opioid dependence. *American Family Physician, 63*(12), 2404-2410.

Krantz, M.J., Lewkowiez, L., Hays, H., et al. (2002). Torsade de pointes associated with very-high-dose methadone. *Annals of Internal Medicine, 137*(6), 501-504.

Li, Y., Kantelip, J.P., Gerritsen-van Schieveen, P., et al. (2008). Interindividual variability of methadone response: Impact of genetic polymorphism. *Molecular Diagnosis Therapy, 12*(2), 109-124.

Lugo, R.A., Satterfield, K.L., & Kern, S.E. (2005). Pharmacokinetics of methadone. *Journal of Pain & Palliative Care Pharmacotherapy, 19*(4), 13-24.

Merrill, J.O., Jackson, T.R., Schulman, B.A., et al. (2005). Methadone medical maintenance in primary care. An implementation evaluation. *Journal of General Internal Medicine, 20*(4), 344-349.

Mintzer, M.Z., & Stitzer, M.L. (2002). Cognitive impairment in methadone maintenance patients. *Drug and Alcohol Dependence, 67*(1), 41-51.

Wilbourne, P., Wallerstedt, C., Dorato, V., et al. (2001). Clinical management of methadone dependence during pregnancy. *Journal of Perinatal Nursing, 14*(4), 26-45.

Wu, L.T., Blazer, D.G., Stitzer, M.L., et al. (2008). Infrequent illicit methadone use among stimulant-using patients in methadone maintenance treatment programs: A national drug abuse treatment clinical trials network study. *American Journal on Addictions, 17*(4), 304-311.

METHAMPHETAMINE

Names

BAN or INN Generic Synonyms: Metamfetamine; d-Deoxyephedrine

Brand/Trade[1]: Desoxyn®

Chemical: (+)-(s)-N, α-Dimethylphenethylamine

Street: *Acelerante*; Amp; *Bambita*; Bathtub Crank; *Batu*; Beans; Billy; Blade; Blue Meth; Blue Mollies; Brain Burners; Chalk; Champagne; Chicken Feed; Chimichanga; Chris; Chrissie; Christina; Christmas Tree Meth; Cinnamon; Clear; Coffee; Crank; Crankenstine; Crink; Cris; Crissie; *Cristina*; Cristine; Cristy; Crosses; Crypto; Crystal; Crystal Glass; Crystal Meth; Crystal Speed; Desocsins; Desogtion; Devil's Dandruff; Dice; Doe; Flash; Fluff; G; Gak; Geek; Geep; Glass; Go; Go Fast; Gonzolez; Go Pills; Goose-Egg; Granulated Orange; Gumption; Hanyak; Hard Crystal; Hawaiian Salt; Hillbilly Crack; Hironpon; Hiropon; Holiday Meth; Hot Ice; Hydro; Ice; Ink; Ish; Jenny Crank; Jet Fuel; Jib; Juice; Kaksonjae; L.A. Glass; L.A. Ice; Lemon Drop; Load of Laundry; Met; Meth[2]; Methedrine; Methlies Quik; Mexican Crack; Mike; Motherdear; Motorcycle Crack; No Doze; OZs; Peanut Butter; Peanut Butter Meth; Pellets; Pep Pills; Poor Man's Cocaine; Quartz; Redneck Cocaine; Red Phosphorus; Rip; Rock Candy; Rocket Fuel; Rudy; Schmiz; *Scootie; Shabu*; Shards; Sketch; Soap Dope; Spackle; Sparkle; Speckled Birds; Speed; Speed Racer; Spoosh; Stove Top; Stove Top Speed; Super Ice; Tangerine; Tasmanian Devil; Tick Tick; Tina; Trash; Tutu; Tweak; Tweek; Ups; Uppers; Velocidad; Wake; Wash; West Coast; White Cross; Working Man's Cocaine; *Yaba*[3]; *Ya Ba*; Yellow Bam; Yellow Powder; Zip

Pharmacologic Classification

Psychostimulant, amphetamine

Brief General Overview

Methamphetamine, first synthesized in Japan in 1919 (see Amphetamines monograph), has psychostimulant actions that are similar to those of cocaine but last much longer. Commonly referred to as "Speed," methamphetamine is now the favorite and most abused of the amphetamine psychostimulants. Methamphetamine has almost always been intravenously injected, but the crystalline form (i.e., "Ice") is now smoked[4] and has gained increased popularity because it allows users to achieve a "high" equal to that obtained with intravenous injection—but more rapidly and without the associated risks (e.g., abscesses; need for needles and syringes; infection, particularly with hepatitis virus and HIV; collapsed or damaged veins; thrombophlebitis). Ice smoking initially gained popularity in Hawaii and California more than two decades ago and has now spread across both urban and rural North America.

Dosage Forms and Routes of Administration

Methamphetamine is licitly produced by pharmaceutical manufacturers in North America and is available in both regular and extended-release oral tablets. Most illicitly produced methamphetamine is produced in Mexico or in the Los Angeles, California, area under the control and direction of Mexican criminal organizations, outlaw motorcycle gangs, and their affiliated youth gangs. Typically, methamphetamine is produced on a large scale in "super labs"—illicit laboratories capable of producing 10 or more pounds of methamphetamine per day. It also is illicitly synthesized in clandestine ("mom and pop") laboratories across North America, ranging from small basement laboratories to sophisticated laboratories on college campuses. Methamphetamine can be relatively easily synthesized from inexpensive over-the-counter ingredients and common supplies[5] and is also produced for personal use in smaller amounts in kitchens, bathrooms, and other home settings.[6]

It is estimated that methamphetamine has been used by more than 5% of adults in North America and that its use is increasing. Although users may be found in all segments of North American society, the highest rate of methamphetamine use is found in adolescent boys and men of European descent. These users generally are high school or college students and young adults, 16 to 40 years of age, who are either employed in nonprofessional jobs or unemployed. A higher rate of methamphetamine abuse is found in Hawaiians, Native Americans, and gay and bisexual men than in the general population. (Also see Note 3 regarding the use of *Yaba*.) Gay and bisexual men use methamphetamine as one of their five main party or club drugs (i.e., cocaine, gamma-hydroxybutyrate [GHB], ketamine, methamphetamine, and methylenedioxymethamphetamine [MDMA, Ecstasy]; see monographs). These drugs are used to facilitate social disinhibition, arouse sexual desire, and enhance sexual experiences among members of the gay and bisexual community.

Mechanism of CNS Action

Methamphetamine is a potent psychostimulant. It appears to elicit its stimulant actions by increasing the release of dopamine and norepinephrine from central adrenergic neurons and inhibiting their transporter-facilitated reuptake. A direct effect on α- and β-adrenergic receptors and inhibition of the enzyme amine oxidase also appear to be involved. However, the exact mechanism of action has not been determined (see Amphetamines monograph).

Pharmacodynamics/Pharmacokinetics

Methamphetamine is rapidly absorbed after oral ingestion. After smoking, the bioavailability of methamphetamine is ~60% and after intranasal sniffing (snorting) it is ~80%. The steady-state volume of distribution is 4.2 L/kg. The primary site of metabolism is the liver. Mean total body clearance is ~270 mL/kg/hr. The mean half-life of elimination is ~11 hours. Both metabolites and unchanged drug are excreted primarily in the urine, and excretion is pH dependent. Thus, in alkaline urine, excretion is significantly decreased and elimination half-life is increased. In acidic urine, excretion is significantly increased and elimination half-life is decreased. Effects are generally noted within 30 seconds to 30 minutes, depending on the method of use (e.g., intravenous injection versus oral ingestion). Psychostimulant effects usually last for 4 to 8 hours but may persist for up to 24 hours.

Current Approved Indications for Medical Use

Attention-deficit/hyperactivity disorder; exogenous obesity; narcolepsy

Desired Action/Reason for Personal Use

Alertness, vigilance or wakefulness; appetite/hunger suppression; arousal of sexual desires; enhance sexual experiences (particularly among gay and bisexual men); energy; euphoria; exhilaration (intense); facilitate sexual activity (particularly among gay and bisexual men); heighten sense of well-being; reduce fatigue; "rush" or "flash"[7]; social disinhibition (particularly among gay and bisexual men)

Toxicity

Acute: Agitation; anorexia; anxiety; bruxism (teeth grinding); cardiac dysrhythmias; dizziness; headache; hyperactivity; hyperexcitability; hypertension; hyperthermia; hyperventilation; insomnia; irritability; mydriasis; myocardial infarction; nervousness (extreme); palpitations; paranoid delusions; perspiration (increased); psychosis[8]; restlessness; seizures; sexual desire (increased); stroke; tachycardia; talkativeness (incessant); tremor

Chronic: Cardiomyopathy, cognitive impairment[9]; damaged veins (with intravenous injection); dermatoses; infections (at injection sites); hepatitis, HIV/AIDS, and other infections (with intravenous injection and associated high-risk sexual behavior)[10]; neurotoxicity[11]; occupational problems; paranoid delusions; physical dependence; psychological dependence; psychosis (particularly with higher dosages and can recur spontaneously); relationship problems; skin abscesses (with intravenous injection); social deterioration; stereotypic behavior (e.g., picking at the skin); tooth wear (particularly of the anterior maxillary teeth); weight loss

Pregnancy & Lactation: FDA Pregnancy Category C (see Appendix B). Safety of methamphetamine use by adolescent girls and women who are pregnant has not been established. Adolescent girls and women who are physically or psychologically dependent on methamphetamine have an increased risk for premature delivery and low birth weight neonates. Neonates also may display signs and symptoms of the methamphetamine withdrawal syndrome, including agitation and lassitude (also see Amphetamines monograph). Adolescent girls and women who are pregnant should not use methamphetamine.

Safety of methamphetamine use by adolescent girls and women who are breast-feeding has not been established. Methamphetamine is excreted in breast milk. Adolescent girls and women who are breast-feeding should not use methamphetamine.

Abuse Potential

Physical dependence: High (USDEA Schedule II; high potential for abuse)
Psychological dependence: High

Withdrawal Syndrome

Abrupt discontinuation of methamphetamine after regular, long-term, high-dosage use may result in the methamphetamine withdrawal syndrome. Signs and symptoms include EEG changes during sleep, fatigue, and mental depression, which is often severe. There is no specific pharmacotherapy for the management of the methamphetamine withdrawal syndrome. Medical management remains symptomatic. See the Amphetamines monograph.

Overdosage

Signs and symptoms of acute methamphetamine overdosage include cardiovascular reactions (e.g., dysrhythmias, hypertension or hypotension, and circulatory collapse), combativeness, confusion, destruction of skeletal muscle (rhabdomyolysis), GI complaints (e.g., abdominal cramps, diarrhea, nausea, and vomiting), hallucinations, hyperpyrexia, hyperreflexia, panic, rapid respirations, restlessness, and tremor. Depression and fatigue generally follow the central stimulation. Fatal methamphetamine overdosage usually terminates in convulsions and coma.

Methamphetamine overdosage requires emergency medical support of body systems with attention to increasing methamphetamine elimination. Increasing methamphetamine elimination is particularly important when the extended-release tablet formulation of methamphetamine has been involved in the overdosage. There is no known antidote.

Notes

1. Also formerly marketed under the brand/trade name Methedrine®.
2. The common street name for many of the drugs and substances of abuse are often used interchangeably and sometimes refer to several different drugs and substances of abuse. In this case, "Meth" also refers to the opiate analgesic methadone.
3. *Yaba* is the Thai name for a mixture of methamphetamine and caffeine. It is produced in the form of small tablets (i.e., about the size of a saccharin or aspartame [Equal®] tablet) intended for oral use. The tablets are primarily produced and imported from Burma for use by Asian Americans, particularly those from Laos or Thailand. However, the tablets are becoming increasingly popular among adolescents and young adults who frequent dance clubs and raves, particularly in California.
4. Historically, it is interesting to note that this change in the preferred pattern of use to smoking also occurred with cocaine. The intranasal sniffing (snorting) of cocaine was commonly replaced by smoking when the crack form of cocaine was introduced (see Cocaine monograph).
5. These ingredients and supplies include acetone, anhydrous ammonia, cold and allergy tablets that contain pseudoephedrine, coffee filters, drain cleaner, isopropyl (rubbing) alcohol, lithium batteries, lye, Mason jars, pillowcases, and toluene. Methamphetamine also can be synthesized from amphetamine, phenylalanine, or phenylpropanolamine. To prevent the diversion of these drugs for the illicit production of methamphetamine, the Comprehensive Methamphetamine Control Act of 1996 was passed. This law placed combination ephedrine drug products, phenylpropanolamine, and pseudoephedrine under regulation as List I chemicals.
6. Children are often exposed to fumes associated with the production of methamphetamine in home settings (e.g., kitchens, family rooms, basements) by their parents or others living in the home. Signs and symptoms of exposure observed in these children may include abdominal pain, amber- or dark-colored urine, blurred vision, chemical burns, chest pain, cognitive impairment, coughing, diarrhea, discharge from the eyes, eye pain, fever, headaches, hallucinations, irritability, jaundice, laryngeal congestion or laryngitis, malnutrition, nausea, neglect, respiratory irritation, skin irritation, sneezing, tachycardia, vomiting, tearing, watery eyes, and weight loss. These children also are

exposed to various levels of abuse and neglect, resulting in behavior problems, malnutrition, and poor hygiene with associated infections (e.g., respiratory and urinary tract) and various infestations (e.g., lice).

7. Usually associated only with intravenous injection or smoking of methamphetamine.

8. The psychosis is often clinically indistinguishable from paranoid schizophrenia and is probably one of the most severe signs and symptoms of intoxication.

9. Cognitive impairment includes deficits in abstract thinking, learning, memory, and psychomotor speed. These deficits appear to be related to neurotoxicity involving the dopamine terminals, particularly in the caudate and putamen. Some of the methamphetamine-induced neurotoxicity may be due to down-regulation (i.e., temporary neuroadaptive changes) and may be reversible with protracted abstinence from methamphetamine use. However, some of the neurotoxic effects may be permanent—in which case, risk for parkinsonism with advancing age increases significantly (also see Note 11).

10. Chronic infection is a serious problem in all injectable methamphetamine users, but it is compounded in gay men, for whom injectable methamphetamine use also has been associated with high-risk sexual behaviors (e.g., anal sex, anonymous sex, low rates of condom use, multiple sex partners, and sexual marathons) that may place them at increased risk of contracting and spreading HIV and other sexually transmitted diseases, as well as other contagious diseases (e.g., hepatitis C).

11. Neurotoxicity has long been associated with methamphetamine-induced damage to dopaminergic neurons in the basal ganglia and reduced dopamine transporter density in the caudate/putamen, nucleus accumbens, and prefrontal cortex. Data currently indicate that long-term, high dosage methamphetamine use selectively damages the nigrostriatal dopamine projection of the brain, resulting in permanent parkinsonian-like symptoms (e.g., pill-rolling tremor, shuffling gait).

References

Anglin, M.D., Burke, C., Perrochet, B., et al. (2000). History of the methamphetamine problem. *Journal of Psychoactive Drugs, 32*(2), 137-141.

Cho, A.K., & Melega, W.P. (2002). Patterns of methamphetamine abuse and their consequences. *Journal of Addictive Diseases, 21*(1), 21-34.

Comer, S.D., Hart, C.L., Ward, A.S., et al. (2001). Effects of repeated oral methamphetamine administration in humans. *Psychopharmacology, 155*(4), 397-404.

Cunningham, J.K., Liu, L.M., & Muramoto, M. (2008). Methamphetamine suppression and route of administration: Precursor regulation impacts on snorting, smoking, swallowing and injecting. *Addiction, 103*(7), 1174-1186.

Davidson, C., Gow, A.J., Lee, T.H., et al. (2001). Methamphetamine neurotoxicity: Necrotic and apoptotic mechanisms and relevance to human abuse and treatment. *Brain Research. Brain Research Reviews, 36*(1), 1-22.

Diaz, R.M., Heckert, A.L., & Sánchez, J. (2005). Reasons for stimulant use among Latino gay men in San Francisco: A comparison between methamphetamine and cocaine users. *Journal of Urban Health, 82*(1, Supplement 1), i71-i78.

Domier, C.P., Simon, S.L., Rawson, R.A., et al. (2000). A comparison of injecting and noninjecting methamphetamine users. *Journal of Psychoactive Drugs, 32*(2), 229-232.

Drug Enforcement Administration (DEA) Justice. (2002). Implementation of the Comprehensive Methamphetamine Control Act of 1996; regulation of pseudoephedrine, phenylpropanolamine, and combination ephedrine drug products and reports of certain transactions to nonregulated persons. Final rule. *Federal Register, 67*(60), 14853-14862.

Durell, T.M., Kroutil, L.A., Crits-Christoph, P., et al. (2008). Prevalence of nonmedical methamphetamine use in the United States. *Substance Abuse Treatment, Prevention, and Policy, 3*, 19.

Freese, T.E., Obert, J., Dickow, A., et al. (2000). Methamphetamine abuse: Issues for special populations. *Journal of Psychoactive Drugs, 32*(2), 177-182.

Gonzalez, C.F., Barrington, E.H., Walton, M.A., et al. (2000). Cocaine and methamphetamine: Differential addiction rates. *Psychology of Addictive Behaviors, 14*(4), 390-396.

Guilarte, T.R. (2001). Is methamphetamine abuse a risk factor for parkinsonism? *Neurotoxicology, 22*(6), 725-731.

Halkitis, P.N., Mukherjee, P.P., & Palamar, J.J. (2007). Multi-level modeling to explain methamphetamine use among gay and bisexual men. *Addiction, 102*(Supplement 1), 76-83.

Halkitis, P.N., Parsons, J.T., & Stirratt, M.J. (2001). A double epidemic: Crystal methamphetamine drug use in relation to HIV transmission among gay men. *Journal of Homosexuality, 41*(2), 17-35.

Hanson, G.R., Rau, K.S., & Fleckenstein, A.E. (2004). The methamphetamine experience: A NIDA partnership. *Neuropharmacology, 47*(Supplement 1), 92-100.

Harris, D.S., Boxenbaum, H., Everhart, E.T., et al. (2003). The bioavailability of intranasal and smoked methamphetamine. *Clinical Pharmacology & Therapeutics, 74*(5), 475-486.

Hart, C.L., Gunderson, E.W., Perez, A., et al. (2008). Acute physiological and behavioral effects of intranasal methamphetamine in humans. *Neuropsychopharmacology, 33*(8), 1847-1855.

Hart, C.L., Ward, A.S., Haney, M., et al. (2003). Methamphetamine attenuates disruptions in performance and mood during simulated night-shift work. *Psychopharmacology, 169*(1), 42-51.

Iritani, B.J., Hallfors, D.D., & Bauer, D.J. (2007). Crystal methamphetamine use among young adults in the USA. *Addiction, 102*(7), 1102-1113.

Kish, S.J. (2008). Pharmacologic mechanisms of crystal meth. *CMAJ: Canadian Medical Association Journal, 178*(13), 1679-1682.

Mahoney, J.J. 3rd, Kalechstein, A.D., De La Garza, R. 2nd, et al. (2008). Presence and persistence of psychotic symptoms in cocaine- versus methamphetamine-dependent participants. *American Journal on Addictions, 17*(2), 83-98.

McCann, U.D., Kuwabara, H., Kumar, A., et al. (2008). Persistent cognitive and dopamine transporter deficits in abstinent methamphetamine users. *Synapse, 62*(2), 91-100.

McKetin, R., McLaren, J., Lubman, D.I., et al. (2006). The prevalence of psychotic symptoms among methamphetamine users. *Addiction, 101*(10), 1473-1478.

McKetin, R., McLaren, J., Lubman, D.I., et al. (2008). Hostility among methamphetamine users experiencing psychotic symptoms. *American Journal on Addictions, 17*(3), 235-240.

Moszczynska, A., Fitzmaurice, P., Ang, L., et al. (2004). Why is parkinsonism not a feature of human methamphetamine users? *Brain, 127*(Part 2), 363-370.

Parsons, J.T., Kelly, B.C., & Weiser, J.D. (2007). Initiation into methamphetamine use for young gay and bisexual men. *Drug and Alcohol Dependence, 90*(2-3), 135-144.

Paulus, M.P., Hozack, N.E., Zauscher, B.E., et al. (2002). Behavioral and functional neuroimaging evidence for prefrontal dysfunction in methamphetamine-dependent subjects. *Neuropsychopharmacology, 26*(1), 53-63.

Rawson, R.A., Anglin, M.D., & Ling, W. (2002). Will the methamphetamine problem go away? *Journal of Addictive Diseases, 21*(1), 5-19.

Richards, J.R., & Brofeldt, B.T. (2000). Patterns of tooth wear associated with methamphetamine use. *Journal of Periodontology, 71*(8), 1371-1374.

Salo, R., Nordahl, T.E., Possin, K., et al. (2002). Preliminary evidence of reduced cognitive inhibition in methamphetamine-dependent individuals. *Psychiatry Research, 111*(1), 65-74.

Sekine, Y., Iyo, M., Ouchi, Y., et al. (2001). Methamphetamine-related psychiatric symptoms and reduced brain dopamine transporters studied with PET. *American Journal of Psychiatry, 158*(8), 1206-1214.

Semple, S.J., Patterson, T.L., & Grant, I. (2002). Motivations associated with methamphetamine use among HIV+ men who have sex with men. *Journal of Substance Abuse Treatment, 22*(3), 149-156.

Shoptaw, S., Reback, C.J., Freese, T.E. (2002). Patient characteristics, HIV serostatus, and risk behaviors among gay and bisexual males seeking treatment for methamphetamine abuse and dependence in Los Angeles. *Journal of Addictive Diseases, 21*(1), 91-105.

Sim, T., Simon, S.L., Domier, C.P., et al. (2002). Cognitive deficits among methamphetamine users with attention deficit hyperactivity disorder symptomatology. *Journal of Addictive Diseases, 21*(1), 75-89.

Simon, S.L., Domier, C.P., Sim, T., et al. (2002). Cognitive performance of current methamphetamine and cocaine abusers. *Journal of Addictive Diseases, 21*(1), 61-74.

Special report: Club drugs & HIV. (2002). Drug treatment best hope for meth-using MSMs. Researchers want to get word out about problem. *AIDS Alert, 17*(11), 137-138, 143.

Volkow, N.D., Chang, L., Wang, G.J., et al. (2001). Low level brain dopamine D2 receptors in methamphetamine abusers: Association with metabolism in the orbitofrontal cortex. *The American Journal of Psychiatry, 158*(12), 2015-2021.

Volkow, N.D., Chang, L., Wang, G.J., et al. (2001). Loss of dopamine transporters in methamphetamine abusers recovers with protracted abstinence. *Journal of Neuroscience, 21*(23), 9414-9418.

Volz, T.J., Hanson, G.R., & Fleckenstein, A.E. (2007). The role of the plasmalemmal dopamine and vesicular monoamine transporters in methamphetamine-induced dopaminergic deficits. *Journal of Neurochemistry, 101*(4), 883-888.

Wermuth, L. (2000). Methamphetamine use: Hazards and social influences. *Journal of Drug Education, 30*(4), 423-433.

Yui, K., Goto, K., Ikemoto, S., et al. (2001). Susceptibility to subsequent episodes of spontaneous recurrence of methamphetamine psychosis. *Drug and Alcohol Dependence, 64*(2), 133-142.

Yui, K., Ikemoto, S., & Goto, K. (2002). Factors for susceptibility to episode recurrence in spontaneous recurrence of methamphetamine psychosis. *Annals of the New York Academy of Sciences, 965*, 292-304.

METHAQUALONE

Names

BAN or INN Generic Synonyms: None

Brand/Trade[1]

Chemical: 2-Methyl-3-o-tolyl-4(3H)-quinazolinone

Street: 714's; Canadian Quail; Cortals; Gorilla Biscuits; Love Drug; LU; Ludes; Luds; Mandies; Q; Quads; Quay; Rues; Soap; Soapers; Soaps; Sopes; Sporos; Vitamin Q; Wallbanger

Pharmacologic Classification

Psychodepressant, sedative-hypnotic: miscellaneous (synthetic quinazolinone [quinazoline])

Brief General Overview

Methaqualone, first synthesized in India in 1955, was introduced to North America as a sedative-hypnotic in 1965. It was touted as a safe alternative to the barbiturates because it was thought to possess little potential for physical or psychological dependence, but it soon became apparent that these claims were not true. During the 1970s the popularity of personal use of methaqualone for its psychodepressant actions increased, and by 1984 licit pharmaceutical production was halted when methaqualone was designated a USDEA Schedule I drug. Currently, methaqualone is not widely used in North America.

Dosage Forms and Routes of Administration

Methaqualone is available in oral tablet form and is usually ingested. Although methaqualone is no longer produced in North America, it is smuggled into Canada and the United States in large quantities, primarily from China, Mexico, and, more recently, South Africa, where its use has increased significantly.[2] In both Africa and India, methaqualone is widely available and the preferred method of use is smoking the crushed tablets, either sprinkled within a tobacco cigarette or heated on a piece of aluminum foil so that the vaporized fumes can be inhaled (i.e., similar to "chasing the dragon;" see Opiate Analgesics monograph).

Mechanism of CNS Action

Valid and reliable data are not available.

Pharmacodynamics/Pharmacokinetics

After oral ingestion, peak serum concentrations occur at ~3 hours. The elimination half-life of methaqualone is ~12 hours. Additional valid and reliable data are not available.

Current Approved Indications for Medical Use

None

Desired Action/Reason for Personal Use

Euphoria (intense); prevention/self-management of the methaqualone withdrawal syndrome

Toxicity

Acute: Cognitive impairment; dizziness; drowsiness; hangover effect; psychomotor impairment; respiratory depression

Chronic: Physical dependence; psychological dependence

Pregnancy & Lactation: Valid and reliable data are not available.

Abuse Potential

Physical dependence: High (USDEA Schedule I; use is prohibited)
Psychological dependence: High

Withdrawal Syndrome

A significant withdrawal syndrome may occur upon abrupt discontinuation of regular, long-term methaqualone use. The syndrome is similar to the barbiturate withdrawal syndrome (see Barbiturates monograph) and has been associated with status epilepticus and death. To prevent or minimize the withdrawal syndrome, regular, long-term use of methaqualone should be discontinued gradually over 1 to 2 weeks.

Overdosage

Signs and symptoms of methaqualone overdosage include ataxia, clonus, coma, drowsiness, hyperreflexia, nystagmus, respiratory depression or arrest, and stupor. Methaqualone overdosage can result in significant respiratory depression and death. Overdosage requires emergency medical support of body systems with attention to maintaining respiratory function. There is no known antidote.

Notes

1. Methaqualone was previously available in North America by the brand/trade names Mandrax®, Parest®, Quaalude®, and Sopor® and is still referred to "on the street" by these names.
2. Methaqualone is currently the illicit synthetic drug of choice among South Africans. In South Africa, the primary users are black adolescent boys and young men, 15 to 30 years of age.

References

Bhana, A., Parry, C.D., Myers, B., et al. (2002). The South African Community Epidemiology Network on Drug Use (SACENDU) project, phases 1-8: Cannabis and Mandrax. *South African Medical Journal, 92*(7), 542-547.

McCarthy, G., Myers, B., & Siegfried, N. (2005). Treatment for methaqualone dependence in adults. *The Cochrane Database of Systematic Reviews, 18*(2), CD004146.

van Zyl, E.F. (2001). A survey of reported synthesis of methaqualone and some positional and structural isomers. *Forensic Science International, 122*(2-3), 142-149.

METHCATHINONE

Names

BAN or INN Generic Synonyms: Ephedrone

Brand/Trade: None

Chemical: 2-(Methylamino)-1-phenylpropan-1-one

Street: Bathtub Speed; Big C; C; Cadillac Express; Cat; Ephedrone; Ephidrine; Ephidrone; Gagers; Gaggers; Gas; Ggob; Goey; Go Fast; Goob; Jeff; Kitty; Meth's Cat; Meth's Kitten; Morning Star; Mulka; Slick Superspeed; Sniff; Star; Stat; The C; Tweeker; Wannabe-Speed; Wild Cat; Wonder Star

Pharmacologic Classification

Psychostimulant, miscellaneous: structural β-ketone analogue of methamphetamine and cathinone

Brief General Overview

Methcathinone, as its name implies, is structurally related to cathinone (see *Catha edulis* monograph).[1] First synthesized in Germany in 1928, it was used as an antidepressant in the former Soviet Union between 1930 and 1980. Although it was considered for use as an appetite suppressant in the United States during the 1950s by the Parke-Davis Pharmaceutical Company, it was never marketed. By the late 1970s, wide personal use of methcathinone began across the former Soviet Union (e.g., Estonia, Latvia, Russia). However, its North American use can be traced to a graduate student in Michigan, working as an intern at Parke-Davis during the late 1980s, who "rediscovered" methcathinone from old research records. It is usually illicitly synthesized from ephedrine or pseudoephedrine, and its personal use has rapidly spread across North

America. Methcathinone produces amphetamine-like effects, and its abuse potential is similar to that of methamphetamine (see monograph).

Dosage Forms and Routes of Administration

Methcathinone is manufactured in clandestine laboratories across North America.[2] Much like amphetamine and cocaine, it is generally available as a water-soluble crystalline hydrochloride salt[3] and is used in much the same way. For example, it can be used in the crystal form by nasal sniffing (snorting), dissolved in an alcoholic beverage and orally ingested, or dissolved in a small amount of water and intravenously injected. North American methcathinone users primarily are men in their early 20s of European descent. These men use methcathinone much like the amphetamines are used, in binges or "runs" lasting 2 to 6 days. Methcathinone use is expected to significantly increase over the next 5 years.

Mechanism of CNS Action

The exact mechanism of methcathinone's psychostimulant actions has not been determined. Methcathinone appears to inhibit monoamine neurotransmitter intracellular accumulation and specifically inhibits the reuptake of serotonin by means of simple competition for the serotonin binding site within the serotonin transporter (SERT). A decrease in dopamine reuptake capacity may also play a role in methcathinone's mechanism of action.

Pharmacodynamics/Pharmacokinetics

Methcathinone's onset of action is within 15 to 30 minutes after oral ingestion, and its psychostimulant actions generally persist for 4 to 6 hours. Physical dependence with tolerance can develop relatively quickly over several days of use. Additional valid and reliable data are not available.

Current Approved Indications for Medical Use

None

Desired Action/Reason for Personal Use

Alertness (increased); burst of energy; euphoria; feelings of invincibility; racing thoughts (speeding of the mind); wakefulness (extended over a period of time)

Toxicity[4]

Acute: Aggressive and violent behavior (increased); anorexia; anxiety; cardiac dysrhythmias; cognitive impairment; dehydration; delusions; depression (following use); epistaxis (associated with intranasal sniffing, or snorting); fever; hallucinations; headaches; hyperventilation; insomnia; mania; muscle twitching; mydriasis (moderate); nausea; nervousness; palpitations; paranoia (potentially severe); perspiration (excessive); restlessness; seizures; stomach pains; tachycardia; talkativeness; tremors

Chronic: Acne vulgaris; nasal septal perforation (associated with intranasal sniffing, or snorting, similar to that associated with snorting cocaine [see monograph]); neurotoxicity[5]; paranoid psychosis; physical dependence; proteinuria; psychological dependence; weight loss (may be extreme)

Pregnancy & Lactation: Valid and reliable data are not available.

Abuse Potential

Physical dependence: High (USDEA Schedule I; use is prohibited)
Psychological dependence: High

Withdrawal Syndrome

Discontinuation of regular, long-term methcathinone use has been associated with a methcathinone withdrawal syndrome characterized by feelings of despair, lack of energy, and sadness progressing to severe depression. Tremors or seizures may occur during withdrawal when higher dosages have been used over several days.

Overdosage

Valid and reliable data are not available. Overdosage deaths involving methcathinone have been reported in the former Soviet Union. Readers are referred to the Methamphetamines monograph "Overdosage" section because of the shared spectrum of pharmacology, including actions and toxicities. There is no known antidote for methcathinone.

Notes

1. It also is a beta-ketone analogue of methamphetamine (see monograph).
2. The chemical synthesis of methcathinone is relatively simple and can be accomplished in a home kitchen using easily obtainable ingredients.
3. The crystalline salt form has a characteristic pleasant odor similar to that of pistachio ice cream.
4. Methcathinone toxicity is largely due to increased serotonin levels. However, significant toxicity may also be due to contaminants and byproducts related to its synthesis and production in illicit laboratories. For example, a popular recipe available over the Internet creates methcathinone from common cold products utilizing permanganate to catalyze the chemical reaction. Manganese can be an unwanted by-product of this synthesis process, and several cases of manganism (i.e., manganese toxicity) have been reported in the literature, in which intravenous users developed signs and symptoms similar to those observed in Parkinson's disease (i.e., apathy, bradykinesia, gait disturbance, and hypophonia). However, unlike Parkinson's disease, manganism is not responsive to levodopa pharmacotherapy.
5. There is ample evidence of persistent reductions in dopamine transporter density, suggesting potential risk for permanent neuropsychiatric disorders, including parkinsonism.

References

Belhadj-Tahar, H., & Sadeg, N. (2005). Methcathinone: A new postindustrial drug. *Forensic Science International, 153*(1), 99-101.

Cozzi, N.V., & Foley, K.F. (2003). Methcathinone is a substrate for the serotonin uptake transporter. *Pharmacology & Toxicology, 93*(5), 219-225.

De Bie, R.M., Gladstone, R.M., Strafella, A.P., et al. (2007). Manganese-induced Parkinsonism associated with methcathinone (Ephedrone). *Archives of Neurology, 64*(6), 886-889.

Huang, C.C. (2007). Parkinsonism induced by chronic manganese intoxication—an experience in Taiwan. *Chang Gung Medical Journal, 30*(5), 385-395.

Paul, B.D., & Cole, K.A. (2001). Cathinone (Khat) and methcathinone (CAT) in urine specimens: A gas chromatographic-mass spectrometric detection procedure. *Journal of Analytical Toxicology, 25*(7), 525-530.

Sanotsky, Y., Lesyk, R., Fedoryshyn, L., et al. (2007). Manganic encephalopathy due to "ephedrone" abuse. *Movement Disorders, 22*(9), 1337-1343.

Stepens, A., Logina, I., Liguts, V., et al. (2008). A Parkinsonian syndrome in methcathinone users and the role of manganese. *The New England Journal of Medicine, 358*(10), 1009-1017.

5-METHOXY-N,N-DIISOPROPYLTRYPTAMINE

Names

BAN or INN Generic Synonyms: None

Brand/Trade: None

Chemical: 5-Methoxy-N,N-diisopropyltryptamine

Street: Foxy; Foxy-Methoxy; 5-MeO-DIPT

Pharmacologic Classification

Psychodelic, LSD-like psychodelic: indole/tryptamine

Brief General Overview

5-Methoxy-N,N-diisopropyltryptamine (5-MeO-DIPT), an intermediate-acting, orally active psychodelic, is synthetically produced. It was first synthesized by Alexander Shulgin in the late 1970s but has only recently (i.e., in the 21st century) become popular among attendees at dance clubs and raves. A number of users report concomitant use of gamma-hydroxybutyrate (GHB; see monograph) to counteract the anxiety and insomnia associated with its use.

Dosage Forms and Routes of Administration

5-MeO-DIPT is available from both legitimate chemical companies (usually through the Internet) and illicit chemical manufacturers. It is becoming increasingly popular at dance clubs and raves on the east and west coasts of North America (e.g., New York and California). 5-MeO-DIPT is generally available in oral capsule or tablet formulations. The oral tablets are often embossed with an "alien" head, fox, or spider logo. 5-MeO-DIPT is almost always orally ingested by users. However, it also can be intranasally sniffed (snorted) and, if available as, or converted to, the freebase form, it can be used by pulmonary inhalation (i.e., smoked).

Mechanism of CNS Action

The exact mechanism of action of 5-MeO-DIPT has not been determined. However, it appears to be largely related to its affinity for the serotonin (5-hydroxytryptamine) receptors, particularly 5-HT2.[1] Dopamine D2-receptor agonism also appears to mediate the psychodelic actions of 5-MeO-DIPT.

Pharmacodynamics/Pharmacokinetics

Onset of action is generally within 20 to 60 minutes after oral ingestion, and effects generally persist for 3 to 6 hours. Three major metabolic pathways have been identified for 5-MeO-DIPT: (1) O-demethylation to form 5-hydroxy-N,N-diisopropyltryptamine (5-OH-DIPT), (2) hydroxylation and methylation to form 6-hydroxy-5-methoxy-N,N-diisopropyltryptamine (6-OH-5-MeO-DIPT), and (3) side-chain degradation to form 5-methoxy-N-isopropyltryptamine (5-MeO-NIPT). Oxidative deamination results in the urinary metabolite 5-methoxy-indole acetic acid (5-MeO-IAA). Additional valid and reliable data are not available.

Current Approved Indications for Medical Use

None

Desired Action/Reason for Personal Use

Arousal of sexual desire and enhance sexual experience; auditory distortions; empathy; energy; enhanced tactile sensations; euphoria; hallucinations (auditory and visual); sense of well-being; social disinhibition

Toxicity

Acute: Agitation; anxiety; diarrhea; insomnia; jaw clenching (mild); muscle tension; mydriasis; nausea; restlessness; rhabdomyolysis (rare); unpleasant smell and taste (strong); vomiting

Chronic: Valid and reliable data are not available.

Pregnancy & Lactation: Valid and reliable data are not available.

Abuse Potential

Physical dependence: None to low (USDEA Schedule I; use is prohibited)
Psychological dependence: Low

Withdrawal Syndrome

A 5-MeO-DIPT withdrawal syndrome has not been reported. However, tolerance lasting several days after use and cross-tolerance with lysergic acid diethylamide (LSD; see monograph) have been reported.

Overdosage

One case of fatal overdosage and several cases of nonfatal overdosage have been reported involving 5-MeO-DIPT. However, these few case reports are insufficient for drawing generalizable conclusions. There is no known antidote. Additional valid and reliable data are needed.

Note

1. This proposed mechanism of action is very similar to that of lysergic acid diethylamide (LSD; see monograph), with which 5-MeO-DIPT shares most of its psychodelic and other actions.

References

Alatrash, G., Majhail, N.S., & Pile, J.C. (2006). Rhabodomyolysis after ingestion of "foxy," a hallucinogenic tryptamine derivative. *Mayo Clinic Proceedings, 81*(4), 550-551.

Kamata, T., Katagi, M., Kamata, H.T., et al. (2006). Metabolism of the psychotomimetic tryptamine derivative 5-methoxy-N,N-diisopropyltryptamine in humans: Identification and quantification of its urinary metabolites. *Drug Metabolism and Disposition, 34*(2), 281-287.

Leinwand, D. (2002, July 22). Dangerous club-drug knockoffs surge. *USA Today.* Available: http://www.usatoday.com/news/nation/2002-07-22-drug-fakes_x.htm.

Meatherall, R., & Sharma, P. (2003). Foxy, a designer tryptamine hallucinogen. *Journal of Analytical Toxicology, 27*(5), 313-317.

Tanaka, E., Kamata, T., Katagi, M., et al. (2006). A fatal poisoning with 5-methoxy-N,N-diisopropyltryptamine, Foxy. *Forensic Science International, 163*(1-2), 152-154.

Wilson, J.M., McGeorge, F., Smolinske, S., et al. (2005). A foxy intoxication. *Forensic Science International, 148*(1), 31-36.

3,4-METHYLENEDIOXYAMPHETAMINE

Names

BAN or INN Generic Synonyms: Tenamfetamine

Brand/Trade: None

Chemical: α-Methyl-3,4-(methylenedioxy)phenethylamine; 3,4-methylenedioxyphenyl-isopropylamine

Street: Adam; Hug Drug; Love Drug; MDA; Mellow Drug of America

Pharmacologic Classification

Psychodelic, amphetamine-like psychodelic: phenethylamine

Brief General Overview

3,4-Methylenedioxyamphetamine (MDA), an amphetamine analogue, was first synthesized in 1910 as an appetite suppressant but was never clinically used for that purpose in North America. An interesting drug, MDA produces psychodelic effects at lower dosages and more amphetamine-like actions at higher dosages. MDA also is a known metabolite of 3,4-methylenedioxymethamphetamine (MDMA; see monograph).

Dosage Forms and Routes of Administration

MDA is synthesized in illicit laboratories. It is generally available in powder or tablet formulations for oral ingestion.

Mechanism of CNS Action

Valid and reliable data are not available.

Pharmacodynamics/Pharmacokinetics

The psychodelic actions of MDA usually are experienced within 30 minutes, peak at ~90 minutes, and last ~8 to 12 hours. The elimination half-life of MDA is ~11.5 hours. MDA appears to undergo significant postmortem redistribution; thus, postmortem blood concentrations of MDA cannot be easily and directly correlated with antemortem blood concentrations. Additional valid and reliable data are not available.

Current Approved Indications for Medical Use

None

Desired Action/Reason for Personal Use

Aesthetic enjoyment; enhanced sociability; euphoria; feelings of closeness to others (increased feelings of empathy); hallucinations (primarily visual and mild); introspection (self-insight); mood elevation; social disinhibition

Toxicity

Acute: Agitation; anorexia; bruxism (grinding of the teeth); dry mouth; hypertension; hyperthermia; muscle spasms; mydriasis; nausea; seizures; sweating (increased); tachycardia; tachypnea; vomiting

Chronic: Psychological dependence; other valid and reliable data are not available

Pregnancy & Lactation: Valid and reliable data are not available.

Abuse Potential

Physical dependence: Low (USDEA Schedule I; use is prohibited)
Psychological dependence: Low to moderate

Withdrawal Syndrome

An MDA withdrawal syndrome has not been reported.

Overdosage

MDA-related fatalities have been documented in the published literature and have been associated with cardiovascular arrest, disseminated intravascular coagulation, hyperthermia, and seizures. Acute MDA overdosage requires emergency medical support of body systems. There is no known antidote.

References

Christophersen, A.S. (2000). Amphetamine designer drugs—An overview and epidemiology. *Toxicology Letters, 112-113,* 127-131.

Elliott, S.P. (2005). MDMA and MDA concentrations in antemortem and postmortem specimens in fatalities following hospital admission. *Journal of Analytical Toxicology, 29*(5), 296-300.

Garcia-Repetto, R., Moreno, E., Soriano, T., et al. (2003). Tissue concentrations of MDMA and its metabolite MDA in three fatal cases of overdose. *Forensic Science International, 135*(2), 110-114.

Kolbrich, E.A., Goodwin, R.S., Gorelick, D.A., et al. (2008). Plasma pharmacokinetics of 3,4-methylenedioxymethamphetamine after controlled oral administration to young adults. *Therapeutic Drug Monitoring, 30*(3), 320-332.

Liu, R.H., Liu, H.C., & Lin, D.L. (2006). Distribution of methylenedioxymethamphetamine (MDMA) and methylenedioxyamphetamine in postmortem and antemortem specimens. *Journal of Analytical Toxicology, 30*(8), 545-550.

3,4-METHYLENEDIOXYETHYLAMPHETAMINE

Names

BAN or INN Generic Synonyms: N-Ethyl MDA

Brand/Trade: None

Chemical: (±)-N-Ethyl-α-methyl-3,4-(methylenedioxy)phenethylamine

Street: Eve; MDE; MDEA

Pharmacologic Classification

Psychodelic, amphetamine-like psychodelic: phenethylamine

Brief General Overview

3,4-Methylenedioxyethylamphetamine (MDEA) is related to 3,4-methylenedioxyamphetamine (MDA) and methylenedioxymethamphetamine (MDMA) and is often used together with these other psychodelics (see respective monographs). Personal use of MDEA for its psychodelic actions first gained popularity in Europe during the 1990s. MDEA use has now spread to North America, where it is primarily associated with attendance at techno-music dance parties or raves and the house-music scene. Typical users are men in their early 20s of European descent. These users generally (1) would not list MDEA as their drug of first choice and (2) concomitantly use other drugs and substances of abuse with MDEA, primarily alcohol and other psychodelics.

Dosage Forms and Routes of Administration

MDEA is illicitly produced in clandestine laboratories across North America. It is generally available as an oral tablet formulation and is orally ingested. MDEA, together with other phenethylamines, or ring-substituted amphetamines (e.g., MDA and MBDB), is often found in products illicitly represented and sold "on the street" as pure MDMA.

Mechanism of CNS Action

Valid and reliable data are not available.

Pharmacodynamics/Pharmacokinetics

Valid and reliable data are not available.

Current Approved Indications for Medical Use

None

Desired Action/Reason for Personal Use

Euphoria; feelings of contentment and peacefulness; feelings of emotional closeness to others; relaxation; social disinhibition

Toxicity

Acute: hallucinations; hypertension; hyperthermia[1]; insomnia; tachycardia

Chronic: Hepatic dysfunction[2]; psychosis

Pregnancy & Lactation: Valid and reliable data are not available.

Abuse Potential

Physical dependence: Low (USDEA Schedule I; use is prohibited)
Psychological dependence: Moderate

Withdrawal Syndrome

An MDEA withdrawal syndrome has not been reported.

Overdosage

The use of MDEA has been occasionally associated with fatal overdosages.[3] Hyperthermia and hepatic failure appear to be the principal contributing factors. MDEA overdosage requires emergency medical support of body systems with attention to MDEA elimination. There is no known antidote.

Notes

1. Hyperthermic reactions may be exacerbated by the generally warm rooms and overcrowding that characterize the venues used for techno-music dance parties and raves.
2. Available data are limited, and alcohol and other drug use (e.g., concomitant use of other psychodelics) or a contaminant produced during the chemical synthesis of MDEA cannot be ruled out as causes of the reported hepatic damage.
3. The exact relationship of MDEA to these reported deaths is difficult to establish, because virtually all of the victims had other drugs and substances of abuse in their bodies at the time of death.

References

Clauwaert, K.M., Van Bocxlaer, J.F., De Letter, E.A, et al. (2000). Determination of the designer drugs 3,4-methylenedioxymethamphetamine, 3,4-methylenedioxyethylamphetamine, and 3,4-methylenedioxyamphetamine with HPLC and fluorescence detection in whole blood, serum, vitreous humor, and urine. *Clinical Chemistry, 46*(12), 1968-1977.

Di Pietra, A.M., Gotti, R., Del Borrello, E., et al. (2001). Analysis of amphetamine and congeners in illicit samples by liquid chromatography and capillary electrophoresis. *Journal of Analytical Toxicology, 25*(2), 99-105.

Freudenmann, R.W., & Spitzer, M. (2004). The neuropsychopharmacology and toxicology of 3,4-methylenedioxy-N-ethylamphetamine (MDEA). *CNS Drug Reviews, 10*(2), 89-116.

Kraemer, T., & Maurer, H.H. (2002). Toxicokinetics of amphetamines: Metabolism and toxicokinetic data of designer drugs, amphetamine, methamphetamine, and their N–alkyl derivatives. *Therapeutic Drug Monitoring, 24*(2), 277-289.

Schifano, F., Corkery, J., Deluca, P., et al. (2006). Ecstasy (MDMA, MDA, MDEA, MBDB) consumption, seizures, related offences, prices, dosage levels and deaths in the UK (1994-2003). *Journal of Psychopharmacology, 20*(3), 456-463.

Zhao, H., Brenneisen, R., Scholer, A., et al. (2001). Profiles of urine samples taken from Ecstasy users at Rave parties: Analysis by immunoassays, HPLC, and GC-MS. *Journal of Analytical Toxicology, 25*(4), 258-269.

3,4-METHYLENEDIOXYMETHAMPHETAMINE

Names

BAN or INN Generic Synonyms: None

Brand/Trade: None

Chemical: (±)-N,α-Dimethyl-3,4-(methylenedioxy)phenethylamine

Street: Adam; Anastasia; *Bacalao*; Batmans; Beans; Bibs; Bickies; Blue Kisses; Blue Lips; Candies; Charity; Clarity; Cowies; Dancing Shoes; Daves; Dead Road; Debs; Decadence; Diamonds; Disco Biscuits; Doctors; Doves; E; Easy; Ebeneezer; E-bombs; Eccies; Ecstacy; Ecstasy; Eddie Bo; Egg Rolls; Egyptians; Em; Empathy; Es; Essence; Eve; Ex; Exciticity; Fizzle; Flipper; Four Leaf Clover; Fuckstasy; Gary Abletts; Garys; Googs; Greenies; Gum; GWM; Happy Drug; Happy Pill; Herbal Bliss; Hug Drug; Jack and Jills; Jiggas; Jills; Kids; *Kiks*; Kix; Kleenex; Letter Biscuits; Light Meth; Lollies; Louie Vuitton; Louis Vuitton; Love Bug; Love Drug; Love Medicine; Love Pill; Love Potion; Lover's Special; Lover's Speed; Madman; Malcolm; Malcolm X; Mandy; MDM; MDMA; Mitsu's; M&M; Mollys; Pingers; Pressies; Rave; Rave Energy; Rib; Ritual Spirit; Rolling; Running;

Scooby Snacks; Skates; Smartees; Smarties; Speed for Lovers; Sweets; Tachas; Thizz; Tutus; Tweety Birds; Ultimate Xphoria; Vitmain E; Vitamin X; Vowels; Wafers; Wheels; White Dove; Wigits; Wingers; X; X-Men; X-Pills; XTC

Pharmacologic Classification

Psychodelic,[1] amphetamine-like psychodelic: phenethylamine

Brief General Overview

3,4-Methylenedioxymethamphetamine (MDMA) is a ring-substituted amphetamine analogue that is closely related to methylenedioxyamphetamine (MDA).[2] It was first synthesized by German pharmaceutical researchers in 1912 as an appetite suppressant, but it was never marketed. MDMA was initially used after being "rediscovered" during the 1970s and early 1980s by some psychiatrists and psychologists as an adjunct to psychotherapy to facilitate patient communication and expression. Personal use of MDMA soon became popular among college students on campuses across North America. MDMA was banned from licit public use in 1985.[3] Today in North America, its use is synonymous with attendance at raves and dance clubs, particularly by young adults of European descent. These users are usually polydrug and substance-users in their mid-20s, although this pattern of use may be seen in some adolescents. MDMA is now considered to be one of the 10 most abused drugs in the world and the second most abused illicit drug, after cannabis, in North America.

Although many young users subjectively report that the use of MDMA allows them to drink as much as they like at parties and remain sober, objective performance measures (i.e., measures of cognitive abilities and psychomotor skills) demonstrate no improvement in alcohol-impaired performance. However, other data appear to lend support to this claim (see "Pharmacodynamics/Pharmacokinetics" section). MDMA use by gay and bisexual men, particularly during circuit party weekends, is highly correlated with unsafe sexual practices, including unprotected intimate sexual contact with men who (knowingly) are HIV positive. Several studies have reported significant correlations between MDMA use by gay and bisexual men and recent history of unprotected anal intercourse. In addition, gay, lesbian, and bisexual college and university students are twice as likely as their heterosexual cohorts to have used MDMA in the past year.

Dosage Forms and Routes of Administration

MDMA is illicitly produced by chemical synthesis in clandestine laboratories across North America.[4] It is generally available in capsule, powder, and tablet formulations and is almost always orally ingested.[5] The purity of MDMA available "on the street" is currently fairly high. However, it is not unusual to find that it has been adulterated with other phenethylamines, such as MBDB, MDA, and MDEA.

Mechanism of CNS Action

MDMA appears to generate its reported actions (i.e., feelings of elation, emotional closeness, and sensory pleasure) by means of stimulating the release of neurotransmitters, primarily serotonin (5-hydroxytryptamine), and preventing their reuptake. This mechanism involves the interaction with 5-HT transporters (SERTs) as substrates.

Pharmacodynamics/Pharmacokinetics

Peak blood concentrations of MDMA occur 2 to 4 hours after oral ingestion and usually produce mild hallucinogenic and stimulant actions that last from 4 to 8 hours. Approximately 10% of an ingested MDMA dose is metabolized to MDA (see monograph). The elimination half-life of MDMA is ~8 hours. Although available data are limited, it appears that (1) MDMA displays nonlinear (i.e., dose-dependent) pharmacokinetics at dosages within the "recreational" range and (2) deficiency in the hepatic microsomal enzyme CYP2D6[6] places "recreational" users at risk for developing acute toxicity at moderate dosages of MDMA. MDMA also appears to undergo postmortem redistribution. Thus, postmortem blood concentrations cannot be easily and directly correlated with antemortem blood concentrations.

MDMA is commonly used concomitantly with alcohol. An average overall increase in MDMA plasma concentration (~15%) and a corresponding decrease in alcohol plasma concentration was demonstrated when subjects consumed MDMA and alcohol simultaneously.[7] Additional valid and reliable pharmacokinetic data are not available.

Current Approved Indications for Medical Use

None

Desired Action/Reason for Personal Use

Arouse sexual desires (particularly among gay and bisexual men); empathy; enhance sexual experiences (particularly among gay and bisexual men); enhanced self-esteem; euphoria; feelings of intimacy; perceptual distortion; social disinhibition (particularly among gay and bisexual men)

Toxicity

Acute: Acute renal failure (rare); anxiety; bruxism (grinding of the teeth); cardiac dysrhythmias; disseminated intravascular coagulation (rare); dysphoria (3 to 5 days after discontinuation of use); hepatitis (drug-induced); hyperkinesia; hypertension; hyperthermia/hyperpyrexia[8]; hyponatremia (MDMA use is often accompanied by excessive ingestion of water or other beverages)[9]; impulsive behavior; mental confusion; mydriasis; perceptual distortion; pneumomediastinum (rare); psychosis (amphetamine-like, occurring rarely with higher dosages); rhabdomyolysis (rare); seizures; sweating (profuse); tachycardia; urinary retention

Chronic[10,11]: Cognitive impairment; fatigue; hepatic impairment (increased risk and incidence with repeated or regular, long-term use of MDMA); insomnia; memory impairment (particularly, verbal memory); neurogenic bladder; neurotoxicity (and resultant neurological impairment, particularly affecting the serotonin system)[12]; psychological dependence; soreness of the jaw muscles (related to teeth clenching or grinding)

Pregnancy & Lactation: MDMA use during pregnancy appears to present little or no risk of teratogenic effects. No data are readily available on the excretion of MDMA in breast milk. In the absence of these data, it is strongly recommended that adolescent girls and women avoid breast-feeding while using MDMA. This caution is predicated upon (1) MDMA's mechanism of action, (2) reports of neurotoxicity in MDMA users, and (3) the potential for toxicity to the developing CNS of the breast-fed neonate or infant. Additional valid and reliable data are needed.

Abuse Potential

Physical dependence: None (USDEA Schedule I; use is prohibited)
Psychological dependence: Moderate

Withdrawal Syndrome

A specific MDMA withdrawal syndrome has not been reported. However, dysphoria lasting 3 to 5 days after an episode of use is commonly reported. It appears to be related to depletion of neurotransmitters in the CNS, particularly serotonin.

Overdosage

Over 300 MDMA-related fatalities have been reported over the past decade in North America. The vast majority of these deaths have involved adolescent boys and men of European descent, 15 to 40 years of age. In many cases, uncharacteristic behavior and vomiting were observed initially, followed by seizures, disorientation or coma, and death. The fatalities are usually associated with acute renal failure, cardiac dysrhythmias, cerebrovascular accidents, disseminated intravascular coagulation, hyperpyrexia, hyponatremic encephalopathy, and rhabdomyolysis. However, because MDMA users are known to be polydrug and substance of abuse users who concomitantly use alcohol, lysergic acid diethylamide (LSD), and other drugs and substances of abuse, it is difficult to obtain a clear picture as to the etiology and sequelae of MDMA overdosage. In addition, several signs and symptoms of fatal MDMA toxicity (e.g., hyponatremic encephalopathy) can be related to several other user risk factors and behaviors (e.g., concurrent consumption of an excessive amount of beer or water). In any case, because of the very serious and potentially fatal consequences of MDMA overdosage, MDMA overdosage should always be treated as a medical emergency. There is no known antidote.

Notes

1. MDMA is often referred to, particularly by users and proponents of its use, as an "entactogen" (i.e., a drug that causes "touching within"). This term originated during the 1970s and 1980s with the clinical work of several mental health professionals who used MDMA and related drugs in clinical practice to facilitate the therapeutic process with their patients. In that context it was claimed, though not scientifically confirmed, that the use of MDMA promoted, indeed generated, feelings of empathy, emotional warmth, openness, and self-acceptance. MDMA users make a similar claim today in the context of use at raves.
2. MDA also is an active metabolite of MDMA.
3. MDMA has been on restricted use in Canada since 1976.
4. In addition, the U.S. Department of Justice estimates that over 2 million MDMA oral tablets are illegally smuggled into the United States each week, primarily from Belgium, Luxembourg, and the Netherlands.

5. A common pattern of MDMA use observed since the late 1990s involves concurrent use of lysergic acid diethylamide (LSD; see monograph). This specific combination and pattern of use is referred to as "candy flipping." Similarly, the use of MDMA and ketamine is referred to as "kitty flipping" and the use of MDMA and mescaline is referred to as "love flipping." MDMA also is increasingly being used in combination with sildenafil (Viagra®). This combination of use is referred to as "sextasy."

6. It is estimated that 10% of people of European descent are genetically deficient in regard to this hepatic microsomal isoenzyme.

7. In addition, subjects reported a subjective feeling of being less intoxicated but appeared to have no significant reduction in psychomotor impairment. Additional valid and reliable data are needed.

8. Can be severe and ultimately result in death (see "Overdosage").

9. MDMA-associated hyponatremia appears to be due to both (1) the syndrome of inappropriate antidiuretic hormone release (SIADH) and (2) free-water intoxication (i.e., as a result of polydipsia).

10. Some research suggests that women may be more susceptible than men to MDMA-induced neurotoxicity. Other research suggests that MDMA neurotoxicity is augmented by the concomitant use of other psychotropic drugs, such as alcohol and cannabis. Additional valid and reliable data are needed.

11. Neurotoxicity appears to be directly related to serotonergic axonal loss in higher brain regions (e.g., corpus striatum). Repeated or regular, long-term use of MDMA is more likely to result in associated functional deficits, including attentional problems and memory deficits. Younger users may be at higher risk for MDMA-related neurotoxicity. Several studies have suggested that many functional neurological impairments associated with MDMA use may be permanent, because they do not appear to abate even after several years of abstinence.

12. Appears to involve progressive degeneration of nerve terminals.

References

Beuerie, J.R., & Barrueto Jr., F. (2008). Neurogenic bladder and chronic urinary retention associated with MDMA abuse. *Journal of Medical Toxicology, 4*(2), 106-108.

Boyd, C.J., McCabe, S.E., & d'Arcy, H. (2003). Ecstasy use among college undergraduates: Gender, race and sexual identity. *Journal of Substance Abuse Treatment, 24*(3), 209-215.

Brvar, M., Kozelj, G., Osredkar, J., et al. (2004). Polydipsia as another mechanism of hyponatremia after "ecstasy" (3,4 methyldioxymethamphetamine) [sic] ingestion. *European Journal of Emergency Medicine, 11*(5), 302-304.

Cherney, D.Z., Davids, M.R., & Halperin, M.L. (2002). Acute hyponatraemia and 'ecstasy': Insights from a quantitative and integrative analysis. *The Quarterly Journal of Medicine, 95,* 475-483.

Christopherson, A.S. (2000). Amphetamine designer drugs—An overview and epidemiology. *Toxicology Letters, 112-113,* 127-131.

Coco, T.J., & Klasner, A.E. (2004). Drug-induced rhabdomyolysis. *Current Opinion in Pediatrics, 16*(2), 206-210.

Colfax, G.N., Mansergh, G., Guzman, R., et al. (2001). Drug use and sexual risk behavior among gay and bisexual men who attend circuit parties: A venue-based comparison. *Journal of Acquired Immune Deficiency Syndromes, 28,* 373-379.

de la Torre, R., Farré, M., Ortuño, J., et al. (2000). Non-linear pharmacokinetics of MDMA ('ecstasy') in humans. *British Journal of Clinical Pharmacology, 49*(2), 104-109.

De Letter, E.A., Clauwaert, K.M., Lambert, W.E., et al. (2002). Distribution study of 3,4-methyl-enedioxymethamphetamine and 3,4-methylenedioxyamphetamine in a fatal overdose. *Journal of Analytical Toxicology, 26,* 113-118.

Delgado, J.H., Caruso, M.J., Waksman, J.C., et al. (2004). Acute, transient urinary retention from combined ecstasy and methamphetamine use. *The Journal of Emergency Medicine, 26*(2), 173-175.

Eiserman, J.M., Diamond, S., & Schensul, J.J. (2005). "Rollin' on E": A qualitative analysis of ecstasy use among inner city adolescents and young adults. *Journal of Ethnicity in Substance Abuse, 4*(2), 9-38.

Farah, R., & Farah, R. (2008). Ecstasy (3,4-methylenedioxymethamphetamine)-induced inappropriate antidiuretic hormone secretion. *Pediatric Emergency Care, 24*(9), 615-617.

Gerra, G., Zaimovic, A., Ferri, M., et al. (2000). Long-lasting effects of (+/–)3,4-methamphetamine (ecstasy) on serotonin system function in humans. *Biological Psychiatry, 47*(2), 127-136.

Gill, J.R., Hayes, J.A., deSouza, I.S., et al. (2002). Ecstasy (MDMA) deaths in New York City: A case series and review of the literature. *Journal of Forensic Sciences, 47*(1), 121-126.

Gobbi, M., Moia, M., Pirona, L., et al. (2002). p-Methylthioamphetamine and 1-(m-chlorophenyl)piperazine, two non-neurotoxic 5-HT releasers in vivo, differ from neurotoxic amphetamine derivatives in their mode of action at 5-HT nerve endings in vitro. *Journal of Neurochemistry, 82*(6), 1435-1443.

Gouzoulis-Mayfrank, E., & Daumann, J. (2006). The confounding problem of polydrug use in recreational ecstasy/MDMA users: A brief overview. *Journal of Psychopharmacology, 20*(2), 188-193.

Gowing, L.R., Henry-Edwards, S.M., Irvine, R.J., et al. (2002). The health effects of ecstasy: A literature review. *Drug and Alcohol Review, 21*(1), 53-63.

Gross, S.R., Barrett, S.P., Shestowsky, J.S., et al. (2002). Ecstasy and drug consumption patterns: A Canadian rave population study. *Canadian Journal of Psychiatry, 47*(6), 546-551.

Hartung, T.K., Schofield, E., Short, A.I., et al. (2002). Hyponatraemic states following 3,4-methylenedioxymethamphetamine (MDMA, 'ecstasy') ingestion. *The Quarterly Journal of Medicine, 95*(7), 431-437.

Hernandez-Lopez, C., Farre, M., Roset, P.N., et al. (2002). 3,4-Methylenedioxymethamphetamine (ecstasy) and alcohol interactions in humans: Psychomotor performance, subjective effects, and pharmacokinetics. *The Journal of Pharmacology and Experimental Therapeutics, 300*, 236-244.

Hwang, I., Daniels, A.M., & Holtzmuller, K.C. (2002). "Ecstasy"-induced hepatitis in an active duty soldier. *Military Medicine, 167*, 155-156.

Inman, D.S., & Greene, D. (2003). The agony and the ecstasy: Acute urinary retention after MDMA abuse. *British Journal of Urology International, 91*(1), 123.

Kalant, K. (2001). The pharmacology and toxicology of "ecstasy" (MDMA) and related drugs. *CMAJ: Canadian Medical Association Journal, 165*, 917-928.

Kalasinsky, K.S., Hugel, J., & Kish, S.J. (2004). Use of MDA (the "love drug") and methamphetamine in Toronto by unsuspecting users of ecstasy (MDMA). *Journal of Forensic Sciences, 49*(5), 1106-1112.

Klitzman, R.L., Greenberg, J.D., Pollack, L.M., et al. (2002). MDMA ("ecstasy") use, and its association with high risk behaviors, mental health, and other factors among gay/bisexual men in New York City. *Drug and Alcohol Dependence, 66*(2), 115-125.

Klitzman, R.L., Pope, H.G. Jr., & Hudson, J.I. (2000). MDMA ("Ecstasy") abuse and high-risk sexual behaviors among 169 gay and bisexual men. *American Journal of Psychiatry, 157*(7), 1162-1164.

Koesters, S.C., Rogers, P.D., & Rajasingham, C.R. (2002). MDMA ('ecstasy') and other 'club drugs'. The new epidemic. *Pediatric Clinics of North America, 49*, 415-433.

Landabaso, M.A., Iraurgi, I., Jimenez-Lerma, J.M., et al. (2002). Ecstasy-induced psychotic disorder: Six month follow-up study. *European Addiction Research, 8*(3), 133-140.

Lawler, L.P., Abraham, S., & Fishman, E.K. (2001). 3,4-Methylenedioxymethamphetamine (ecstasy)-induced hepatotoxicity: multidetector CT and pathology findings. *Journal of Computer Assisted Tomography, 25*(4), 649-652.

Leung, K.S., & Cottler, L.B. (2008). Ecstasy and other club drugs: A review of recent epidemiologic studies. *Current Opinion in Psychiatry, 21*(3), 234-241.

Logan, B.K., & Couper, F.J. (2001). 3,4-methylenedioxymethamphetamine (MDMA, ecstasy) and driving impairment. *Journal of Forensic Sciences, 46*(6), 1426-1433.

Mattison, A.M., Ross, M.W., Wolfson, T., et al. (2001). Circuit party attendance, club drug use, and unsafe sex in gay men. *Journal of Substance Abuse, 13*(1-2), 119-126.

Mazur, S., & Hitchcock, T. (2001). Spontaneous pneumomediastinum, pneumothorax and ecstasy abuse. *Emergency Medicine, 13*(1), 121-123.

Milani, R.M., Parrott, A.C., Schifano, F., et al. (2005). Pattern of cannabis use in ecstasy polydrug users: Moderate cannabis use may compensate for self-rated aggression and somatic symptoms. *Human Psychopharmacology: Clinical and Experimental, 20*(4), 249-261.

Montoya, A.G., Sorrentino, R., Lukas, S.E., et al. (2002). Long-term neuropsychiatric consequences of "ecstasy" (MDMA): A review. *Harvard Review of Psychiatry, 10*(4), 212-220.

Morgan, M.J., McFie, L., Fleetwood, H., et al. (2002). Ecstasy (MDMA): Are the psychological problems associated with its use reversed by prolonged abstinence? *Psychopharmacology, 159*(3), 294-303.

Obrocki, J., Schmoldt, A., Buchert, R., et al. (2002). Specific neurotoxicity of chronic use of ecstasy. *Toxicology Letters, 127*(1-3), 285-297.

Parrott, A.C. (2002). Recreational ecstasy/MDMA, the serotonin syndrome, and serotonergic neurotoxicity. *Pharmacology, Biochemistry, and Behavior, 71*(4), 837-844.

Parrott, A.C. (2006). MDMA in humans: Factors which affect the neuropsychobiological profiles of recreational ecstasy users, the integrative role of bioenergetic stress. *Journal of Psychopharmacology, 20*(2), 147-163.

Parott, A.C., Gouzoulis-Meyfrank, E., Rodgers, J., et al. (2004). Ecstasy/MDMA and cannabis: The complexities of their interactive neuropsychobiological effects. *Journal of Psychopharmacology, 18*(4), 572-575.

Parrott, A.C., Sisk, E., & Turner, J.J. (2000). Psychobiological problems in heavy "ecstasy" (MDMA) polydrug users. *Drug and Alcohol Dependence, 60*(1), 105-110.

Pentney, A.R. (2001). An exploration of the history and controversies surrounding MDMA and MDA. *Journal of Psychoactive Drugs, 33*(3), 213-221.

Pham, J.V., & Puzantian, T. (2001). Ecstasy: Dangers and controversies. *Pharmacotherapy, 21*(12), 1561-1565.

Rejali, D., Glen, P., & Odom, N. (2002). Pneumomediastinum following Ecstasy (methyl-enedioxymethamphetamine, MDMA) ingestion in two people at the same "rave". *The Journal of Laryngology and Otology, 116*(1), 75-76.

Reneman, L., Booiji, J., de Bruin, K., et al. (2001). Effects of dose, sex, and long-term abstention from use on toxic effects of MDMA (ecstasy) on brain serotonin neurons. *Lancet, 358*(9296), 1831-1832.

Rosenson, J., Smollin, C., Sporer, K.A., et al. (2007). Patterns of ecstasy-associated hyponatremia in California. *Annals of Emergency Medicine, 49*(2), 164-171.

Samyn, N., De Boeck, G., Wood, M., et al. (2002). Plasma, oral fluid and sweat wipe ecstasy concentrations in controlled and real life conditions. *Forensic Science International, 128*(1-2), 90-97.

Schechter, M.D. (1998). 'Candyflipping': Synergistic discriminative effect of LSD and MDMA. *European Journal of Pharmacology, 341*(2-3), 131-134.

Schifano, F., Corkery, J., Deluca, P., et al. (2006). Ecstasy (MDMA, MDA, MDEA, MBDB) consumption, seizures, related offences, prices, dosage levels and deaths in the UK (1994-2003). *Journal of Psychopharmacology, 20*(3), 456-463.

Schilt, T., de Win, M.M., Koeter, M., et al. (2007). Cognition in novice ecstasy users with minimal expo-sure to other drugs: A prospective cohort study. *Archives of General Psychiatry, 64*(6), 728-736.

Sim, T., Jordan-Green, L., Lee, J., et al. (2005). Psychosocial correlates of recreational ecstasy use among college students. *Journal of American College Health, 54*(1), 25-29.

Strote, J., Lee, J.E., & Wechsler, H. (2002). Increasing MDMA use among college students: Results of a national survey. *The Journal of Adolescent Health, 30*(1), 64-72.

Teter, C.J., & Guthrie, S.K. (2001). A comprehensive review of MDMA and GHB: Two common club drugs. *Pharmacotherapy, 21*(12), 1486-1513.

Thomasius, R., Zapletalova, P., Petersen, K., et al. (2006). Mood, cognition and serotonin transporter availability in current and former ecstasy (MDMA) users: The longitudinal perspective. *Journal of Psychopharmacology, 20*(2), 211-225.

Traub, S.J., Hoffman, R.S., & Nelson, L.S. (2002). The "ecstasy" hangover: Hyponatremia due to 3,4-methylenedioxymethamphetamine. *Journal of Urban Health, 79*(4), 549-555.

Verheyden, S.L., Hadfield, J., Calin, T., et al. (2002). Sub-acute effects of MDMA (+/-3,4-methyl-enedioxymethamphetamine, "ecstasy") on mood: Evidence of gender differences. *Psychopharmacology, 161*(1), 23-31.

Wish, E.D., Fitzelle, D.B., O'Grady, K.E., et al. (2006). Evidence for significant polydrug use among ecstasy-using college students. *Journal of American College Health, 55*(2), 99-104.

Wolff, K., Tsapakis, E.M., Winstock, A.R., et al. (2006). Vasopressin and oxytocin secretion in response to the consumption of ecstasy in a clubbing population. *Journal of Psychopharmacology, 20*(3), 400-410.

Yacoubian, G.S. Jr. (2002). Assessing the temporal relationship between race and ecstasy use among high school seniors. *Journal of Drug Education, 32*(3), 213-225.

N-METHYL-1-(3,4-METHYLENEDIOXYPHENYL)-2-BUTANAMINE

Names

BAN or INN Generic Synonyms: None

Brand/Trade: None

Chemical: N-Methyl-1-1-(3,4-methylenedioxyphenyl)-2-aminobutane

Street: Eden; Euro; Fido-Dido[1]; MBDB; MDP-2-MB; Methyl-J; Mibi Dibi

Pharmacologic Classification

Psychodelic, amphetamine-like psychodelic: phenethylamine

Brief General Overview

N-methyl-1-(3,4-methylenedioxyphenyl)-2-butanamine (MBDB) is a synthetic phenethylamine. Personal use of MBDB and other phenethylamines (e.g., methylenedioxyethylamphetamine [MDEA], methylenedioxymethamphetamine [MDMA, Ecstasy]) is generally associated with the current "dance scene" and raves.[2] MDBD was first synthesized during the early 1980s as a nonhallucinogenic analogue of MDMA (Ecstasy).[3] It was classified by its synthesizers as an "entactogen" (i.e., a drug or substance that causes inner contact with oneself and feelings of empathy toward others). However, MBDB was found to generally produce less intense and, reportedly, fewer desired effects than MDMA (see monograph). Over the past decade, MBDB use has been commonly reported in the European literature. However, its use in North America continues to be relatively low.

Dosage Forms and Routes of Administration

MBDB is synthesized in illicit chemical laboratories primarily in Israel and Spain. It is generally available for use in oral tablet form[4] and is orally ingested.

Mechanism of CNS Action

The exact mechanism of MBDB's psychodelic action has not been determined. However, it is believed to be similar to that of MDMA (see monograph).

Pharmacodynamics/Pharmacokinetics

MBDB is well absorbed following oral ingestion. Peak blood concentrations occur ~2 hours after oral ingestion, and actions generally last for 4 to 6 hours. MBDB is metabolized in the liver to several metabolites, including 3,4-methylenedioxyphenyl-2-butanamine (BDB). Both MBDB and BDB have been detected in several body fluids, including blood, saliva, sweat, and urine. Additional valid and reliable data are not available.

Current Approved Indications for Medical Use

None

Desired Action/Reason for Personal Use

Alteration of consciousness; pleasant sense of introspection; sense of empathy toward others

Toxicity

Acute: Clenched jaw; dry mouth; headache (usually during "coming down" phase); mydriasis; nystagmus; sweating; tachycardia

Chronic: Valid and reliable data are not available.

Pregnancy & Lactation: Valid and reliable data are not available.

Abuse Potential[5]

Physical dependence: None to low (USDEA Schedule I; use is prohibited)
Psychological dependence: Low

Withdrawal Syndrome

An MBDB withdrawal syndrome has not been reported.

Overdosage

MBDB overdosage has been fatal. Acute MBDB overdosage requires emergency medical support of body systems with attention to MBDB elimination. There is no known antidote. Additional valid and reliable data are needed.

Notes

1. Fido-Dido is a cartoon character used in the advertisement of a common soft-drink.
2. As a deliberate marketing or sales ploy, MBDB is almost always represented and sold as MDMA (Ecstasy).
3. It is actually the α-ethyl homologue of MDMA (Ecstasy) and is deliberately designed and produced (i.e., it cannot be accidentally produced as a byproduct of MDMA synthesis).
4. It occasionally is available as a powder or oral capsule.
5. Abuse potential has been somewhat difficult to characterize, because MBDB is usually available with (and used in combination with) other psychodelics, notably 4-bromo-2,5-dimethoxyphenethylamine (2C-B), lysergic acid diethylamide (LSD), or methylenedioxymethamphetamine (MDMA, Ecstasy) (see respective monographs).

References

Carter, N., Rutty, G.N., Milroy, C.M., et al. (2000). Deaths associated with MBDB misuse. *International Journal of Legal Medicine, 113*(3), 168-170.

Kavanagh, P., Dunne, J., Feely, J., et al. (2001). Phenylalkylamine abuse among opiate addicts attending a methadone treatment programme in the Republic of Ireland. *Addiction Biology, 6*(2), 177-181.

Schifano, F., Corkery, J., Deluca, P., et al. (2006). Ecstasy (MDMA, MDA, MDEA, MBDB) consumption, seizures, related offences, prices, dosage levels and deaths in the UK (1994-2003). *Journal of Psychopharmacology, 20*(3), 456-463.

METHYLPHENIDATE

Names

BAN or INN Generic Synonyms: Methylphenidylacetate

Brand/Trade: Biphentin®; Concerta®; Metadate®; Methylin®; Ritalin®; Ritalin-SR®

Chemical: Methyl-α-phenyl-2-piperidine acetate

Street: JIF; MPH; R-Ball; Rs; Skippy; The Smart Drug; Vitamin R; West Coast

Pharmacologic Classification

Psychostimulant, miscellaneous: synthetic

Brief General Overview

Methylphenidate is commonly prescribed for the symptomatic management of attention-deficit/hyperactivity disorder (ADHD). It also is personally used nonmedically by several population groups for its psychostimulant actions. For example, adolescents and young adults have the highest rate of personal use, with approximately 3% reporting unprescribed use in the previous year and males outnumbering females three to one. Virtually all of these adolescents and young adults use methylphenidate orally, although it may be used intranasally or intravenously. A growing percentage of this group over the past decade has been adolescents whose ADHD is medically managed with methylphenidate. In addition, college and university students of European descent, particularly men and those who are polydrug users, are increasingly using methylphenidate.

Dosage Forms and Routes of Administration

Methylphenidate is legally produced by several pharmaceutical manufacturers in North America. It is available in both regular and extended-release oral tablets, which are usually orally ingested. However, the tablets may also be crushed, dissolved in a small amount of water, and filtered through a cigarette filter[1] for intranasal or intravenous use. Intranasal use of methylphenidate was common in the past and now appears to be increasingly common again, particularly among college students and adults with ADHD.

Methylphenidate is obtained for illicit use solely through diversion from legal sources. These sources include burglary of pharmacies, theft from pharmaceutical deliveries to clinics or hospitals, forged prescriptions, and, increasingly, theft from children and adolescents for whom it was legally prescribed. In regard to the latter, the perpetrators are usually age-cohorts of the child or adolescent who obtain the methylphenidate through bullying and threats. It also may be obtained from children and adolescents through positive inducements, such as paying for it, trading desirable items or other drugs and substances for it, or exchanging sex for it. Also, parents may obtain prescriptions for methylphenidate from their child's or adolescent's prescriber by falsely reporting associated signs and symptoms, and then using the methylphenidate themselves.[2]

Mechanism of CNS Action

The exact mechanism of methylphenidate's psychostimulant action has not been determined. However, it appears to primarily involve stimulation of the CNS by activation of the brain stem arousal system and cortex. Dopamine (D2) receptors and dopamine transporter (DAT) appear to be involved in this action, which results in amplification of dopamine's signals. Methylphenidate also inhibits the norepinephrine transporter. Although methylphenidate is generally compounded as a racemic mixture, the dextro enantiomer appears to be principally responsible for its observed pharmacologic actions.

Pharmacodynamics/Pharmacokinetics

Methylphenidate is rapidly and well absorbed after oral ingestion and achieves mean peak plasma concentrations at ~2 hours. However, bioavailability is low ($F = 0.3$), and peak blood concentrations vary because of extensive first-pass hepatic metabolism. Compared with regular methylphenidate oral tablets (i.e., Ritalin®), methylphenidate oral extended-release tablets (i.e., Ritalin-SR®) are absorbed more slowly, but to the same extent. Methylphenidate is only slightly bound to plasma proteins (i.e., ~15%) and has an apparent volume of distribution of 2.25 L/kg. Methylphenidate is excreted mainly in the urine as metabolites, with less than 1% excreted in unchanged form. Methylphenidate has a mean elimination half-life of ~2 hours and its mean total body clearance is ~10 L/hour/kg.

Current Approved Indications for Medical Use

Attention-deficit/hyperactivity disorder; narcolepsy

Desired Action/Reason for Personal Use

Appetite/hunger suppression and associated maintenance or reduction of weight; decrease feelings of fatigue or tiredness; increase alertness, vigilance, and wakefulness

Toxicity

Acute: Aggressive behavior; agitation; alopecia; anorexia; anxiety; arthralgia; blurred vision; dizziness; dyskinesia; fever; hallucinations; headache; hypertension; insomnia; nausea; nervousness; painful menstruation; palpitations; pruritus; psychosis (particularly with intravenous use); rash; seizures[3]; stomach pain; sudden death[4]; tachycardia; tics; Tourette's disorder; vomiting

Chronic: Growth retardation among children; physical dependence; psychological dependence; weight loss

Pregnancy & Lactation: FDA Pregnancy Category C (see Appendix B). Safety of methylphenidate use by adolescent girls and women who are pregnant has not been established. Valid and reliable data are needed.

Safety of methylphenidate use by adolescent girls and women who are breast-feeding has not been established. Valid and reliable data are required.

Abuse Potential

Physical dependence: Moderate to high (USDEA Schedule II; high potential for abuse)
Psychological dependence: High

Withdrawal Syndrome

A specific methylphenidate withdrawal syndrome has not been reported. However, severe depression can be unmasked upon abrupt discontinuation of regular, long-term use.

Overdosage

Signs and symptoms of acute methylphenidate overdosage are associated with its psychostimulant and sympathomimetic actions. These signs and symptoms may include agitation, cardiac dysrhythmias, confusion, convulsions, delirium, dryness of the mouth and mucous membranes, euphoria, flushing, hallucinations, headache, hyperpyrexia/hyperthermia (body temperature above 41° C [106° F]), hyperreflexia, hypertension, muscle twitching, mydriasis, palpitations, sweating, tremors, tachycardia, and vomiting. Acute methylphenidate overdosage requires emergency medical support of body systems with attention to increasing methylphenidate elimination, particularly when overdosage involves oral extended-release tablets. There is no known antidote. Although uncommon, the potential for death with intranasal sniffing (snorting) of methylphenidate does exist; several cases of such deaths among adolescents have been reported.

Notes

1. The solution is filtered to remove any particulate matter ("chalk") that may have been used in formulating the tablets. Intravenous injection of solutions that contain particulate matter may result in pain at the injection site and phlebitis.
2. In our clinical experience, it is generally the child's mother, who usually has a history of drug and substance abuse, who falls into this category.
3. Seizure frequency is increased among methylphenidate users, particularly those who have a preexisting seizure disorder.
4. Sudden death has been reported in children and adolescents prescribed methylphenidate pharmacotherapy at usual recommended dosages for the medical management of ADHD. Preexisting structural cardiac abnormalities and other serious cardiac conditions appear to have placed these children and adolescents at particular risk for sudden death. Additional valid and reliable data are needed. However, given these findings, methylphenidate should not be used by children and adolescents with preexisting cardiac abnormalities or other serious cardiac conditions.

References

Arria, A.M., Caldeira, K.M., O'Grady, K.E., et al. (2008). Nonmedical use of prescription stimulants among college students: Associations with attention-deficit-hyperactivity disorder and polydrug use. *Pharmacotherapy, 28*(2), 156-169.

Babcock, Q., & Byrne, T. (2000). Student perceptions of methylphenidate abuse at a public liberal arts college. *Journal of American College Health, 49*(3), 143-145.

Bright, G.M. (2008). Abuse of medications employed for the treatment of ADHD: Results from a large-scale community survey. *Medscape Journal of Medicine, 10*(5), 111.

Coetzee, M., Kaminer, Y., & Morales, A. (2002). Megadose intranasal methylphenidate (Ritalin) abuse in adult attention deficit hyperactivity disorder. *Substance Abuse, 23*(3), 165-169.

Foley, R., Mrvos, R., & Krenzelok, E.P. (2000). A profile of methylphenidate exposures. *Journal of Toxicology. Clinical Toxicology, 38*(6), 625-630.

Forrester, M.B. (2006). Methylphenidate abuse in Texas, 1998-2004. *Journal of Toxicology and Environmental Health. Part A: Current Issues, 69*(12), 1145-1153.

Heil, S.H., Holmes, H.W., Bickel, W.K., et al. (2002). Comparison of the subjective, physiological, and psychomotor effects of atomoxetine and methylphenidate in light drug users. *Drug and Alcohol Dependence, 67*(2), 149-156.

Klein-Schwartz, W. (2002). Abuse and toxicity of methylphenidate. *Current Opinion in Pediatrics, 14*(2), 219-223.

Kollins, S.H., MacDonald, E.K., & Rush, C.R. (2001). Assessing the abuse potential of methylphenidate in nonhuman and human subjects: A review. *Pharmacology, Biochemistry, and Behavior, 68*(3), 611-627.

Markowitz, J.S., & Patrick, K.S. (2008). Differential pharmacokinetics and pharmacodynamics of methylphenidate enantiomers: Does chirality matter? *Clinical Psychopharmacology, 28*(Supplement 2), S54-S61.

McCabe, S.E., & Teter, C.J. (2007), Drug use related problems among nonmedical users of prescription stimulants: A web-based survey of college students from a Midwestern university. *Drug and Alcohol Dependence, 91*(1), 69-71.

McCabe, S.E., Teter, C.J., & Boyd, C.J. (2004). The use, misuse and diversion of prescription stimulants among middle and high school students. *Substance Use & Misuse, 39*(70), 1095-1116.

McCabe, S.E., Teter, C.J., & Boyd, C.J. (2006). Medical use, illicit use and diversion of prescription stimulant medication. *Journal of Psychoactive Drugs, 38*(1), 43-56.

Meririnne, E., Kankaanpaa, A., & Seppala, T. (2001). Rewarding properties of methylphenidate: Sensitization by prior exposure to the drug and effects of dopamine D1- and D2-receptor antagonists. *The Journal of Pharmacology and Experimental Therapeutics, 298*(2), 539-550.

Rush, C.R., & Baker, R.W. (2001). Behavioral pharmacological similarities between methylphenidate and cocaine in cocaine abusers. *Experimental and Clinical Psychopharmacology, 9*(1), 59-73.

Schenk, J.O. (2002). The functioning neuronal transporter for dopamine: Kinetic mechanisms and effects of amphetamines, cocaine and methylphenidate. *Progress in Drug Research, 59*, 111-131.

Still, A., Gordon, M., Mercer, J., et al. (2002). Ritalin: Drug of abuse. Two case reports of intra-arterial injection. *New Zealand Medical Journal, 114*(1144), 521-522.

Volkow, N.D., Fowler, J.S., Wang, G., et al. (2002). Mechanism of action of methylphenidate: Insights from PET imaging studies. *Journal of Attention Disorders, 6*(Supplement 1), S31-S43.

Volkow, N.D., Fowler, J.S., Wang, G.J., et al. (2002). Role of dopamine in the therapeutic and reinforcing effects of methylphenidate in humans: Results from imaging studies. *European Neuropsychopharmacology, 12*(6), 557-566.

Weiner, A.L. (2000). Emerging drugs of abuse in Connecticut. *Connecticut Medicine, 64*(1), 19-23.

Wilens, T.E., Adler, L.A., Adams, J., et al. (2008). Misuse and diversion of stimulants prescribed for ADHD: A systematic review of the literature. *Journal of the American Academy of Child & Adolescent Psychiatry, 47*(1), 21-31.

Wilens, T.E., Gignac, M., Swezey, A., et al. (2006). Characteristics of adolescents and young adults with ADHD who divert or misuse their prescribed medications. *Journal of the American Academy of Child & Adolescent Psychiatry, 45*(4), 408-414.

4-METHYLTHIOAMPHETAMINE

Names

BAN or INN Generic Synonyms: Para-Methylthioamphetamine

Brand/Trade: None

Chemical: α-Methyl-4-methylthiophenethylamine; 1-(4-methylthiophenyl)-2-aminopropane

Street: 4-MT; 4-MTA; Dominator; Flatliners; Golden Eagle; p-MTA; S5

Pharmacologic Classification

Psychodelic, amphetamine-like psychodelic: phenethylamine

Brief General Overview

4-Methylthioamphetamine (4-MTA) is structurally and pharmacologically similar to methylenedioxyamphetamine (MDA; see monograph). It was originally synthesized as a "serotonin-releasing drug" for research purposes by a professor in Indiana during the early 1990s. 4-MTA has been used in Europe since the mid-1990s, but it has not yet gained much popularity in North America. In Europe, 4-MTA is primarily used in association with attendance at raves and techno-dance parties and clubs.

Dosage Forms and Routes of Administration

4-MTA is illicitly produced in clandestine laboratories, primarily located in Belgium, the Netherlands, Switzerland, and the United Kingdom. Generally available as tablets that are orally ingested, 4-MTA is smuggled into North America.

Mechanism of CNS Action

The psychodelic actions of 4-MTA appear to be predominantly due to its effect on the neurotransmitter serotonin (5-HT). 4-MTA increases the release of serotonin from neurons and blocks its reuptake. It appears to be several times more potent in this regard than either MDA or methylenedioxymethamphetamine (MDMA; see monograph). 4-MTA also reversibly inhibits the enzyme monoamine oxidase A (MAO-A).

Pharmacodynamics/Pharmacokinetics

4-MTA is minimally metabolized in the liver. The main metabolite is 4-methylthiobenzoic acid. The mean elimination half-life of 4-MTA is ~7 hours. The euphoria associated with 4-MTA, which is generally mild, reportedly can persist for up to 12 hours. Additional valid and reliable data are not available.

Current Approved Indications for Medical Use

None

Desired Action/Reason for Personal Use

Euphoria (mild); stimulant actions, including wakefulness (mild)

Toxicity

Acute: Anorexia; hyperthermia; increased intraocular pressure (particularly when higher dosages are used); insomnia; thirst

Chronic[1]: Weight loss. Additional valid and reliable data are not available.

Pregnancy & Lactation: Valid and reliable data are not available.

Abuse Potential

Physical dependence: Low (USDEA Schedule I; use is prohibited)
Psychological dependence: Moderate

Withdrawal Syndrome

A 4-MTA withdrawal syndrome has not been reported.

Overdosage

4-MTA overdosage has resulted in several deaths in Europe and the United Kingdom. In most of these cases, the victim was also concomitantly using other drugs and substances of abuse, usually MDMA. Related signs and symptoms of 4-MTA overdosage resemble those of the serotonin syndrome and can include exaggerated reflex responses, involuntary muscle contractions, muscle twitching, restlessness, sweating (excessive), shivering, tremor, and, ultimately, seizures, coma, and death. 4-MTA overdosage requires emergency medical support of body systems. There is no known antidote.

Note

1. Neurotoxicity, such as that associated with the use of other psychodelics (e.g., MDMA), has *not* been reported with 4-MTA.

References

Carmo, H., Hengstler, J.G., de Boer, D., et al. (2004). Comparative metabolism of the designer drug 4-methylthioamphetamine by hepatocytes from man, monkey, dog, rabbit, rat and mouse. *Naunyn-Schmiedeberg's Archives of Pharmacology, 369*(2), 198-205.

Decaestecker, T., De Letter, E., Clauwaert, K., et al. (2001). Fatal 4-MTA intoxication: Development of liquid chromatographic-tandem mass spectrometric assay for multiple matrices. *Journal of Analytical Toxicology, 25*(8), 705-710.

De Letter, E.A., Coopman, V.A., Cordonnier, J.A., et al. (2001). One fatal and seven non-fatal cases of 4-methylthioamphetamine (4-MTA) intoxication: Clinico-pathological findings. *International Journal of Legal Medicine, 114*(6), 352-356.

Elliott, S.P. (2000). Fatal poisoning with a new phenylethylamine: 4-Methylthioamphetamine (4-MTA). *Journal of Analytical Toxicology, 24*(2), 85-89.

Elliott, S.P. (2001). Analysis of 4-methylthioamphetamine in clinical specimens. *Annals of Clinical Biochemistry, 38*(part 4), 339-347.

Ewald, A.H., Peters, F.T., Weise, M., et al. (2005). Studies on the metabolism and toxicological detection of the designer drug 4-methylthioamphetamine (4-MTA) in human urine using gas chromatography-mass spectrometry. *Journal of Chromatography B Analytical Technologies in the Biomedical Life Sciences, 824*(1-2), 123-131.

Staack, R.F., & Maurer, H.H. (2005). Metabolism of designer drugs of abuse. *Current Drug Metabolism, 6*(3), 259-274.

Winstock, A.R., Wolff, K., & Ramsey, J. (2002). *Drug and Alcohol Dependence, 67*(2), 111-115.

World Health Organization. (2001). WHO Expert Committee on Drug Dependence. Thirty-second report. *World Health Organization Technical Report Series, 903*, i-v, 1-26.

MIDAZOLAM (See Benzodiazepines)

MITRAGYNINE (See *Kratom*)

MIXED AMPHETAMINES

Names

BAN or INN Generic Synonyms: Mixed Amfetamines

Brand/Trade: Adderall®; Adderall XR®

Chemical: See "Dosage Forms and Routes of Administration"

Street[1]: Addies; Blueberries; Oranges; Tic-Tacs

Pharmacologic Classification

Psychostimulant, amphetamine

Brief General Overview

A specific pharmaceutical formulation of mixed amphetamines for the medical management of ADHD was developed and marketed in the mid 1990s. Thus, compared with the other amphetamines, this formulation has a relatively short history of both clinical and personal use as a psychostimulant.[2] Soon after the introduction of mixed amphetamines into clinical practice in North America, several patterns of personal use developed that are now well established. These patterns include use by college and university students[3] to help them stay awake to study ("cram") for examinations or prepare term papers and other assignments. These users, both men and women,[4] are generally of European descent. Another pattern of use predominantly involves women 20 to 40 years of age of European descent. These women use the mixed amphetamines as a "pick-me-up" and as an aid to maintaining or reducing body weight. Interestingly, adolescents whose ADHD is being medically managed with mixed amphetamines generally do not use it for other indications or in ways other than as prescribed. These adolescents, who often have comorbid substance use disorders, preferentially use other drugs and substances of abuse, including alcohol, cannabis, and cocaine (see respective monographs).[5]

Dosage Forms and Routes of Administration

The mixed amphetamines formulation is produced for medical use through chemical synthesis by licit pharmaceutical manufacturers in North America. It is a combination product of different amphetamines, different amphetamine salts, and different isomers (amphetamine aspartate, amphetamine sulfate, dextroamphetamine saccharate, and dextroamphetamine sulfate, as illustrated in Table 6). The formulation is available in tablets and in extended-release capsules that contain short-acting and long-acting beads or pellets, in several dosages ranging from 5 mg to 30 mg.

TABLE 6
Amphetamine Salt Content of Mixed Amphetamines 10 mg and 20 Tablets

Ingredient[a]	10 mg Tablet[b]	20 mg Tablet[b]
Amphetamine aspartate	2.5 mg	5 mg
Amphetamine sulfate	2.5 mg	5 mg
Dextroamphetamine saccharate	2.5 mg	5 mg
Dextroamphetamine sulfate	2.5 mg	5 mg
Total amphetamine base equivalent	6.3 mg	12.6 mg

[a]In Canada, Adderall XR® contains dextroamphetamine and levoamphetamine salts in a 3:1 ratio. Adderall XR® was withdrawn from the Canadian market in 2005 because of concern about reports of sudden deaths (see "Toxicity: Acute"). It was subsequently returned to the market, but in a revised formulation. In the United States, the original product was never withdrawn from the market or reformulated.
[b]Contains a mixture of the amphetamine salts listed, with an overall 3:1 ratio of dextro- to levo- isomers.

Users generally obtain their mixed amphetamines through diversion of legitimate prescriptions. In this regard, it is not unusual for mothers to simply help themselves to the mixed amphetamines tablets or extended-release capsules that were prescribed for the symptomatic management of their child's or adolescent's ADHD. Brothers and sisters commonly take their younger sibling's mixed amphetamines "pills" for themselves, while older adolescents, including those for whom the drug was prescribed, have been reported to sell some of their supply to friends and classmates for profit.[6] In addition, the mixed amphetamines oral tablets and capsules are readily available for purchase on-line over the Internet.

Although most users orally ingest the mixed amphetamines oral capsules, an increasing number of adolescent and college- or university-age users are intranasally sniffing (snorting) the capsule contents.[7]

Mechanism of CNS Action

The mixed amphetamines formulation belongs to the amphetamine group of sympathomimetic amines that have CNS stimulant action. Peripheral actions include elevation of systolic and diastolic blood pressures and weak bronchodilator and respiratory stimulant action. The mixed amphetamines appear to elicit their stimulant actions primarily by increasing the release of norepinephrine from presynaptic storage vesicles in central adrenergic neurons. A direct effect on α- and β-adrenergic receptors, inhibition of the enzyme amine oxidase,[8] and the release of dopamine also may be involved. The amphetamines bind to the dopamine transporter (DAT) and thus reduce its ability to transport or "clear" dopamine from the synaptic cleft (i.e., they prevent transport back into the presynaptic neuron). (See also the Amphetamines monograph.)

Pharmacodynamics/Pharmacokinetics

The mixed amphetamines formulation is well absorbed after oral ingestion. Food significantly reduces oral bioavailability. The time to maximal blood concentrations following oral ingestion is ~7 hours. The mixed amphetamines undergo extensive metabolism, partially mediated by the hepatic isoenzyme CYP2D6. Approximately 30% of the mixed amphetamines is eliminated in unchanged form in the urine. However, alkalinization of the urine significantly reduces renal elimination; thus, modification of urinary pH can change the amount excreted in unchanged form in the urine (i.e., from 1% to 75%). The mean half-life of elimination is ~10 hours. Substantial intersubject variability has been reported. This finding, together with the use of different amphetamines, salts, and isomers within the combination mixed amphetamines product, make pharmaco-kinetic characterization extremely difficult.

Current Approved Indications for Medical Use

Attention-deficit/hyperactivity disorder; sleep disorders: narcolepsy

Desired Action/Reason for Personal Use

Appetite/hunger suppression and associated weight loss or maintenance; CNS stimulation (i.e., enhance alertness and vigilance or wakefulness); euphoria/exhilaration (intense); facilitate academic performance; get "high" or "party"; increase feelings of confidence; increase physical endurance; reduce fatigue

Toxicity

Acute: Abdominal cramps; anorexia; anxiety; blurred vision; cardiac dysrhythmias; chills; CNS stimulation; constipation; death (secondary to amphetamine-related accident or homicide); diarrhea; dizziness; dry mouth; flushing; headache; hypertension; increased sexual desire; insomnia; mydriasis; nausea; nervousness; palpitations; restlessness; seizures; stroke; sudden death (occurring generally in children and adolescents with structural heart abnormalities); tachycardia; tics; tremor; unpleasant taste; urinary retention

Chronic: Agitation; asthenia; cardiomyopathy; dermatoses (severe); dopamine trans-porter reduction; growth suppression in children; hallucinations; hepatitis; hyperactivity; insomnia (marked); irritability; neurological impairment (working memory impairment); paranoia; physical dependence; psychological dependence; psychosis; tics (motor and phonic, particularly in children and adolescents with preexisting Tourette's syndrome); tolerance; urinary tract infection; weight loss

Pregnancy & Lactation: FDA Pregnancy Category C (see Appendix B). Safety of mixed amphetamines use by adolescent girls and women who are pregnant has not been established. Neonates born to mothers who are physically dependent on amphetamines have an increased risk for premature delivery and low birth weight. During the neonatal period, these neonates also may display signs and symptoms of the amphetamine withdrawal syndrome, including agitation or lassitude. Adolescent girls and women who are pregnant should not use the mixed amphetamines.

Safety of mixed amphetamines use by adolescent girls and women who are breast-feeding has not been established. However, amphetamines are excreted in breast milk. Adolescent girls and women who are breast-feeding should not use the mixed amphetamines.

Abuse Potential

Physical dependence: High (USDEA Schedule II; high potential for abuse)
Psychological dependence: High

Withdrawal Syndrome

A mixed amphetamines withdrawal syndrome has not been reported. However, abrupt discontinuation of the mixed amphetamines after regular, long-term personal use of high dosages may result in extreme fatigue, mental depression, and sleep pattern changes on EEG. (See "Pregnancy and Lactation.") (See also Amphetamines monograph.)

Overdosage

Because mixed amphetamines is a combination amphetamine product, signs and symptoms of overdosage are the same as in any acute amphetamine overdosage. Those signs and symptoms include aggressiveness, assaultiveness, cardiovascular reactions (e.g., circulatory collapse, dysrhythmias, hypertension or hypotension), confusion, gastrointestinal complaints (e.g., abdominal cramps, diarrhea, nausea, and vomiting), hallucinations, hyperpyrexia, hyperreflexia, hyperventilation, panic, restlessness, rhabdomyolysis, and tremor. Depression and fatigue usually follow the central stimulation. Fatal amphetamine overdosage is usually preceded by convulsions and coma. Mixed amphetamines overdosage requires emergency symptomatic medical support of body systems with attention to increasing mixed amphetamines elimination, particularly when the extended-release formulations have been used. There is no known antidote.

Notes

1. See the Amphetamines monograph for a list of general "street" names for the various amphetamines.
2. For a general overview of other amphetamines (i.e., dextroamphetamine and methamphetamine), see the Amphetamines monograph.
3. Up to one-third of college and university students report having used psychostimulants prescribed for the medical management of ADHD (primarily methylphenidate [see monograph] and the mixed amphetamines) to facilitate their academic performance. In addition, up to 20% of this group reports having used the mixed amphetamines to "party" or "get high."

   Increasingly, high school seniors are emulating this pattern of college and university student use by using the mixed amphetamines to help them study for college entrance examinations. This behavior is often based on the behavior they observe in their older college and university siblings.

4. The equal gender representation is in stark contrast to the gender representation of children and adolescents diagnosed with ADHD (i.e., boys with ADHD outnumber girls by a ratio of 10 to 1).
5. However, up to 25% report having "overused" their mixed amphetamines on at least one occasion.
6. Some studies have reported that up to one-third of school-age children and adolescents with ADHD have been approached to give up, sell, or trade their mixed amphetamines.
7. In this context, the immediate-release tablets are preferred over the extended-release capsules because they are ground more easily into a dry powder amenable for intranasal snorting (i.e., grinding the time-release beads or pellets that are emptied from the extended-release capsules produces a "gummy" mixture).
8. The amphetamines, particularly in higher dosages, inhibit monoamine oxidase A and B (i.e., enzymes that metabolize dopamine, epinephrine, norepinephrine, and serotonin).

References

Arria, A.M., Caldeira, K.M., O'Grady, K.E., et al. (2008). Nonmedical use of prescription stimulants among college students: Association with attention-deficit-hyperactivity disorder and polydrug use. *Pharmacotherapy, 28*(2), 156-169.

Auiler, J.F., Liu, K., Lynch, J.M., et al. (2002). Effect of food on early drug exposure from extended-release stimulants: Results from the Concerta, Adderall XR Food Evaluation (CAFE) Study. *Current Medical Research and Opinion, 18*(5), 311-316.

Bright, G.M. (2008). Abuse of medications employed for the treatment of ADHD: Results from a large-scale community survey. *The Medscape Journal of Medicine, 10*(5), 111.

Bukstein, O. (2008). Substance abuse in patients with attention-deficit/hyperactivity disorder. *The Medscape Journal of Medicine, 10*(1), 24.

Cheng, A., Tithecott, G.A., Edwards, W.E., et al. (2007). The impact of the withdrawal of Adderall XR (long-acting mixed amphetamine salts) from the Canadian market on paediatric patients and their families. *Paediatrics & Child Health, 12*(5), 373-378.

Clausen, S.B., Read, S.C., & Tulloch, S.J. (2005). Single- and multiple-dose pharmacokinetics of an oral mixed amphetamine salts extended-release formulation in adults. *CNS Spectrums, 10*(12, Supplement 20), 6-15.

Cody, J.T., Valtier, S., & Nelson, S.L. (2003). Amphetamine enantiomer excretion profile following administration of adderall. *Journal of Analytical Toxicology, 27*(7), 485-492.

Cody, J.T., Valtier, S., & Nelson, S.L. (2004). Amphetamine excretion profile following multidose administration of mixed salt amphetamine preparation. *Journal of Analytical Toxicology, 28*(7), 563-574.

DeSantis, A.D., Webb, E.M., & Noar, S.M. (2008). Illicit use of prescription ADHD medications on a college campus: A multimethodological approach. *Journal of American College Health, 57*(3), 315-324.

Ermer, J.C., Shojaei, A., Pennick, M., et al.(2007). Bioavailability of triple-bead mixed amphetamine salts compared with a dose-augmentation strategy of mixed amphetamine salts extended release plus mixed amphetamine salts immediate release. *Current Medical Research and Opinion, 23*(5), 1067-1075.

Faraone, S.V., & Wilens, T.E. (2007). Effect of stimulant medications for attention-deficit/hyperactivity disorder on later substance use and the potential for stimulant misuse, abuse, and diversion. *Journal of Clinical Psychiatry, 68*(Supplement 11), 15-22.

Forrester, M.B. (2007). Adderall abuse in Texas, 1998-2004. *Journal of Toxicology and Environmental Health, Part A: Critical Issues, 70*(7), 658-664.

Greenhill, L.L., Swanson, J.M., Steinhoff, K., et al. (2003). A pharmacokinetic/pharmacodynamic study comparing a single morning dose of adderall to twice-daily dosing in children with ADHD. *Journal of the American Academy of Child & Adolescent Psychiatry, 42*(10), 1234-1241.

Gualtieri, C.T., & Johnson, L.G. (2008). Medications do not necessarily normalize cognition in ADHD patients. *Journal of Attention Disorders, 11*(4), 459-469.

Kollins, S.H. (2008). A qualitative review of issues arising in the use of psycho-stimulant medications in patients with ADHD and co-morbid substance use disorders. *Current Medical Research and Opinion, 24*(5), 1345-1357.

Kramer, W.G., Read, S.C., Tran, B.V., et al. (2005). Pharmacokinetics of mixed amphetamine salts extended release in adolescents with ADHD. *CNS Spectrums, 10*(10, Supplement 15), 6-13.

Marks, D.H. (2008). Cardiomyopathy due to ingestion of Adderall. *American Journal of Therapeutics, 15*(3), 287-289.

McGough, J.J., Biederman, J., Greenhill, L.L., et al. (2003). Pharmacokinetics of SLI381 (ADDERALL XR), an extended-release formulation of Adderall. *Journal of the American Academy of Child & Adolescent Psychiatry, 42*(6), 684-691.

Schubiner, H. (2005). Substance abuse in patients with attention-deficit hyperactivity disorder: Therapeutic implications. *CNS Drugs, 19*(8), 643-655.

Surles, L.K., May, H.J., & Garry, J.P. (2002). Adderall-induced psychosis in an adolescent. *Journal of the American Board of Family Practice, 15*(6), 498-500.

Teter, C.J., McCabe, S.E., LaGrange, K., et al. (2006). Illicit use of specific prescription stimulants among college students: Prevalence, motives, and routes of administration. *Pharmacotherapy, 26*(10), 1501-1510.

Thomas, S., & Upadhyaya, H. (2002). Adderall and seizures. *Journal of the American Academy of Child & Adolescent Psychiatry, 41*(4), 365.

Tulloch, S.J., Zhang, Y., McLean, A., et al. (2002). SLI381 (Adderall XR), a two-component, extended-release formulation of mixed amphetamine salts: Bioavailability of three test formulations and comparison of fasted, fed, and sprinkled administration. *Pharmacotherapy, 22*(11), 1405-1415.

Weisler, R.H. (2005). Safety, efficacy and extended duration of action of mixed amphetamine salts extended-release capsules for the treatment of ADHD. *Expert Opinion on Pharmacotherapy, 6*(6), 1003-1018.

Wilens, T.E. (2006). Mechanism of action of agents used in attention-deficit/hyperactivity disorder. *Journal of Clinical Psychiatry, 67*(Supplement 8), 32-38.

Wilens, T.E., Adler, L.A., Adams, J., et al. (2008). Misuse and diversion of stimulants prescribed for ADHD: A systematic review of the literature. *Journal of the American Academy of Child & Adolescent Psychiatry, 47*(1), 21-31.

MODAFINIL

Names

BAN or INN Generic Synonyms: None

Brand/Trade: Alertec®; Provigil®; Sparlon®

Chemical: 2-[(Diphenylmethyl)sulfinyl] acetamide

Street: None

Pharmacologic Classification

Psychostimulant, miscellaneous

Brief General Overview

Modafinil is a novel CNS stimulant, or analeptic, that was introduced into clinical practice in North America in 1994 for the treatment of hypersomnia and narcolepsy. In 2007, its "r" isomer (i.e., armodafinil; see monograph) was approved by FDA.

Dosage Forms and Routes of Administration

Modafinil is available from licit pharmaceutical manufacturers in oral tablet form. When abused, it is usually ingested. Over the past 5 years, modafinil has been increasingly referred to as a "lifestyle" drug and is being increasingly used in this capacity by hard-working and hard-partying young adults, including college or university students and young professionals.

Mechanism of CNS Action

Modafinil's mechanism of action appears to be distinct from those of other psycho-stimulants, such as cocaine and dextroamphetamine. The exact mechanism of modafinil's CNS stimulant action as related to its use for symptomatic management of narcolepsy has not been determined. However, it appears to primarily involve (1) stimulation of α_1-adrenergic receptors, (2) increase in the metabolism (turnover rate) of serotonin (5-HT), and (3) inhibition of the activity of GABA neurons. On EEG, modafinil increases high-frequency alpha waves and decreases delta and theta waves (i.e., produces EEG changes consistent with measures of increased mental alertness). At therapeutic dosages, it also appears to significantly improve memory. Modafinil also displays weak peripheral sympathomimetic activity.

Pharmacodynamics/Pharmacokinetics

Modafinil is well absorbed at a moderate rate after oral ingestion. Peak blood concentrations are achieved in ~3 hours. Ingestion of food may slightly decrease the rate, but not the extent, of modafinil absorption. Modafinil is moderately bound to plasma proteins (about 60%) and has an apparent mean volume of distribution of ~66 L (i.e., 0.94 L/kg). It is metabolized extensively in the liver, primarily by means of amide hydrolysis, and is excreted primarily as inactivated metabolites (i.e., modafinil acid and modafinil sulfone) in the urine. High-dose or long-term modafinil use may induce the production of hepatic microsomal enzymes (i.e., CYP3A4), resulting in an increase in the metabolism of other drugs and autoinduction (i.e., stimulation of its own metabolism). Less than 10% is excreted in unchanged form in the urine. Modafinil has a mean elimination half-life of 10 to 15 hours, and its total body clearance is ~5 L/hour.

Current Approved Indications for Medical Use[1]

Hypersomnia, idiopathic; narcolepsy; obstructive sleep apnea/hypopnea syndrome (adjunctive pharmacotherapy); shift-work sleep disorder

Desired Action/Reason for Personal Use

CNS stimulation (i.e., enhanced alertness or vigilance and wakefulness); euphoria; feelings of confidence

Toxicity

Acute: Anorexia; anxiety; chest pain; diarrhea; dizziness; dry mouth; dyspepsia; epistaxis; headache; hypertension; insomnia; nausea; nervousness; palpitations; restlessness; rhinitis; tachycardia; tremors; visual disturbance

Chronic: Psychological dependence

Pregnancy & Lactation: FDA Pregnancy Category C (see Appendix B). Safety of modafinil use by adolescent girls and women who are pregnant has not been established. However, because modafinil crosses the placental barrier in humans, adolescent girls and women who are pregnant should not use modafinil.

Safety of modafinil use by adolescent girls and women who are breast-feeding has not been established. Additional valid and reliable data are needed.

Abuse Potential[2]

Physical dependence: Low (USDEA Schedule IV; low potential for abuse)
Psychological dependence: Low

Withdrawal Syndrome

A modafinil withdrawal syndrome has not been reported.

Overdosage

Signs and symptoms of acute modafinil overdosage are associated with its CNS stimulant and sympathomimetic actions. These signs and symptoms may include agitation, anxiety, confusion, diarrhea, disorientation, excitation, headache, hypertension (systolic), hypertonia, insomnia, irritability, palpitations, tachycardia, and tremor. Acute modafinil overdosage requires emergency medical support of body systems, with attention to increasing modafinil elimination. There is no known antidote.

Notes

1. The U.S. military uses modafinil, as well as dextroamphetamine (see monograph), as "go pills" to improve alertness, vigilance, and wakefulness among soldiers and pilots during active duty. Modafinil was used in this regard by U.S. military combat soldiers during both Gulf wars.
2. Available data suggest that the potential for causing physical or psychological dependence is significantly lower for modafinil than for other psychostimulants, such as the amphetamines and cocaine.

References

Balon, J.S., & Feifel, D. (2006). A systematic review of modafinil: Potential clinical uses and mechanisms of action. *Journal of Clinical Psychiatry, 67*(4), 554-566.

Jasinski, D.R. (2000). An evaluation of the abuse potential of modafinil using methylphenidate as a reference. *Journal of Psychopharmacology, 14*(1), 53-60.

Jasinski, D.R., & Kovacevic-Ristanovic, R. (2000). Evaluation of the abuse liability of modafinil and other drugs for excessive daytime sleepiness associated with narcolepsy. *Clinical Neuropharmacology, 23*(3), 149-156.

Keating, G.M., & Raffin, M.J. (2005). Modafinil: A review of its use in excessive sleepiness associated with obstructive sleep apnoea/hypopnoea syndrome and shift work sleep disorder. *CNS Drugs, 19*(9), 785-803.

Minzenberg, M.J., & Carter, C.S. (2008). Modafinil: A review of neurochemical actions and effects on cognition. *Neuropsychopharmacology, 33*(7), 1477-1502.

Myrick, H., Malcolm, R., Taylor, B., et al. (2004). Modafinil: Preclinical, clinical, and post-marketing surveillance—A review of abuse liability issues. *Annals of Clinical Psychiatry, 16*(2), 101-109.

Randomized trial of modafinil as a treatment for the excessive daytime somnolence of narcolepsy: US Modafinil in Narcolepsy Multicenter Study Group. (2000). *Neurology, 54*(5), 1166-1175.

Robertson, P. Jr., & Hellriegel, E.T. (2003). Clinical pharmacokinetic profile of modafinil. *Clinical Pharmacokinetics, 42*(2), 123-137.

Rush, C.R., Kelly, T.H., Hays, L.R., et al. (2002). Acute behavioral and physiological effects of modafinil in drug abusers. *Behavioural Pharmacology, 13*(2), 105-115.

Rush, C.R., Kelly, T.H., Hays, L.R., et al. (2002). Discriminative-stimulus effects of modafinil in cocaine-trained humans. *Drug and Alcohol Dependence, 67*(3), 311-322.

Stoops, W.W., Lile, J.A., Fillmore, M.T., et al. (2005). Reinforcing effects of modafinil: Influence of dose and behavioral demands. *Psychopharmacology, 182*(1), 186-193.

Swanson, J.M., Greenhill, L.L., Lopez, F.A., et al. (2006). Modafinil film-coated tablets in children and adolescents with attention-deficit/hyperactivity disorder: Results of a randomized, double-blind, placebo-controlled, fixed-dose study followed by abrupt discontinuation. *Journal of Clinical Psychiatry, 67*(1), 137-147.

Wesensten, N.J. (2006). Effects of modafinil on cognitive performance and alertness during sleep deprivation. *Current Pharmaceutical Design, 12*(20), 2457-2471.

MORPHINE

Names

BAN or INN Generic Synonyms: None

Chemical: (5α,6α)-7,8-Didehydro-4,5-epoxy-17-methylmorphinan-3,6-diol

Brand/Trade: Duramorph®; Kadian®; M-Eslon®; Morphitec®; M.O.S.®; MS Contin®; MSIR®; Oramorph SR®; ratio-Morphine SR®; Roxanol®

Street: Aunt Emma; Big M; Cecil; Dope; Dream; Dreamer; Drugstore Dope; Eli Lilly; Emsel; First Line; Glad Stuff; God's Drug; G.O.M.; Good Ole M; Hardcore; Hospital Heroin; Hows; Hydrogen Bomb; Lydia; M; Miss Emma; Miss Morph; Mister Blue; Mojo; Monkey; Morf; Morph; Morphi; Morphia; *Morphina*; Morpho; Morphy; M.S.; Mother; Murphy; Old Steve; Racehorse Charley; Red Cross; Sister; Stuff; Sweet Morpheus; Unkie; Unkie White; White Angel; White Goddess; White Merchandize; White Nurse; White Stuff[1]

Pharmacologic Classification

Psychodepressant, opiate analgesic: pure agonist (natural)

Brief General Overview

Morphine was named after the Greek and Roman gods of dreams (i.e., Morpheus). It is naturally derived from the resin obtained from the opium poppy (*Papaver somniferum*), which contains approximately 10% morphine by weight. Isolated from opium resin in France over 200 years ago, morphine has been widely used by physicians for the management of moderate to severe pain and personally used for its desired psychodepressant actions. Morphine also is produced synthetically.

Three distinct groups of morphine users can be identified: (1) users whose physical pain was improperly medically managed and who are, as a result, now opiate analgesic dependent; (2) health care professionals who use morphine in an attempt to self-medicate chronic back pain, migraine pain, or job pressures, and now, physically dependent, continue to use it because of its ready availability to them in the workplace; and (3) people who use morphine because they know that the pharmaceutical ampul or vial they illicitly obtained is "sterile" and "pure" (i.e., it has not been tampered with) and contains high quality morphine at a specific concentration. They also may be users who are dependent on opiate analgesics and whose usual opiate analgesic (e.g., heroin) is unavailable or too costly to buy. For the first group, the usual source of morphine is legitimate prescriptions. For the second group, it is self-prescription of morphine or, more commonly, diversion from the work setting (e.g., hospital unit, pharmacy, or directly from patients in their care). Finally, for the third group, the usual source is diversion from a health care setting, or for the second group, pharmacy burglaries, obtaining prescriptions from multiple providers (i.e., "double-doctoring"), and illicit purchase.[2]

Dosage Forms and Routes of Administration

Morphine is legally produced by several pharmaceutical manufacturers in North America. It is available in a wide variety of dosage formulations, including intramuscular, intravenous, and subcutaneous injectables; oral concentrates; regular and extended-release capsules; solutions; syrups; tablets; and rectal suppositories. The preferred method of morphine use is intravenous injection. However, oral and other formulations are used when intravenous morphine is unavailable, particularly when the drug is needed to prevent or self-manage the morphine withdrawal syndrome (see section). Increasingly, as with a number of other drugs and substances of abuse, intranasal sniffing (snorting) of morphine is becoming increasingly popular.

Generally, morphine users, including those who maintain normal work schedules and those who have opted into treatment for their morphine dependency, may be confronted with mandatory urine testing for drug and substance use (e.g., court-ordered condition of release or parole; employment-required testing; condition of methadone maintenance program enrollment). Several effective adulterants for avoiding detection of current morphine use are available, including Stealth®. This product is available primarily over the Internet and is reportedly quite effective at interfering with the detection of morphine by sophisticated analytical tools, including gas chromatography–mass spectrometry (GC-MS). However, if the concentration of morphine is moderate to high, the sample will still generally test positive on immunoassay.

Mechanism of CNS Action

Morphine acts at specific opiate receptor sites (e.g., mu) in the CNS, producing desired psychodepressant actions, particularly analgesia. Analgesia is achieved not by raising the pain threshold but by modifying a person's perception of the pain experience. Thus, the pain is still experienced, but it is not as aversive, and any anxiety or stress associated with it also is markedly reduced. Unfortunately, tolerance to morphine's analgesic actions occurs with regular, long-term use. Increasingly higher doses of morphine are required to manage the pain and, if the drug is not used regularly, a morphine withdrawal syndrome may be precipitated (see "Withdrawal Syndrome"). In addition to its analgesic and other desired psychodepressant actions, morphine causes nausea and vomiting, primarily by direct stimulation of the chemoreceptor trigger zone (CTZ), and respiratory depression, primarily by suppressing the response of the respiratory center to carbon dioxide. (Also see "Toxicity" and the Opiate Analgesics monograph.)

Pharmacodynamics/Pharmacokinetics

Morphine is fairly well absorbed after oral ingestion. However, only ~40% reaches the systemic circulation because of significant first-pass hepatic metabolism. Thus, morphine is less potent after oral ingestion than after intramuscular or subcutaneous injection. Plasma protein binding is low (approximately 36%). The mean apparent volume of distribution is ~3 L/kg (range, 1 to 5 L/kg). In elderly people, the volume of distribution is considerably smaller, and initial concentrations of morphine are thus correspondingly higher. Peak analgesic action occurs within 20 minutes after intravenous injection and within 1 hour after intramuscular, oral, rectal, or subcutaneous administration. Morphine is metabolized rapidly and extensively, primarily in the liver by glucuronidation to morphine-3-glucuronide and morphine-6-glucuronide. A small amount (i.e., generally <2%) is metabolized to hydromorphone (see monograph). Less than 10% of an administered morphine dose is eliminated in unchanged form in the urine. Morphine's total body clearance ranges from 900 to 1200 mL/minute. The elimination half-life is ~2 to 4 hours. Morphine's duration of action is 3 to 5 hours when it is ingested orally or injected intramuscularly, intravenously, or subcutaneously.

Current Approved Indications for Medical Use

Pain, acute (moderate to severe); pain, chronic cancer (moderate to severe)

Desired Action/Reason for Personal Use

Euphoria; prevention/self-management of the opiate analgesic withdrawal syndrome; "rush"; sleepy, trancelike state ("nod") during which visions or vivid daydreams may occur

Toxicity

Acute: Apnea; cognitive impairment; constipation; dizziness; drowsiness; flushing; headache; hypotension; lightheadedness; miosis; nausea; pruritus; respiratory depression; sedation; stomach upset; sweating, excessive; urinary difficulty; urticaria; vomiting

Chronic: Physical dependence with tolerance; psychological dependence

Pregnancy & Lactation: FDA Pregnancy Category C (see Appendix B). Safety of morphine use by adolescent girls and women who are pregnant has not been established. Although morphine use during pregnancy has not been associated with congenital malformations, regular high-dosage use near term may result in neonatal morphine dependence (with the possibility of respiratory depression at birth) and, subsequently, the neonatal morphine withdrawal syndrome. Adolescent girls and women who are pregnant should not use morphine.

Safety of morphine use by adolescent girls and women who are breast-feeding has not been established. Morphine is excreted in breast milk. The concentration of morphine in breast milk is generally higher than the concentration in maternal blood. Expected pharmacologic actions (e.g., CNS or respiratory depression, constipation) may occur in breast-fed neonates and infants, who also may develop signs and symptoms of physical dependence—and withdrawal if breast-feeding is abruptly discontinued. Adolescent girls and women who are breast-feeding should not use morphine.

Abuse Potential

Physical dependence: High (USDEA Schedule II; high potential for abuse)
Psychological dependence: High

Withdrawal Syndrome

Regular long-term use of morphine is associated with physical and psychological dependence. Thus, abrupt discontinuation of regular, long-term use may result in the morphine withdrawal syndrome. The morphine withdrawal syndrome also may be precipitated in regular, long-term users of morphine (an opiate analgesic agonist) when an opiate analgesic antagonist (e.g., naloxone [Narcan®]) or a mixed opiate analgesic agonist/antagonist (e.g., pentazocine [Talwin®]) is used.

Acute signs and symptoms of the morphine withdrawal syndrome include abdominal pain, anorexia, body aches, chills, diarrhea, fever (unexplained), insomnia, nausea, nervousness, piloerection (gooseflesh), restlessness, rhinitis, shivering, sneezing, stomach cramps, sweating (excessive), tachycardia, tremors, weakness, and yawning. Although not usually life-threatening, the morphine withdrawal syndrome requires appropriate medical management. It may be avoided with a gradual discontinuation of morphine use.

Overdosage

Signs and symptoms of morphine overdosage include respiratory depression (i.e., decrease in respiratory rate and tidal volume, Cheyne-Stokes respiration, cyanosis), extreme somnolence progressing to stupor or coma, miosis, skeletal muscle flaccidity, and cold, clammy skin. Bradycardia and hypotension also may occur. Severe morphine overdosage may result in apnea, cardiac arrest, circulatory collapse, and death.

Morphine overdosage requires emergency medical support of body systems, with attention to increasing morphine elimination. The opiate analgesic antagonist naloxone (Narcan®) is the specific antidote for respiratory depression. Usual dosages of naloxone precipitate the morphine withdrawal syndrome in users who are physically dependent on morphine. The severity of the syndrome depends on the degree of the user's physical dependence, the amount of morphine used, and the dose of naloxone administered. For these users, 10% to 20% of the usual naloxone dosage should be administered initially and the dosage then adjusted (increased) according to individual response.

Notes

1. The commonly available salt forms of morphine (i.e., morphine hydrochloride and morphine sulfate) are both white, bitter-tasting crystalline powders.
2. For example, cases have been reported to us on numerous occasions over the years of nurses, usually women, administering normal saline to patients in their care in lieu of the ordered morphine (or meperidine) dose, and injecting the diverted morphine doses into an empty normal saline multidose vial, which is usually kept in their uniform pocket to take home for their personal use or to give to a family member (i.e., son) or boyfriend to keep him "out of jail."

References

Cody, J.T., Valtier, S., & Kuhlman, J. (2001). Analysis of morphine and codeine in samples adulterated with Stealth. *Journal of Analytical Toxicology, 25*(7), 572-575.

Cone, E.J., Caplan, Y.H., Moser, F., et al. (2008). Evidence that morphine is metabolized to hydromorphone but not to oxymorphone. *Journal of Analytical Toxicology, 32*(4), 319-323.

Haemmig, R.B., & Tschacher, W. (2001). Effects of high-dose heroin versus morphine in intravenous drug users: A randomized double-blind crossover study. *Journal of Psychoactive Drugs, 33*(2), 105-110.

Johnson, F., Wagner, G., Sun, S., et al. (2008). Effect of concomitant ingestion of alcohol on the in vivo pharmacokinetics of KADIAN (morphine sulfate extended-release) capsules. *Journal of Pain, 9*(4), 330-336.

McDonough, P.C., Levine, B., Vorce, S., et al. (2008). The detection of hydromorphone in urine specimens with high morphine concentrations. *Journal of Forensic Sciences, 53*(3), 752-754.

Rook, E.J., Huitema, A.D., van den Brink, W., et al. (2006). Population pharmacokinetics of heroin and its major metabolites. *Clinical Pharmacokinetics, 45*(4), 401-417.

MUSHROOMS (See *Amanita muscaria;* Psilocin; and Psilocybin)

NALBUPHINE

Names

BAN or INN Generic Synonyms: None

Brand/Trade: Nubain®

Chemical: 17-(Cylobutylmethyl)-4,5α-epoxymorphinan-3,6α,14-triol

Street: Nubian

Pharmacologic Classification

Psychodepressant, opiate analgesic: mixed agonist/antagonist (synthetic)

Brief General Overview

Nalbuphine is chemically related to oxymorphone. Although it was thought to present a very low risk for physical or psychological dependence, reports emerged during the late 1990s of its increased personal use. The principal population of nalbuphine users was men between 20 and 30 years of age, usually bodybuilders or weightlifters and sometimes professional athletes. Generally, their nalbuphine use began as either prescribed pharmacotherapy or self-medication for acute, severe pain from injuries related to weightlifting. Virtually all of these users also reported illicit use of anabolic/androgenic steroids.[1]

Dosage Forms and Routes of Administration

Nalbuphine is licitly produced by a pharmaceutical manufacturer in North America. It is available for injectable use only and can be injected intramuscularly, intravenously, or subcutaneously. In North America, most users inject nalbuphine intravenously. However, bodybuilders and professional athletes who inject anabolic/androgenic steroids intramuscularly will also inject nalbuphine intramuscularly.

Mechanism of CNS Action

Nalbuphine elicits its analgesic, other psychodepressant, and respiratory depressant actions primarily by binding to endorphin receptors, particularly kappa and mu sites, in the CNS. It appears to function as an agonist at the kappa sites and as an antagonist at the mu sites. However, the exact mechanism of nalbuphine's action has not been determined. (See also the Opiate Analgesics monograph.)

Pharmacodynamics/Pharmacokinetics

Nalbuphine has limited oral bioavailability (~20%). Thus, administration by injection is required for optimal bioavailability. Onset of action occurs within 3 minutes after intravenous injection and within 15 minutes after intramuscular or subcutaneous injection. Analgesic actions generally persist for 3 to 6 hours after onset. The mean apparent volume of distribution is 4 L/kg. Nalbuphine is metabolized in the liver, and less than 5% is excreted in unchanged form in the urine. The mean elimination half-life is ~5 hours, and the mean total body clearance is 1.5 L/minute.

Current Approved Indications for Medical Use

Pain disorders (acute or chronic pain, moderate to severe)

Desired Action/Reason for Personal Use

Euphoria; prevention/self-management of the opiate analgesic withdrawal syndrome[2]; self-management of acute or chronic pain, moderate to severe

Toxicity

Acute: Blurred vision; chills; cognitive impairment; constipation; dizziness; dry mouth; dyspnea; headache; hypertension; itching (severe); lightheadedness; mental depression; nausea; pain at injection site; psychomotor impairment; respiratory depression (moderate)[3]; sedation; sweating (excessive); sweaty, clammy feeling; tachycardia; vomiting

Chronic: Physical dependence; psychological dependence

Pregnancy & Lactation: FDA Pregnancy Category B (see Appendix B). Safety of nalbuphine use by adolescent girls and women who are pregnant has not been established. Nalbuphine rapidly crosses the placenta and may achieve fetal blood concentrations approximately equivalent to maternal blood concentrations. Associated fetal and neonatal effects have been reported, including fetal bradycardia and neonatal bradycardia and respiratory depression. Adolescent girls and women who are pregnant should not use nalbuphine.

Safety of nalbuphine use by adolescent girls and women who are breast-feeding has not been established. However, nalbuphine is excreted in breast milk in relatively low concentrations of less than 100 ng/mL (i.e., generally <1% of the total administered maternal dose). Additional valid and reliable data are needed.

Abuse Potential

Physical dependence: Moderate to severe (USDEA: not a scheduled drug)[4]
Psychological dependence: Moderate to severe

Withdrawal Syndrome

Regular, long-term use of nalbuphine is associated with the development of physical and psychological dependence. Abrupt discontinuation after regular, long-term use may result in a nalbuphine withdrawal syndrome, reportedly a milder form of the opiate analgesic withdrawal syndrome, with signs and symptoms that include abdominal cramps, anxiety, fever, lacrimation, nausea, piloerection, restlessness, rhinorrhea, and vomiting. Nalbuphine also may precipitate signs and symptoms of the opiate analgesic withdrawal syndrome among regular, long-term users of pure opiate analgesic agonists (e.g., fentanyl, morphine, and oxymorphone; see respective monographs), because it has mixed opiate analgesic agonist/antagonist actions (also see Opiate Analgesics monograph).

Overdosage

Signs and symptoms of nalbuphine overdosage are similar to the signs and symptoms of other opiate analgesic overdosages, although respiratory depression reportedly is less severe. Nalbuphine overdosage requires emergency medical support of body systems, with attention to increasing nalbuphine elimination. Naloxone (Narcan®) is a specific and effective antidote.[5]

Notes

1. A noted exception is the small number of health care professionals who personally use nalbuphine.
2. Because nalbuphine is a mixed agonist/antagonist, its use can precipitate the opiate analgesic withdrawal syndrome in people who are currently using, and are physically dependent on, pure opiate analgesic agonists (e.g., morphine).
3. Severe respiratory impairment is generally not observed as the dosage is increased, because of a "ceiling effect" related to nalbuphine's mixed agonist/antagonist activity.
4. Nalbuphine is one of the few opiate analgesics in the United States (also see Tramadol and Zipeprol monographs) that is *not* controlled under the Controlled Substances Act.
5. Particular caution is indicated with naloxone use for people who are physically dependent on nalbuphine, because of the potential for precipitation of the nalbuphine withdrawal syndrome.

References

Gharagoziou, P., Hashemi, E., DeLorey, T.M., et al. (2006). Pharmacological profiles of opioid ligands at kappa opioid receptors. *BMC Pharmacology, 6*, 3.

Jacqz-Aigrain, E., Serreau, R., Boissinot, C., et al. (2007). Excretion of ketoprofen and nalbuphine in human milk during treatment of maternal pain after delivery. *Therapeutic Drug Monitoring, 29*(6), 815-818.

Oliveto, A., Sevarino, K., McCance-Katz, E., et al. (2002). Butorphanol and nalbuphine in opiate-dependent humans under a naloxone discrimination procedure. *Pharmacology, Biochemistry, and Behavior, 71*(1-2), 85-96.

NICOTINE

Names

BAN or INN Generic Synonyms: None

Brand/Trade[1]: Habitrol®; Nicoderm®; Nicorette®; Nicotrol NS®; Prostep®

Chemical: (s)-3-(1-Methyl-2-pyrrolidinyl)pyridine

Street[2]: Alfalfa; Bacco; Baccy; Bad Boys; Bidis[3]; Bogeys; Brad; Burn; Butt; Cancer Sticks; Chew; Chew-Bacca; Cig; Cigar; Cigarette; Cigarillo; Ciggies; Cigs; Coffin Nails; Cowboy Killers; Death Stick; Deck; Dings; Dip; Drag; Fags; Freedom Sticks; Grant; Indian Drug; Jacks; Jewport; Joes; Lady Nicotine; Lamps; Leaf; Lung Darts; Magic Dragons; Nackles; Nail; Nic Stick; Niggerport; Nigger Sticks; Obama Sticks; Old Rope; Pipe Tobacco; Plug; Refries; Rollies; Ronnies; Seegar; Short; Sin Stick; Smoke; Smurt; Snuff; Spit; Splurge; Square; Stogies; Stokes; Straights; Strikes; Suicide Drug; Sweet Cancer; Tabacky; Tailors; TM; Tobacco; Troggs

Pharmacologic Classification

Psychostimulant, miscellaneous

Brief General Overview

Nicotine is a natural liquid alkaloid found in the leaf of the tobacco plant (*Nicotiana tabacum*).[4] Smoking tobacco usually contains 1% to 2% nicotine. It is only one of approximately 4000 chemicals present in tobacco smoke and, although less toxic than several of the other chemicals, it is the chemical responsible for the development of physical and psychological dependence on tobacco. Tobacco smoking is the largest single preventable cause of illness and disease in North America and the largest single cause of premature death in developed countries worldwide.[5]

Use of nicotine in the form of smoking tobacco in cigarettes, cigars, and pipes is widespread in North American society and appears to be increasing in certain population groups (i.e., adolescent girls) despite wide publicity of the adverse effects (e.g., lung cancer, oral cancer). The use of smokeless tobacco products (e.g., chewing tobacco, snuff) is likewise prevalent, with 8% of young men, particularly of European descent, now reporting the use of snuff.

Tobacco smokers cannot be defined as belonging preferentially to any single ethnic, racial, or social group. They currently include approximately one-fourth of the adult population of North America.[6] Most users begin to smoke tobacco before they are 14 years of age,[7] and it is estimated that every day of the year more than 3000 North American children and adolescents begin to smoke tobacco. Youth who have attentional or emotional disorders are more likely to smoke tobacco, in an unconscious effort to self-medicate these disorders.

Increasingly, adolescents and immigrants from India smoke "bidis"—hand-rolled, unfiltered cigarettes imported from India (see Note 3). The tobacco in bidi cigarettes contains 25% to 50% more nicotine per gram than do conventional North American cigarettes. In addition, North American adolescents and young adults, along with recent immigrants from the Middle East, are increasingly chewing "quid," *areca* nut, alone or in combination with tobacco, or tobacco alone wrapped in *betel* leaves (see *Betel cutch* monograph). The plant substances and *betel* leaves are chewed and retained in the mouth for maximal buccal absorption of their major psychotropic constituents.

Another adolescent smoking phenomenon that has significantly increased over the past 5 years, particularly among boys, is the use of cigarillos.[8] These products appear to have been intentionally designed for this market, with popular brand names that include Black & Mild®,[9] Cheroots®, and Prime Time®. In addition, they are attractive to young users because they are (1) small and thus easier to handle and smoke than a larger cigar, (2) commonly sold individually or in "kiddy packs" (i.e., packages containing 3 to 8 cigarillos) and less expensive than typical packages of 20 cigarettes, and (3) flavored.[10] Cigarillos typically contain from 5 to 12 times the nicotine present in regular cigarettes and, when smoked, they deliver significantly higher concentrations of hydrogen cyanide and cancer-causing nitrosamines.

Although cigarette smoking has declined slightly or remained stable across all jurisdictions in North America over the past decade,[11] the use of cigars has increased by up to 50% and the use of cigarillos by up to 150%.

Dosage Forms and Routes of Administration

Nicotine is available in tobacco products (e.g., chewing tobacco, tobacco cigarettes and cigars, pipe tobacco, and tobacco snuff[12,13]) and in refined pharmaceutical products. The pharmaceutical products, which were developed to help tobacco smokers discontinue their use of nicotine, are available in three major dosage formulations: (1) nicotine chewing gum, formulated for buccal absorption; (2) nicotine nasal spray, formulated for intranasal absorption; and (3) transdermal nicotine delivery systems, formulated for transdermal absorption. Tobacco smoking remains the most convenient and economical method of nicotine use, both in North America and worldwide.

Mechanism of CNS Action

Pharmacologically, nicotine appears to exert its psychostimulant action secondarily to direct stimulation of nicotinic acetylcholine (cholinergic) receptors (nAChRs). There are several distinct subtypes of nicotinic receptors that are widely distributed in the CNS.[14] Nicotinic receptors, which are ligand-gated ion channels, are structurally diverse and have varied roles. Activation of these channels causes a rapid increase in cellular permeability to sodium and potassium ion depolarization and excitation. Nicotinic receptors in the CNS are composed of two subunits, α and β,[15] which are found in discrete regions of the brain. The nicotinic receptors in the CNS are undefined in relation to response. However, nicotinic receptors in autonomic ganglia affect depolarization and firing of postganglionic neurons, and those in the adrenal medulla affect secretion of catecholamines, which results in the opening of the cation channel in nAChRs.

Nicotine stimulates the CNS at all levels, including the cerebral cortex, where its action causes increased cognitive activity. The psychostimulation is followed by depression. The effect of nicotine on the motor neurons leads to a marked reduction in muscle tone. Its action here also may be associated with the feelings of relaxation that can accompany smoking. Cigarette smoking typically produces an increase in hand tremor and an alerting pattern on the EEG. At the same time, however, there is decreased tone in some skeletal muscles (e.g., quadriceps femoris) and a decrease in deep-tendon reflexes. These effects may involve stimulation of the Renshaw cells in the spinal cord.

The major action of nicotine is CNS stimulation. This action, which is modulated primarily in the cortex via the locus ceruleus, produces increased alertness and cognitive performance. A CNS reward system modulated primarily by dopamine release in the limbic system produces a pleasurable sensation. Nicotine binds to nAChRs, which are found in various body organs and tissues, including the CNS and neuromuscular junctions. Nicotine also has cardiovascular actions associated with its stimulation of sympathetic ganglia and the adrenal medulla and its activation of aortic and carotid chemoreceptors. These actions result in tachycardia, vasoconstriction, and increased blood pressure. The pharmacologic action of nicotine is dose dependent. Lower doses stimulate autonomic ganglia, whereas higher doses block autonomic ganglia. The action on autonomic ganglia also varies according to the degree of tolerance that a user has developed to nicotine. The nicotine replacement products work simply by providing nicotine in dosage formulations that are associated with significantly less morbidity and mortality than tobacco smoking.

Pharmacodynamics/Pharmacokinetics

Nicotine absorption after oral ingestion is low (i.e., $F = 0.3$). The pharmacokinetics of nicotine favor buccal absorption, which is rapid and avoids first-pass hepatic metabolism that would result in immediate and rapid inactivation.[16] Buccally absorbed chewing gum formulations (e.g., Nicorette®) provide nicotine blood concentrations that approximate those obtained by inhaling the smoke from a tobacco cigarette (i.e., $F = 0.9$). The nicotine, which is in the form of a natural extract from the tobacco plant, is bound to an ion-exchange resin and is released only during chewing. Thus, the rate of nicotine release and the resultant blood concentrations are related to the rate and vigor with which the gum is chewed. Nicotine is only slightly bound to plasma proteins (i.e., <5%). The volume of distribution is approximately 2 to 3 L/kg. Nicotine is primarily metabolized in the liver by hepatic microsomal enzyme CYP2A6 to the inactive metabolite cotinine and subsequently to 3'-hydroxycotinine. Its hepatic clearance rate is ~1.2 L/minute. Nicotine clearance displays significant interindividual variability, primarily in regard to the genetic polymorphism of CYP2A6, that is highly correlated with age, gender, and racial factors. Over 20 different metabolites of nicotine have been identified, all of which are less pharmacologically active than the parent compound. Both nicotine and its metabolites are rapidly excreted in the urine (~15% in unchanged form). Elimination is affected by urinary pH. Alkaline urine can decrease nicotine elimination, whereas acidic urine can increase elimination (i.e., acidification of the urine to below a pH of 5 can result in up to 30% of the dose being eliminated in unchanged form). The mean elimination half-life is 2 hours.

Current Approved Indications for Medical Use

Symptomatic management of the nicotine withdrawal syndrome associated with cessation of tobacco smoking in people who are physically and psychologically dependent on nicotine.[17]

Desired Action/Reason for Personal Use

Alertness and attention (nicotine has been found to facilitate memory by improving attentional performance); euphoria; prevention/self-management of the nicotine withdrawal syndrome; weight loss or control (nicotine prevents weight gain by suppressing the appetite for sweet-tasting food and increasing energy expenditure both at rest and during exercise); well-being

Toxicity[18]

Acute: Acute adverse effects, usually manifested by cortical stimulation or local effects of smoking, include cough (due to irritation from tobacco smoke); dizziness; euphoria; fluid retention; flushing; GI cramps; headache; hypertension; insomnia; itching; lightheadedness; nausea; palpitations; rash; seizures; tachycardia; tinnitus; tremor; vomiting

Chronic: Aging of the skin (premature)[19]; cancers, various[20]; chronic obstructive pulmonary disease (COPD; due to direct effects of tobacco smoke); heart disease[21]; lung cancer; pancreatic cancer (related to tobacco smoking); physical dependence with tolerance; psychological dependence; SIDS (in offspring)[22]

Pregnancy & Lactation: FDA Pregnancy Category D (see Appendix B). Although nicotine replacement products may be safer for the fetus than tobacco smoking (i.e., the fetus is not exposed to additional chemicals that are present in tobacco smoke), the use of nicotine products has been associated, as has tobacco smoking, with spontaneous abortion. Long-term tobacco smoking or the use of nicotine replacement products also may result in expected pharmacologic actions among neonates, including physical dependence and the signs and symptoms of the nicotine withdrawal syndrome. Adolescent girls and women who are pregnant should not smoke tobacco and should avoid the use of nicotine replacement products. These products should be used during pregnancy only if the risk to the mother and embryo, fetus, or neonate is justified by the risk posed by continued maternal tobacco smoking. If nicotine replacement pharmacotherapy is required, pregnant adolescent girls and women should be advised of the potential benefits and possible risks to themselves and the embryo, fetus, or neonate.

Nicotine, whether obtained from tobacco smoking or from nicotine replacement products, is excreted in breast milk. Concentrations of nicotine and its metabolite cotinine in breast milk may be as much as three times the concentrations present in maternal blood. Breast-fed neonates and infants may display signs and symptoms of nicotine ingestion, including diarrhea, increased heart rate, restlessness, and vomiting. Adolescent girls and women who are breast-feeding should be advised of the potential risks to their neonates and infants. If tobacco smoking is continued or if nicotine products are required, breast-feeding should be discontinued.

Abuse Potential

Physical dependence: High (USDEA: not a scheduled drug)
Psychological dependence: High

Tolerance to the actions of nicotine has been well established in humans. Tolerance develops to most (e.g., dizziness, nausea, vomiting), but not all of the effects of nicotine. For example, after one or two cigarettes, even a chronic smoker exhibits an increase in blood pressure, pulse rate, and hand tremor. Smokers appear to metabolize nicotine more rapidly than nonsmokers, but it is likely that tolerance is due primarily to pharmacodynamic changes (e.g., neuroadaptation of nicotinic receptors) rather than to pharmacokinetic changes. There are conflicting reports on the duration of tolerance. In human smokers, some aspects of tolerance wax and wane rapidly. Thus, the first cigarette of the day produces a much greater cardiovascular and subjective response than subsequent cigarettes.

Withdrawal Syndrome[23,24]

Many people who use nicotine for its psychostimulant effects find that after a period of continued use they are unable to discontinue use easily, and they often seek professional help (e.g., from a counselor, nurse, pharmacist, physician, or psychologist). Approximately two-thirds of these people are able to discontinue nicotine use for a few days, but of these, only 20% to 30% remain abstinent 12 months later. People who have been advised by a physician to discontinue nicotine use because of serious health problems (e.g., myocardial infarction, lung cancer) also complain of difficulty discontinuing use for longer than a few days or weeks.

A nicotine withdrawal syndrome has been clearly identified. Signs and symptoms of nicotine withdrawal syndrome (as defined by *DSM-IV-TR*) vary in intensity during the course of withdrawal and can be seen as long as 14 days after the use of tobacco products has been discontinued. Associated signs and symptoms include anxiety, bradycardia, depression, fatigue, headaches, hunger, inability to concentrate, insomnia, irritability, lack of energy, restlessness, and weight gain. The nicotine withdrawal syndrome may intensify over 2 to 4 days and then gradually dissipate over 1 to 3 weeks. The aversive aspects of nicotine withdrawal appear to contribute significantly to the continuing use of nicotine. Signs and symptoms of nicotine withdrawal can be alleviated by use of nicotine from smoking tobacco or from replacement products, such as nicotine chewing gum or nicotine transdermal delivery systems (patches). Both central and peripheral groups of nicotinic acetylcholine receptors are involved in mediating the affective and somatic signs and symptoms of nicotine withdrawal.

To aid nicotine withdrawal, several pharmacotherapeutic approaches have been developed and approved, including both nicotine-containing products, such as Nicoderm® and Nicorette®, and non-nicotine-containing products, such as bupropion (Zyban®) and varenicline (Chantix®).

Overdosage

Overdosage has not generally been associated with regular use of smoking tobacco, except when tobacco products have been unintentionally ingested by infants and children or pets. Overdosage associated with nicotine replacement products has been related to simultaneously chewing, or chewing in rapid succession, more than the recommended number of chewing gum squares. It also has been reported with inadvertent access of young children to transdermal delivery systems. The risk for overdosage associated with swallowing chewing gum products is low, because absorption without chewing is slow and incomplete. In addition, any absorbed nicotine undergoes extensive first-pass hepatic metabolism. The toxicity associated with overdosage may be minimized by the associated early nausea and vomiting that occurs with excessive nicotine use. The signs and symptoms of acute nicotine overdosage can be mild to moderate, or moderate to severe. Mild to moderate signs and symptoms are abdominal pain, cold sweat, confusion, diarrhea, diaphoresis, dizziness, headache, hearing and vision disturbances, nausea, pallor, salivation (excessive), vomiting, and weakness (marked). Moderate to severe signs and symptoms are breathing difficulty; confusion; circulatory collapse; faintness and prostration; hypotension; rapid, weak, irregular pulse; and terminal convulsions, with death occurring within minutes because of respiratory failure due to paralysis of the muscles of respiration.

There have been reports of patients simultaneously applying several transdermal nicotine delivery systems or swallowing these systems. Signs and symptoms of overdosage associated with transdermal delivery systems are the same as those with other nicotine overdosage. Hypotension, prostration, and respiratory failure may be observed with severe overdosage. Convulsions and death may follow as a result of peripheral or central respiratory paralysis or, less frequently, cardiac failure. In cases of overdosage, the use of any nicotine product should be discontinued immediately; this includes immediate removal of the transdermal delivery system. After removal of the transdermal system, the skin should be flushed with water. Soap must not be used, because it may increase nicotine absorption from the skin site. Nicotine will continue to be delivered into the bloodstream for several hours after removal of the system, because of the depot of nicotine that is formed in the skin as part of the pharmacologic bioavailability of the transdermal system.

The minimal single acute lethal dose of ingested nicotine in adults is approximately 50 mg. However, amounts of nicotine that are tolerated by adult tobacco smokers can be fatal if ingested by children or pets. Suspected or actual nicotine overdosage requires emergency medical support of body systems, with attention to maintaining adequate respiratory function and ventilation, and increasing nicotine elimination. There is no known specific antidote. People who are using nicotine replacement products should be cautioned to (1) keep these products safely stored out of the reach of children and pets and (2) properly dispose of these products to prevent inadvertent access. They also should be cautioned against concurrent tobacco smoking while using nicotine replacement products.

Notes

1. In addition, there are hundreds of brand names for cigarettes, cigarillos, cigars, chewing tobacco, pipe tobacco, and snuff.
2. Some of these street names refer to specific nicotine delivery systems (e.g., cigarettes).
3. Bidis are small, brown, imported, unfiltered, hand-rolled cigarettes. They are made, primarily in India, from tobacco wrapped in a tendu or temburni leaf (*Diospyros melanoxylon*). Bidis are often available in different flavors (e.g., cherry, chocolate, and mango). They are particularly popular among

adolescents as an alternative to traditional cigarettes and are obtained from some convenience stores and tobacco-selling Internet sites.

4. Another plant, *Nicotiana rustica*, also contains nicotine, but it is less well known and is grown only in parts of India and Russia.

5. It is currently estimated that tobacco smoking is responsible for, or contributes in a significant way to, over 1000 deaths every day in North America.

6. This rate is down significantly from ~50% after World War II.

7. Traditionally, underage tobacco smokers obtained their "smokes" from older siblings, stole them from their parents, or purchased them at local convenience stores. Over the past decade, a significant new source of supply has become available: the Internet. Internet cigarette vendors are located in over half of the 50 states in the United States and are often on Indian reservations or reserves. These sites ship cigarettes, cured tobacco leaf, and bidis to purchasers across North America.

8. Cigarillos, small or "mini" cigars, are differentiated from cigarettes because, like larger cigars, the tobacco they contain is wrapped in tobacco leaves rather than rolled in cigarette papers.

9. The Black & Mild® brand of cigarillos is particularly popular among adolescent boys of African descent.

10. Flavors that have been marketed include apple, "appletini," cherry, chocolate, chocolate mint, coconut, cranberry, grape, mint, peach, piña colada, raspberry, rum, strawberry, tangerine, and vanilla.

11. At approximately 25%.

12. Snuff is made by grinding dried tobacco leaves into a fine powder that is nasally insufflated (snorted). Various aromatic and flavoring agents are added to the snuff to produce a preferred type, or blend, similar to pipe tobaccos. The use of snuff, or dried snuff as it was called, was popular during the 16th through 18th centuries after the introduction of tobacco to Europe. However, it is now relatively uncommon.

13. Use of wet snuff or "smokeless tobacco," as it is labeled by producers, or "spit tobacco," as it is referred to by users and others, remains at a constant low level. North American users, or "dippers," are primarily adolescent boys and men of European descent who reside in rural (e.g., farming) communities. Historically, baseball players have had a significantly higher than average use rate for spit tobacco. Ostensibly, it is used to enhance athletic performance, but this effect has not been demonstrated in published studies. The use of smokeless tobacco would be expected to cause a slight psychostimulant action, with increased blood pressure, increased heart rate, and prevention of the nicotine withdrawal syndrome, in regular long-term users.

14. Nicotinic acetylcholine receptors have been identified in other organ systems, including lymphocytes and nasal mucosa. The nAChRs in lymphocytes may play a role in regulating immune function. The nAChRs in nasal mucosa may be involved in producing the nasal reactions (e.g., sensitivity) to tobacco smoke and to nicotine nasal spray products that are observed in some people.

15. Eight different α and three different β subunits have been identified in vertebrate nervous systems. This number of subunits allows for the possibility of several subtypes of nAChRs, defined by their constituent subunits (e.g., α4β2-subtype, α7-subtype).

16. Holding an average amount of smokeless tobacco, or snuff, in the mouth (depending upon the nicotine level of the brand used) for approximately 30 minutes reportedly provides as much nicotine as smoking three tobacco cigarettes.

17. This indication for use is generally referred to as "nicotine replacement therapy," and a variety of nicotine products and dosage formulations are used, including nicotine chewing gums, intranasal sprays, oral inhalers, oral lozenges, and transdermal delivery systems (patches).

18. Nicotine is most often obtained from smoking tobacco products. Thus, the toxicity associated with this pattern of use (e.g., chronic obstructive lung disease, lung cancer, and respiratory tract irritation) also must be considered. When considered from this perspective, it is clear that tobacco smoking is the leading cause of preventable death in the entire world.

19. Due to nicotine-induced vasoconstriction of blood vessels in the skin.

20. Cancers involving a number of body organs (i.e., bladder, esophagus, head, kidney, larynx, lung, neck, oral cavity, and stomach) have been correlated with tobacco smoking. For many of these cancers, a direct cause-and-effect relationship with tobacco use remains tentative. Research increasingly suggests a significant genetic contribution to the relationship between tobacco smoking and cancer.

21. Due to both the direct effects of the nicotine and the carbon monoxide produced while smoking tobacco products.

22. Neonates and infants who sleep (i.e., "bed share") with mothers who smoke tobacco are at significant

risk of sudden infant death syndrome (SIDS). However, because most reports in the literature have noted that the mothers had used alcohol or an illicit drug or substance of abuse in addition to smoking tobacco, the exact contributory effect of tobacco smoke to SIDS remains speculative.

23. Faster metabolizers of nicotine report greater and more frequent signs and symptoms of nicotine withdrawal. Therefore, they are more likely to self-medicate (i.e., smoke another cigarette) to provide relief of these signs and symptoms.

24. Nicotine withdrawal also has been reported to cause delirium in patients who have acute brain injuries.

References

Balfour, D.J. (2002). The neurobiology of tobacco dependence: A commentary. *Respiration, 69*(1), 7-11.

Benowitz, N.L. (2008). Clinical pharmacology of nicotine: Implications for understanding, preventing, and treating tobacco addiction. *Clinical Pharmacology & Therapeutics, 83*(4), 531-541.

Caggiula, A.R., Donny, E.C., White, A.R., et al. (2001). Cue dependency of nicotine self-administration and smoking. *Pharmacology, Biochemistry, and Behavior, 70*(4), 515-530.

Cigarillo smoking in Canada: A review of results from CTUMS, Wave 1, 2007. (2008, February). Physicians for a Smoke-free Canada. Available: http://www.smoke-free.ca/pdf_1/cigarillos-2008.pdf.

Dani, J.A., & De Biasi, M. (2001). Cellular mechanisms of nicotine addiction. *Pharmacology, Biochemistry, and Behavior, 70*(4), 439-446.

Dani, J.A., Ji, D., & Zhou, F.M. (2001). Synaptic plasticity and nicotine addiction. *Neuron, 31*(3), 349-352.

Domino, E.F. (2001). Nicotine and tobacco dependence: Normalization or stimulation? *Alcohol, 24*(2), 83-86.

Fisher, L. (2000). Bidis—the latest trend in U.S. teen tobacco use. *Cancer Causes and Control, 11*(6), 577-578.

Gehricke, J.G., Loughlin, S.E., Whalen, C.K., et al. (2007). Smoking to self-medicate attentional and emotional dysfunctions. *Nicotine & Tobacco Research, 9*(Supplement 4), S523-S536.

Ho, M.K., & Tyndale, R.F. (2007). Overview of the pharmacogenomics of cigarette smoking. *The Pharmacogenomics Journal, 7*(2), 81-98.

James, C., Klenka, H., & Manning, D. (2003). Sudden infant death syndrome: Bed sharing with mothers who smoke. *Archives of Disease in Childhood, 88*(2), 112-113.

Jones, D.L., & Mobley, C.C. (2000). Treatment of nicotine addiction. *Texas Dental Journal, 117*(6), 26-32.

Juliano, L.M., & Brandon, T.H. (2002). Effects of nicotine dose, instructional set, and outcome expectancies on the subjective effects of smoking in the presence of a stressor. *Journal of Abnormal Psychology, 111*(1), 88-97.

Kalman, D. (2002). The subjective effects of nicotine: Methodological issues, a review of experimental studies, and recommendations for future research. *Nicotine & Tobacco Research, 4*(1), 25-70.

Kenny, P.J., & Markou, A. (2001). Neurobiology of the nicotine withdrawal syndrome. *Pharmacology, Biochemistry, and Behavior, 70*(4), 531-549.

Kuper, H., Boffetta, P., & Adami, H.O. (2002). Tobacco use and cancer causation: Association by tumour type. *Journal of Internal Medicine, 252*(3), 206-224.

MacLeod, S.L., & Chowdhury, P. (2006). The genetics of nicotine dependence: Relationship to pancreatic cancer. *World Journal of Gastroenterology, 12*(46), 7433-7439.

Malaiyandi, V., Sellers, E.M., & Tyndale, R.F. (2005). Implications of CYP2A6 genetic variation for smoking behaviors and nicotine dependence. *Clinical Pharmacology & Therapeutics, 77*(3), 145-158.

Malson, J.L., & Pickworth, W.B. (2002). Bidis—hand-rolled, Indian cigarettes: Effects on physiological, biochemical and subjective measures. *Pharmacology, Biochemistry, and Behavior, 72*(1-2), 443-447.

Malson, J.L., Sims, K., Murty, R., et al. (2001). Comparison of the nicotine content of tobacco used in bidis and conventional cigarettes. *Tobacco Control, 10*(2), 181-183.

Mayer, S.A., Chong, J.Y., Ridgway, E., et al., (2001). Delirium from nicotine withdrawal in neuro-ICU patients. *Neurology, 57*(3), 551-553.

Mwenifumbo, J.C., & Tyndale, R.F. (2007). Genetic variability in CYP2A6 and the pharmacokinetics of nicotine. *Pharmacogenomics, 8*(10), 1385-1402.

Nakajima, M. (2007). Smoking behavior and related cancers: The role of CYP2A6 polymorphisms. *Current Opinion in Molecular Therapeutics, 9*(6), 538-544.

Page, J.B., & Evans, S. (2004). Cigars, cigarillos, and youth: Emergent patterns in subcultural complexes. *Journal of Ethnicity in Substance Abuse, 2*(4), 63-76.

Pagliaro, A.M. (2002). Abusable psychotropic use among children and adolescents. In L.A. Pagliaro & A.M. Pagliaro (Eds.), *Problems in pediatric drug therapy* (4th ed., pp. 347-385). Washington, DC: American Pharmaceutical Association.

Perkins, K.A., Gerlach, D., Broge, M., et al. (2001). Dissociation of nicotine tolerance from tobacco dependence in humans. *The Journal of Pharmacology and Experimental Therapeutics, 296*(3), 849-856.

Peters R.J. Jr., Kelder, S.H., Prokhorov, A.V., et al. (2005). Beliefs and social norms about smoking onset and addictions among urban adolescent cigarette smokers. *Journal of Psychoactive Drugs, 37*(4), 449-453.

Picciotto, M.R., Brunzell, D.H., & Caldarone, B.J. (2002). Effect of nicotine receptors on anxiety and depression. *Neuroreport, 13*(9), 1097-1106.

Ribisl, K.M., Kim, A.E., & Williams, R.S. (2001). Web sites selling cigarettes: How many are there in the USA and what are their sales practices? *Tobacco Control, 10*(4), 352-359.

Robbins, L.T. (2001). Flavored cigarettes (bidis) popular among youth. *NCSL Legisbrief, 9*(45), 1-2.

Rubinstein, M.L., Benowitz, N.L., Auerback, G.M., et al. (2008). Rate of nicotine metabolism and withdrawal symptoms in adolescent light smokers. *Pediatrics, 122*(3), e643-e647.

Rubinstein, M.L., Thompson, P.J., Benowitz, N.L., et al. (2007). Cotinine levels in relation to smoking behavior and addiction in young adolescent smokers. *Nicotine & Tobacco Research, 9*(1), 129-135.

Warren, C.W., Jones, N.R., Peruga, A., et al. (2008). Global youth tobacco surveillance, 2000-2007. *MMWR: Surveillance Summaries, 57*(1), 1-28.

NITRAZEPAM

Names

BAN or INN Generic Synonyms: N-Desmethylnimetazepam

Brand/Trade: Mogadon®; Nitrazadon®

Chemical: 1,3-Dihydro-7-nitro-5-phenyl-2H-1,4-benzodiazepin-2-one

Street: Don; Dons; Moggies; Moogles; Nitro's; NTZ

Pharmacologic Classification

Psychodepressant, sedative-hypnotic: benzodiazepine

Brief General Overview

Nitrazepam possesses hypnotic as well as anticonvulsant activity.

Dosage Forms and Routes of Administration

Nitrazepam is produced by licit pharmaceutical manufacturers in North America[1] and is available as an oral tablet formulation. It is personally used for its psychodepressant actions. It is usually orally ingested, but rarely the tablets may be pulverized to a powder that is intranasally snorted. Nitrazepam is readily available over the Internet.

Mechanism of CNS Action

The exact mechanism of nitrazepam's hypnotic action has not yet been fully determined. However, it appears to be mediated by, or work in concert with, the inhibitory neurotransmitter GABA (see Benzodiazepines monograph). Nitrazepam's anticonvulsant actions may be related to its binding to voltage-dependent sodium channels, where it slows their recovery from inactivation (i.e., depolarization).

Pharmacodynamics/Pharmacokinetics

Nitrazepam is rapidly absorbed from the GI tract after oral ingestion and has good bioavailability ($F=0.80$). Although concurrent ingestion of food may delay the peak concentration by ~1 hour, it does not significantly affect bioavailability. Onset of action is generally within 1 hour, and peak blood concentrations occur ~3 hours after ingestion. Nitrazepam is moderately bound to plasma proteins (i.e., ~87%) and has an apparent volume of distribution of ~3 L/kg. It is extensively metabolized in the liver, primarily by nitroreduction, to several inactive metabolites, including 7-aminonitrazepam, that are predominantly excreted in the urine. Less than 1% of nitrazepam is excreted in unchanged form in the urine. Total body clearance is ~75 mL/minute, and the mean elimination half-life is ~25 hours.

Current Approved Indications for Medical Use[2]

Sleep disorders: insomnia (short-term symptomatic management)

Desired Action/Reason for Personal Use

Alcohol-like disinhibitory euphoria or "high" (relatively mild); anxiety/stress reduction

Toxicity

Acute: Ataxia; cognitive impairment; confusion; dizziness; drowsiness; fatigue; falls; lethargy; lightheadedness; memory impairment; nausea; psychomotor impairment

Chronic: Abnormal behavior; learning impairment; mental depression; nightmares (associated with suppression of REM sleep); physical dependence; psychological dependence

Pregnancy & Lactation: FDA Pregnancy Category "not established." Safety of nitrazepam use by adolescent girls and women who are pregnant has not been established. Nitrazepam rapidly crosses the placental barrier and, although not directly related to nitrazepam, teratogenic effects have been associated with other benzodiazepines (see Benzodiazepines monograph). Adolescent girls and women who are pregnant should not use nitrazepam.

Safety of nitrazepam use by adolescent girls and women who are breast-feeding has not been established. Nitrazepam is excreted in breast milk at an average concentration that is equal to 25% of the maternal nitrazepam blood concentration. Adolescent girls and women who are breast-feeding should not use nitrazepam.

Abuse Potential

Physical dependence: Low to Moderate (USDEA Schedule IV; low potential for abuse)
Psychological dependence: Moderate

Withdrawal Syndrome

A nitrazepam withdrawal syndrome has been reported upon abrupt discontinuation of nitrazepam after regular, long-term use. Signs and symptoms of withdrawal resemble those of withdrawal from other benzodiazepines (see Benzodiazepines monograph).

Overdosage

Signs and symptoms of nitrazepam overdosage include bradycardia, coma, confusion, diminished reflexes, drowsiness, hypotension, and increased sedation. Nitrazepam overdosage has been fatal. Acute nitrazepam overdosage requires emergency medical support of body systems, with attention to increasing nitrazepam elimination. The benzodiazpine antagonist flumazenil (Anexate®, Romazicon®) may be required.[3]

Notes

1. Nitrazepam (Mogadon®) is manufactured and approved for legitimate medical indications in Canada, but not in the United States.
2. Nitrazepam also has been used with some therapeutic success in the pharmacologic management of childhood epileptic syndromes, such as Lennox-Gastaut syndrome and West syndrome, which are often refractory to conventional anticonvulsant pharmacotherapy.
3. Caution is required, because flumazenil antagonism may precipitate the nitrazepam withdrawal syndrome in people who are physically dependent on nitrazepam.

References

Carlsten, A., Waern, M., Holmgren, P., et al. (2003). The role of benzodiazepines in elderly suicides. *Scandinavian Journal of Public Health, 31*(3), 224-228.

Dündar, Y., Dodd, S., Strobl, J., et al. (2004). Comparative efficacy of newer hypnotic drugs for the short-term management of insomnia: A systematic review and meta-analysis. *Human Psychopharmacology, 19*(5), 305-322.

Honeychurch, K.C., Smith, G.C., & Hart, J.P. (2006). Voltammetric behavior of nitrazepam and its determination in serum using liquid chromatography with redox mode dual–electrode detection. *Analytical Chemistry, 78*(2), 416-423.

Hosain, S.A., Green, N.S., Solomon G.E., et al. (2003). Nitrazepam for the treatment of Lennox-Gastaut syndrome. *Pediatric Neurology, 28*(1), 16-19.

Kitabayashi, Y., Ueda, H., Narumoto, J., et al. (2008). Chronic high-dose nitrazepam dependence: ^{123}I-IMP SPECT and EEG studies. *Addiction Biology, 6*(3), 257-261.

Mikati, M.A., Lepejian, G.A., & Holmes, G.L. (2002). Medical treatment of patients with infantile spasms. *Clinical Neuropharmacology, 25*(2), 61-70.

Moriya, F., & Hashimoto, Y. (2003). Tissue distribution of nitrazepam and 7-aminonitrazepam in a case of nitrazepam intoxication. *Forensic Science International, 131*(2-3), 108-112.

Prasad, P.S., Ray, R., Jain, R., et al. (2001). Abuse liability of nitrazepam: A study among experienced drug users. *Indian Journal of Pharmacology, 33*, 357-362.

Yamazaki, A., Kumagai, Y., Fujita, T., et al. (2007). Different effects of light food on pharmacokinetics and pharmacodynamics of three benzodiazepines, quazepam, nitrazepam and diazepam. *The Journal of Clinical Pharmacy and Therapeutics, 32*(1), 31-39.

NITROUS OXIDE

Names

BAN or INN Generic Synonyms: Dinitrogen Monoxide

Brand/Trade: Generally available by generic name

Chemical: Nitrous oxide

Street: Balloons; Breeze; Buzz Bomb; Cartridges; Factitious Air; Gas; Hippie Crack; Laughing Gas; N-2; N_2O; Nitrous; Pan; Shoot the Breeze; Tanks; Whippets; Whippits

Pharmacologic Classification

Psychodepressant, volatile solvents & inhalants: inhalant gas, general anesthetic

Brief General Overview

Nitrous oxide is a weak anesthetic gas (i.e., minimal alveolar concentration = 105%) that is colorless, odorless, and nonflammable. It has been used clinically as a surgical anesthetic since the late 19th century.[1] However, because of the availability of other, more potent, general anesthetics, the clinical use of nitrous oxide is now primarily limited to the practice of dentistry.

Nitrous oxide is personally used for its psychodepressant actions. However, published data on its patterns of use are relatively scarce. On the basis of a review of the limited data available and our own clinical experience with people who used nitrous oxide, we classify North American users into five groups: (1) adolescents who are experimenting with a number of solvents and inhalants, including nitrous oxide,[2] (2) men of European descent between 18 and 35 years of age, (3) medical and dental students in a "social" setting, (4) health care professionals, primarily dentists and anesthesia technicians,[3] and (5) homosexual and bisexual men of either African or European descent.[4] An emerging group of users is young women in their 20s of European descent, who are increasingly using nitrous oxide as a party drug.

Dosage Forms and Routes of Administration

Nitrous oxide is available from a number of licit chemical or medicinal gas suppliers. Users also can purchase nitrous oxide that is intended for other uses, including (1) whippits, which are intended for use in whipped cream charging bottles,[5] and (2) gas tanks containing nitrous oxide.[6] Finally, some users of nitrous oxide produce their own supply of the gas by means of thermal decomposition of ammonium nitrate.[7]

Mechanism of CNS Action

The exact mechanism of the CNS action of nitrous oxide has not been determined. It appears to cause psychodepression by suppressing activity in the ascending reticular activating system. As with other general anesthetic gases, its activity is presumed to be related to its degree of lipid solubility and not to its specific structure. However, current research suggests that antagonistic action at the N-methyl-D-aspartate (NMDA) receptor and resultant effect on the glutamate-gated cation (principally calcium) channel may play a significant role in nitrous oxide's mechanism of action.

Pharmacodynamics/Pharmacokinetics

Nitrous oxide's onset of action is rapid, and effects begin to dissipate within a few minutes of discontinuing use. Nitrous oxide is not metabolized but is excreted in unchanged form (>99%) through the lungs.[8] Additional valid and reliable data are not available.

Current Approved Indications for Medical Use

General anesthesia

Desired Action/Reason for Personal Use

Alcohol-like disinhibitory euphoria; disorientation; hallucinations

Toxicity

Acute: Asphyxiation[9]; cognitive impairment; dizziness; frostbite, particularly of the lips, mouth, nose, pharynx, and larynx (associated with breathing cold gas from pressurized tanks); hangover effect; headache; hypoxia; laughter (generally following asphyxia phase); memory loss (anterograde)[10]; nausea; paranoia; psychomotor impairment; unconsciousness (due to inadequate oxygen supply)

Chronic: Homocysteine blood concentrations (elevated); psychological dependence; vitamin B_{12} (cyanocobalamin) deficiency and resultant pernicious anemia and neurological impairment (e.g., ataxia, dystaxia, hyporeflexia, myeloneuropathy, paresthesia, peripheral neuropathy)[11]; psychosis (secondary to vitamin B_{12} deficiency)

Pregnancy & Lactation: Safety of nitrous oxide use by adolescent girls and women who are pregnant has not been established. Early reports of increased risk of spontaneous abortion in health care providers (e.g., dentists and dental assistants) occupationally exposed to nitrous oxide while pregnant have not been substantiated. However, isolated case reports persist, and it is known that chronic use of nitrous oxide can lead to vitamin B_{12} deficiency. Therefore, until safety has been demonstrated, pregnant adolescent girls and women should be cautioned not to use, and to avoid occupational exposure to, nitrous oxide. Additional valid and reliable data are needed.

Safety of nitrous oxide use by adolescent girls and women who are breast-feeding has not been established. Additional valid and reliable data are needed.

Abuse Potential

Physical dependence: None to low (USDEA: not a scheduled drug)
Psychological dependence: Low to moderate

Withdrawal Syndrome

A nitrous oxide withdrawal syndrome has not been reported.

Overdosage

Nitrous oxide is relatively nontoxic (i.e., its use has not been associated with respiratory depression or hepatic or renal damage). However, improper use, such as that associated with some patterns of personal use, can cause hypoxia and related sequelae. In this regard, overdosage of nitrous oxide requires emergency medical support, with attention to maintaining respiratory function (e.g., providing manual or mechanical resuscitation and supplemental oxygen, as required). Medical attention to related sequelae, such as aspiration, cardiac dysrhythmias, coma, and seizures, may also be required. There is no known antidote.

Notes

1. Nitrous oxide must be administered in combination with at least 20% oxygen to avoid hypoxia during the induction of general anesthesia. In addition, in order to avoid "diffusional hypoxia," it has been recommended that 100% oxygen be administered instead of air when nitrous oxide pharmacotherapy is discontinued.
2. These adolescents are of either gender and are predominantly of European descent. Adolescents of Hispanic descent are the next largest group of users. Use is lowest among adolescents of African descent.
3. People in this group generally use the available medicinal grade of nitrous oxide, often in the clinical area of practice (e.g., dental office after hours, empty medical or surgical suite). Not much has been published in this area; however, our own experience in treating these professional users suggests that, overwhelmingly, they are men of European descent.
4. These men typically use nitrous oxide and other drugs and substances of abuse, such as alcohol, to cognitively suppress their fear of risk for HIV infection and AIDS while engaging in high-risk sexual behavior with multiple partners.
5. Whippits are small nitrous oxide cartridges or containers (e.g., EZ Whip®). The nitrous oxide is discharged into either a balloon using a "cracker" or a whipped cream charging bottle. A cracker is a metal or plastic device specifically manufactured to facilitate nitrous oxide abuse. It is available for purchase at "head" shops or stores that sell drug paraphernalia, as well as through the Internet. Whipped cream charging bottles are available for purchase from most upscale cooking supply stores. The nitrous oxide is inhaled directly from these secondary containers.
6. The gas tanks are usually stolen from chemistry laboratories or purchased from chemical supply houses and specialty automobile racing stores. The tanks are then filled with either medicinal grade or auto grade nitrous oxide. The latter tanks contain hydrogen sulfide and the gas must be filtered, usually with sodium bicarbonate (i.e., baking soda), before use.
7. This method of obtaining nitrous oxide is not used frequently because (1) heating ammonium nitrate can result in an explosive reaction and (2) nitrogen dioxide, a potential byproduct, is extremely toxic, particularly to lung tissue.
8. A small amount (i.e., <1%) is diffused through the skin or degraded by interaction with cyanocobalamin (vitamin B_{12}) in the intestinal bacteria.
9. Generally associated with breathing pure nitrous oxide gas through an attached face mask without mixing it with oxygen (see Note 1).
10. This effect is a therapeutically desired property of a general anesthetic.
11. Nitrous oxide inactivates cyanocobalamin (i.e., vitamin B_{12}). In some cases of nitrous oxide-induced neurotoxicity Schilling test results are normal, but clinical improvement is seen with both discontinuation of nitrous oxide use and pharmacotherapy with cyanocobalamin.

References

Blanton, A. (2006). Nitrous oxide abuse: Dentistry's unique addiction. *The Journal of the Tennessee Dental Association, 86*(4), 30-31.

Brouette, T., & Anton, R. (2001). Clinical review of inhalants. *The American Journal on Addictions, 10*(1), 79-94.

Butzkueven, H., & King, J.O. (2000). Nitrous oxide myelopathy in an abuser of whipped cream bulbs. *Journal of Clinical Neuroscience, 7*(1), 73-75.

Cartner, M., Sinnott, M., & Silburn, P. (2007). Paralysis caused by "nagging" [sic: "bagging"]. *The Medical Journal of Australia, 187*(6), 366-367.

Diamond, A.L., Diamond, R., Freedman, S.M., et al. (2004). "Whippets"-induced cobalamin deficiency manifesting as cervical myelopathy. *Journal of Neuroimaging, 14,* (3), 277-280.

Iwata, K., O'Keefe, G.B., & Karanas, A. (2001). Neurologic problems associated with chronic nitrous oxide abuse in a non-healthcare worker. *The American Journal of the Medical Sciences, 322*(3), 173-174.

Malamed, S.F., & Clark, M.S. (2003). Nitrous oxide-oxygen: A new look at a very old technique. *Journal of the California Dental Association, 31*(5), 397-403.

McKirnan, D.J., Vanable, P.A., Ostrow, D.G., et al. (2001). Expectancies of sexual "escape" and sexual risk among drug and alcohol-involved gay and bisexual men. *Journal of Substance Abuse, 13*(1-2), 137-154.

Miller, M.A., Martinez, V., McCarthy, R., et al. (2004). Nitrous oxide "whippit" abuse presenting as clinical B12 deficiency and ataxia. *The American Journal of Emergency Medicine, 22*(2), 124.

Sethi, N.K., Mullin, P., Torgovnick, J., et al. (2006). Nitrous oxide "whippit" abuse presenting with cobalamin responsive psychosis. *Journal of Medical Toxicology, 2*(2), 71-74.

Shulman, R.M., Geraghty, T.J., & Tadros, M. (2007). A case of unusual substance abuse causing myeloneuropathy. *Spinal Cord, 45*(4), 314-317.

Singer, M.A., Lazaridis, C., Nations, S.P., et al. (2008). Reversible nitrous oxide-induced myeloneuropathy with pernicious anemia: Case report and literature review. *Muscle & Nerve, 37*(1), 125-129.

Waclawik, A.J., Luzzio, C.C., Juhasz-Pocsine, K., et al. (2003). Myeloneuropathy from nitrous oxide abuse: Unusually high methylmalonic acid and homocysteine levels. *Wisconsin Medical Journal, 102*(4), 43-45.

Waters, M.F., Kang, G.A., Mazziotta, J.C., et al. (2005). Nitrous oxide inhalation as a cause of cervical myelopathy. *Acta Neurologica Scandanavica, 112*(4), 270-272.

Wu, M.S., Hsu, Y.D., Lin, J.C., et al. (2007). Spinal myoclonus in subacute combined degeneration caused by nitrous oxide. *Acta Neurologica Taiwanica, 16*(2), 102-105.

N,N-DIMETHYLTRYPTAMINE (See Dimethyltryptamine)

N-METHYL-1-(3,4-METHYLENEDIOXYPHENYL)-2-BUTANAMINE (See Methyl-1-(3,4-methylenedioxyphenyl)-2-butanamine)

NUTMEG

Names

BAN or INN Generic Synonyms: None

Brand/Trade: None

Chemical: See "Brief General Overview"

Street: Idiot Juice[1]; Magic; Muskatbaum; *Noz Moscada*

Pharmacologic Classification

Psychodelic, amphetamine-like psychodelic: phenethylamine

Brief General Overview

Nutmeg, a commonly used cooking spice, has psychoactive properties for which it is personally used. It is obtained from the dried seed of the *Myristica fragrans* tree, which is indigenous to the Moluccas (formerly, the Spice Islands), part of Indonesia.[2] The natural psychoactive alkaloidal substances found in nutmeg (i.e., elemicin, isoelemicin, myristicin [methoxysafrole], and safrole, among others) are 3,4-methylenedioxyamphetamine-like (MDA-like) compounds that have been used for their psychodelic and traditional ethnomedical actions for over 3000 years in India and Egypt.

Although generally available and legal to purchase, nutmeg has not become a popular substance of abuse because of its associated toxicity. Most users are preadolescent or adolescent boys who are experimenting with various means of altering their consciousness. Adults occasionally report using nutmeg for its psychoactive actions, but never as a drug or substance of abuse of first choice. There also have been rare reports about prison inmates using nutmeg to get "high." However, as the availability of other drugs and substances of abuse increases in North American jails and prisons, which has occurred logarithmically over the past two decades, this once rather common pattern of nutmeg use has virtually disappeared—except around Christmas time.

Dosage Forms and Routes of Administration

Nutmeg is the naturally occurring kernel of the fruit of the *Myristica fragrans* tree. The kernel is removed from the fruit and dried in the sun for approximately 2 months, during which time it is turned daily. The dried kernel is then ground, in the same manner as for use as a cooking spice, and is generally eaten or drunk as a tea.[3]

Mechanism of CNS Action

On the basis of the anticholinergic toxicity profile of nutmeg, its mechanism of action appears to involve the cholinergic system. Additional valid and reliable data are not available.

Pharmacodynamics/Pharmacokinetics

After ingestion, the onset of CNS action begins slowly over 2 to 3 hours, generally peaks in 4 to 6 hours, and persists for 12 to 18 hours. Physical hangover effects may occur and last for a few days. The concurrent ingestion of food slows the absorption of nutmeg and, subsequently, the time to reach its desired actions. During this time, the active ingredients in nutmeg undergo extensive hepatic metabolism, resulting in several metabolites that are excreted in the urine: O-demethyl-elemicin, O-demethyl-dihydroxy-elemicin, demethylenyl-myristicin, dihydroxy-myristicin, and demethylenyl-safrole. Additional valid and reliable data are not available.

Current Approved Indications for Medical Use

None[4]

Desired Action/Reason for Personal Use

Arousal of sexual desire (purported); detachment from reality; euphoria; hallucinations (uncommon); illusions (primarily visual distortions); perceived distortions in time or space; sleepless stupor

Toxicity

Acute: Anxiety; ataxia; blurred vision; dehydration; diarrhea (followed by constipation); dizziness; drowsiness; dry mouth; eye pain; fatigue; feelings of impending doom; fever; hallucinations; hangover effect (may persist for 1 to 2 days); headache (generally transient); laughing or giggling; lethargy; muscle weakness; muscular aches; nystagmus; nausea; palpitations; red eyes; tachycardia; urinary retention

Chronic: Hepatic dysfunction[5]; psychosis (rare)

Pregnancy & Lactation: Valid and reliable data are not available.

Abuse Potential

Physical dependence: None (USDEA: not a scheduled drug)
Psychological dependence: Low[6]

Withdrawal Syndrome

A nutmeg withdrawal syndrome has not been reported.

Overdosage

Nutmeg overdosage may cause acute anticholinergic hyperstimulation and has resulted in death. Typically, users present with signs and symptoms of acute psychosis and anticholinergic toxicity. Treatment consists of appropriate supportive medical care. There is no known antidote.

Notes

1. Refers to a mixture of ground nutmeg and water used by some prison inmates.
2. The encased covering of the nutmeg seed or kernel is used for the production of mace. Nutmeg is currently cultivated primarily in the West Indies. It is commonly imported from the islands of Grenada and Trinidad.
3. Intranasal sniffing (i.e., snorting) of ground nutmeg, often mixed with other ingredients (e.g., *betel* nut), has been popular for centuries in such countries as India and Indonesia. However, this form of use has been relatively uncommon in North America.
4. In its country of origin, it is still used by healers, midwives, and vendors of herbal remedies for such medicinal purposes as the treatment of diarrhea, mouth sores, and insomnia.
5. Safrole, a nonpsychoactive constituent of nutmeg, is hepatotoxic.
6. Classified as such because of the primarily negative features associated with the abuse of nutmeg (see "Toxicity").

References

Beyer, J., Ehlers, D., & Maurer, H.H. (2006), Abuse of nutmeg (Myristica fragrans Houtt.): Studies on the metabolism and the toxicologic detection of its ingredients elemicin, myristicin, and safrole in rat and human urine using gas chromatography/mass spectrometry. *Therapeutic Drug Monitoring, 28*(4), 568-575.

Demetriades, A.K., Wallman, P.D., McGuiness, A., et al. (2005). Low cost, high risk: Accidental nutmeg intoxication. *Emergency Medicine Journal, 22*(3), 223-225.

Forrester, M.B. (2005). Nutmeg intoxication in Texas, 1998-2004. *Human & Experimental Toxicology, 24*(11), 563-566.

McKenna, A., Nordt, S.P., & Ryan, J. (2004). Acute nutmeg poisoning. *European Journal of Emergency Medicine, 11*(4), 240-241.

Sangalli, B.C., & Chiang, W. (2000). Toxicology of nutmeg abuse. *Journal of Toxicology. Clinical Toxicology, 38*(6), 671-678.

Stein, U., Greyer, H., & Hentschel, H. (2001). Nutmeg (myristicin) poisoning—report on a fatal case and a series of cases recorded by a poison information centre. *Forensic Science International, 118*(1), 87-90.

OPIATE ANALGESICS[1]

Names

BAN or INN Generic Synonyms: None

Brand/Trade: See individual monographs

Chemical: See individual monographs

Street: See individual monographs

Pharmacologic Classification[2]

Psychodepressants, opiate analgesics

Brief General Overview

The opiate analgesics are a group of natural (e.g., morphine) and synthetic (e.g., meperidine) derivatives of opium. The natural forms of the opiate analgesics are obtained from opium resin, which is harvested from the unripe seed pod of the plant *Papaver somniferum*—the "poppy that causes sleep."[3] The plant is harvested 1 to 3 weeks after flowering. *Papaver somniferum* is classified as an herb and is indigenous to southeastern Europe and western Asia. The opium poppy has been widely cultivated for millennia in these areas. It also has been introduced to other countries throughout the world by travelers and immigrants, but climatic conditions similar to those of southeastern Europe and western Asia are required for its cultivation.

Traditionally, most of the opium grown was controlled and marketed in the Golden Triangle, which comprises Burma (i.e., Union of Myanmar), Laos, and Thailand. The Golden Triangle produces over 1,000 tons of opium annually and, until the 1970s, supplied most of the opium used to produce heroin for use in the United States. Burma remains the world's second largest producer of licit opium (i.e., over 300 tons in 2008). The Golden Crescent (i.e., Afghanistan,[4] Iran, and Pakistan) also is a traditional area of opium production and marketing. It produces over 10,000 tons of opium per year. In addition, India produces approximately 2,000 tons per year—90% of the world's licit medical requirements for opium.

Currently, approximately 40% of the heroin that reaches North America comes from the opium grown in Afghanistan, Burma, Iran, and Pakistan. Most of this opium is processed into heroin in these countries, with the remainder being processed in Italy, primarily in Sicily. Since the early 1990s, the bulk of the remaining heroin that reaches the streets of the United States (about 40%) has come from opium grown in the western hemisphere, primarily from Colombia and Mexico. Mexico alone supplies a significant and increasing proportion (about 30%) of heroin (primarily, Black Tar heroin) to users in the United States (see Heroin monograph).

The dried resin of the opium poppy contains opium and the isoquinoline alkaloids codeine, morphine, noscapine, papaverine, and thebaine.[5] Some semisynthetic opiate analgesics are derived from the natural products (e.g., heroin is derived from morphine, and hydrocodone [Lortab®] and oxycodone [OxyContin®]) are derived from codeine and thebaine). Others, such as meperidine (Demerol®) and pentazocine (Talwin®), are totally chemically synthesized. All of the opiate analgesics have a propensity to cause physical and psychological dependence.

Dosage Forms and Routes of Administration

Opiate analgesics are produced both by licit pharmaceutical manufacturers in North America and by illicit chemists throughout the world. They are available through drug diversion and purchase over the Internet in a variety of dosage formulations, including (1) injectables for intramuscular, intravenous, and subcutaneous use; (2) intranasal sprays; (3) oral tablets (regular and extended-release), elixirs, and solutions (regular and highly concentrated); (4) rectal suppositories; and (5) transdermal drug delivery systems. People who personally use opiate analgesics use one or more of these dosage formulations and various routes of administration. Users tend to be adolescents, 16 years of age or older, and young, middle-aged, and elderly adults. Historically, opiate analgesic users were more likely to be men, but today men and women are equally represented overall, with increasing numbers of younger adult users being men and older adult users being women. The vast majority (i.e., ~80%) of opiate analgesic users in the United States are of European descent. However, opiate analgesics users can be found, across North America as well as worldwide, among every cultural, ethnic, and socioeconomic group. And high rates of opium and heroin use are found in virtually every opium-producing country.

Mechanism of CNS Action

Opiate analgesics act primarily on the CNS. The perception of and emotional response to pain are modified when opiate analgesics bind to stereospecific receptors in the CNS. Five major groups of opiate, or endorphin, receptors have been identified: delta, epsilon, kappa, mu, and sigma. Opiate analgesic activity occurs at the mu, kappa, and sigma receptors. These receptors are found in the highest concentrations in the brain stem, cortex, hypothalamus, limbic system, midbrain, spinal cord, and thalamus.[6] Pure opiate analgesic agonists (e.g., morphine) exert their actions mainly at the mu receptors.

The opiate analgesics decrease presynaptic neurotransmitter release. In addition to analgesia, opiate agonists suppress the cough reflex, alter mood (i.e., produce euphoria or dysphoria), and cause mental clouding, nausea, vomiting, and respiratory depression. Nausea and vomiting probably are caused by stimulation of the chemoreceptor trigger zone (CTZ). Mixed agonists/antagonists (e.g., butorphanol [Stadol®], nalbuphine [Nubain®], pentazocine [Talwin®]) appear to act primarily at the kappa receptors.

Pharmacodynamics/Pharmacokinetics

Opiate analgesics, available in a variety of dosage formulations, can be used in several ways, which may affect bioavailability and pharmacotherapeutics. For example, opiate analgesics can be orally ingested as capsules (e.g., propoxyphene [Darvon®]), liquids (e.g., methadone), or tablets (e.g., codeine); injected intravenously ("mainlined"; e.g., heroin, pentazocine [Talwin®]) or subcutaneously ("popped" under the skin; e.g., heroin); inhaled into the pulmonary system (smoked; e.g., heroin, opium); intranasally sniffed (snorted; e.g., heroin, hydrocodone); placed in the mouth (sucked; e.g., fentanyl [Actiq®]); and applied to the skin (e.g., fentanyl [Duragesic®]). Traditionally, over the past century, the oral and intravenous methods of use have been the most common. More recently, subcutaneous injection of heroin has been used, primarily by weekend users (i.e., occasional users and those who do not want their heroin use to interfere with their workweek). This pattern of use, particularly during the 1970s and 1980s, was known as "chipping." However, since the early 1990s, smoking (i.e., "chasing the dragon") has increased significantly.

Absorption: Absorption of the various opiate analgesics generally depends on the dosage formulation used (e.g., oral tablet or transdermal delivery system), its purity (i.e., pharmaceutical grade, adulterated, or misrepresented), and its method of use (e.g., oral ingestion, intranasal sniffing [snorting]). When opiate analgesics are intravenously injected, absorption is immediate and complete. The opiate analgesic also reaches the bloodstream rapidly after intramuscular or subcutaneous injection, but absorption is less rapid and more variable than after intravenous injection. Pulmonary inhalation likewise is rapid, as is intranasal sniffing. When the drug is orally ingested, absorption from the GI tract, largely from the intestine, is slow and considerably less complete than with the other methods of use; absorption is also less consistent (i.e., it tends to be more erratic and unpredictable from dose to dose) and may be affected by the concomitant ingestion of food. Blood concentrations of orally ingested opiate analgesics are usually only half, or less than half, those achieved after injection. Opiate analgesics dosage formulations are commonly used in ways for which they were not designed, which also can affect absorption patterns. For example, some transdermal dosage forms are cut into small pieces and swallowed, affecting the usual extended-release delivery of the opiate analgesic. Similarly, some oral tablets are crushed and then mainlined, smoked, or intranasally snorted, or are administered intact per rectum.

Distribution: The various opiate analgesics demonstrate different distribution characteristics after absorption into the bloodstream. For example, morphine, which is not as lipid soluble as codeine, heroin, or methadone, does not cross the blood–brain barrier as readily, so its onset of psychodepressant action is not as rapid. These characteristics may contribute to the reportedly lower desirability of morphine among intravenous opiate analgesic users, who generally prefer heroin.

Metabolism and Excretion: Opiate analgesics are largely metabolized by the liver before they are excreted by the kidneys. Small amounts of codeine and most of the administered dose of heroin are metabolized into morphine, which is further metabolized into inactive products that are finally excreted by the kidneys. The metabolism of most opiate analgesics is relatively rapid. Thus, their duration of action is, on average, 4 to 5 hours, a fact of considerable importance to physically dependent opiate analgesic users, who must continually seek and use the opiate analgesic at intervals as short as 3 to 5 hours to prevent precipitation of the opiate analgesics withdrawal syndrome.

Urine screening for opiate analgesic use usually detects codeine and morphine (either as free drug or as conjugated metabolite), as well as dihydrocodeine, dihydromorphine, and hydromorphone. Heroin use is suspected when both morphine and codeine are detected in the urine, because heroin is metabolized to morphine, which is metabolized to codeine. Thus, rapid screening assays cannot be used to differentially determine whether heroin, codeine, or morphine has been used. Furthermore, codeine is widely available in cough and cold products and combination analgesic products. Poppy seeds also contain small amounts of morphine, and morphine can be detected in the urine for 2 to 4 days after they are consumed. Thus, the ingestion of codeine-containing cough and cold or analgesic products or a sufficient quantity of poppy seeds can yield positive urine screens for morphine and codeine in nonusers—and false positive results for illicit use. Increasingly, specific adulterants (e.g., Stealth®) are being used to produce false negative urine test results to avoid detection of opiate analgesic use. These products are widely advertised and are easily obtained, even by children and adolescents, over the Internet.

Pharmacodynamics: Various endogenous opiate analgesic receptors were discovered during the 1970s and have since been increasingly studied. Naturally occurring opiate analgesic-like substances in the brain (e.g., dynorphins, endorphins, enkephalins) also were identified. Although the receptor classification system that evolved from this research remains incomplete, at least five major groups of receptors are now reasonably well characterized pharmacologically: delta, epsilon, kappa, mu, and sigma. Three of these "G-protein-coupled" receptors (i.e., delta, kappa, and mu) are central to the analgesic activity of the opiate analgesics. The highest concentrations of these receptors are found in the hypothalamus, limbic system, midbrain (mesencephalon), spinal cord, and thalamus. Similarities and differences in the pharmacologic and toxicologic characteristics of individual opiate analgesics are due primarily to their similarities and differences in selectivity for, and binding to, the various groups of opiate analgesic receptors.

Pure opiate analgesic agonists (e.g., morphine) exert their analgesic action primarily at the mu receptor. The mu receptors are associated with analgesia, respiratory depression, euphoria, and physical dependence. The kappa receptors are associated with spinal analgesia, miosis, and sedation. Mixed opiate analgesic agonist–antagonists (e.g., butorphanol, nalbuphine, pentazocine) act primarily at the kappa receptors. The sigma receptors, which are located primarily in the limbic system, are associated with dysphoria, hallucinations, and other psychotomimetic effects that are occasionally encountered by people who use some opiate analgesics (e.g., meperidine [Demerol®]).

The opiate analgesics that stimulate any of these receptors have been designated as agonists (i.e., codeine, fentanyl, heroin, hydromorphone [Dilaudid®], meperidine [Demerol®], methadone [Dolophine®], morphine, oxymorphone [Numorphan®]), while those that block the receptors have been designated as antagonists (i.e., naloxone [Narcan®], Naltrexone [Trexan®]). Opiate analgesics that stimulate one receptor and block another have been designated as mixed agonist–antagonists (i.e., buprenorphine [Buprenex®], butorphanol [Stadol®], nalbuphine [Nubain®], pentazocine [Talwin®]). Naloxone binds to and blocks all opiate analgesic receptors, but its affinity for mu receptors is at least 10-fold higher than its affinity for kappa receptors. This increased affinity for mu receptors perhaps explains why naloxone-induced reversal of respiratory depression occurs with only minimal reversal of the analgesia that results from stimulation of kappa receptors in the spinal cord.

Current Approved Indications for Medical Use[7]

Pain disorders: acute pain, moderate to severe; cancer pain, moderate to severe

Desired Effect/Reason for Personal Use

Dreams ("pipe dreams"); euphoria; pain relief; prevention/self-management of the opiate analgesic withdrawal syndrome; "rush"; sleepy, dreamlike state ("nod")

Toxicity

Several significant complications are associated with *intravenous use* of the opiate analgesics: HIV infection and AIDS; abscesses and infections at injection sites; cardiovascular abnormalities, including scarred and collapsed veins; respiratory abnormalities, including talc granulomas; hepatitis; and tetanus. These complications are not caused by the opiate analgesics themselves, but by the adulterants used to "cut" the opiate analgesic, by nonsterile or shared needles and syringes, and by improper injection techniques. It is important to note that if opiate analgesics were ingested, or even smoked, none of these more serious complications would occur.

Similarly, *intranasal use* of the opiate analgesics, which became increasingly prevalent during the 1990s, has been associated with several adverse effects, including erosion of the lateral nasal walls, nasopharynx, and soft palate; fungal invasion of the nasal surfaces and rhinosinusitis; infection of the nasal surfaces and resultant mucopurulent exudate; and nasal septal perforation. In addition, severe, life-threatening asthma attacks have been associated with intranasal sniffing (i.e., snorting) of heroin by people who have preexisting asthma. Additional toxicities related to the actions of the opiate analgesics are listed below.

Acute[8]: Bradycardia; cardiac arrest; circulatory depression; cognitive impairment; constipation; dilation of superficial blood vessels and resultant warming of the skin; drowsiness; dry mouth; flushing; headache; impotence; laryngospasm; miosis; nausea; pain at injection site (intramuscular, subcutaneous, or intravenous injection); perspiration (increased); phlebitis; postural (orthostatic) hypotension; pruritus; respiratory arrest; respiratory depression; sedation; sexual desire (reduced); shock; syncope; urinary retention; urticaria; vomiting

Chronic: Anemia; constipation; menstrual irregularities; physical dependence; psychological dependence; sex drive, reduced; sphincter of Oddi dysfunction

Pregnancy & Lactation: FDA Pregnancy Category C (see Appendix B). Although opiate analgesics have been used to provide pain relief during labor and delivery, safety of their use by adolescent girls and women who are pregnant has not been established. Opiate analgesics cross the placental barrier; thus, their use prior to labor and delivery may result in drowsiness, lethargy, or other expected pharmacologic actions (e.g., respiratory depression, constipation) in neonates. Although opiate analgesic use during pregnancy has not been directly associated with congenital malformations, long-term maternal opiate analgesic use may result in the neonatal opiate analgesic withdrawal syndrome as neonatal opiate analgesic blood concentrations decrease after birth.

Signs and symptoms of the neonatal opiate analgesic withdrawal syndrome include excessive crying and irritability, fever, hyperactive reflexes, increased respiratory rate, increased number of stools, sneezing, tremors, vomiting, and yawning. The intensity of these signs and symptoms does not always reflect the amount or duration of maternal opiate analgesic use during pregnancy. Although the opiate analgesics methadone and morphine are widely used for the treatment of the neonatal opiate analgesic withdrawal syndrome, there is no consensus as to the best approach for the medical management of this syndrome.

Safety of opiate analgesic use by adolescent girls and women who are breast-feeding has not been established. Opiate analgesics have been detected in breast milk in amounts that can result in expected pharmacologic actions (e.g., CNS and respiratory depression, constipation) and the development of physical dependence in breast-fed neonates and infants. These infants experience the opiate analgesic withdrawal syndrome when maternal opiate analgesic use or breast-feeding is abruptly discontinued. Adolescent girls and women who are breast-feeding should not use opiate analgesics.

Abuse Potential[9]

Physical dependence: High (USDEA Schedule II; high potential for abuse)
Psychological dependence: High

Withdrawal Syndrome

Long-term, regular use of opiate analgesics is associated with the development of physical and psychological dependence. Thus, abrupt discontinuation of regular, long-term opiate analgesic use may result in the opiate analgesic withdrawal syndrome. The opiate analgesic withdrawal syndrome also may occur in people who are physically dependent on pure opiate analgesic agonists (e.g., morphine) when an opiate analgesic antagonist (e.g., naloxone [Narcan®]) or a mixed opiate analgesic agonist/antagonist (e.g., pentazocine [Talwin®]) is used.

Signs and symptoms of the acute opiate analgesic withdrawal syndrome include abdominal cramps and pain, anorexia, anxiety, backache and other body aches, chills, diarrhea, dysphoria, hypertension, insomnia, increased respiratory rate, irritability, nausea, nervousness, piloerection (gooseflesh), restlessness, rhinitis, rhinorrhea, sensitivity to pain (increased), shivering, sneezing, stomach cramps, sweating (excessive), tachycardia, tremors, unexplained fever, weakness, and yawning. Although the opiate analgesic withdrawal syndrome is not usually life threatening, the appropriate use of opiate analgesic withdrawal pharmacotherapy and monitoring are helpful in its management. Gradual discontinuation of regular, long-term use will prevent or minimize these signs and symptoms. Relapse to resumption of opiate analgesic use during as well as after withdrawal is common.

Overdosage

Signs and symptoms of opiate analgesic overdosage (see Table 7) include respiratory depression with reduced respiratory rate and tidal volume; Cheyne-Stokes respirations; cyanosis; extreme somnolence progressing to stupor or coma; skeletal muscle flaccidity; cold, clammy skin; and sometimes hypotension and bradycardia. Severe opiate analgesic overdosage may result in apnea, circulatory collapse, cardiac arrest, and death. Abnormal dilation of the pupils, or mydriasis, may occur with terminal narcosis or severe hypoxia or as a toxic reaction associated with meperidine (Demerol®). The signs and symptoms of severe propoxyphene (Darvon®) overdosage include focal and generalized seizures. Nephrogenic diabetes insipidus and ECG abnormalities also may occur.

TABLE 7

Common Signs and Symptoms of Acute Opiate Analgesic Overdosage

Body System or Organ	Signs and Symptoms
Cardiovascular system	Hypotension, shock
CNS	Stupor or coma; however, with meperidine or propoxyphene, convulsions may occur[a]
Eyes	Generally, pupils are constricted (miosis); however, with meperidine, or extreme hypoxia, pupils may be dilated (mydriasis)
Gastrointestinal system	Constipation
Reflexes	Diminished or absent
Respiratory system	Decreased or absent respirations with cyanosis; pulmonary edema
Thermoregulation	Subnormal body temperature

[a]Convulsions also may occur with anoxia.
Source: Adapted from Pagliaro, L.A., & Pagliaro, A.M. (2004). *Pagliaros' comprehensive guide to drugs and substances of abuse.* Washington, DC: American Pharmacists Association.

Opiate analgesic overdosage requires emergency medical support, particularly of respiratory function, with attention to increasing opiate analgesic elimination. Naloxone (Narcan®), a pure opiate analgesic antagonist, is a specific antidote for the respiratory depression associated with opiate analgesic agonist and mixed opiate analgesic agonist/antagonist overdosages. However, the usual dosage of the opiate analgesic antagonist precipitates the opiate analgesic withdrawal syndrome in people who are physically dependent on opiate analgesics. The severity of the withdrawal syndrome depends on the severity of physical dependence and the dose of the antagonist administered. The use of opiate analgesic antagonists in people who are physically dependent on opiate analgesics should be avoided, if possible. If an opiate analgesic antagonist is required for the medical management of serious respiratory depression in people who are physically dependent on opiate analgesics, lower dosages and cautious dosage titration are recommended.

Notes

1. The opiate analgesics include opium, its derivatives (e.g., codeine, morphine), and several synthetic modifications of morphine (e.g., fentanyl, heroin, hydromorphone, meperidine, methadone, and oxycodone) that possess opiate analgesic-like chemical structures and pharmacologic actions. All of the opiate analgesics have a moderate to high potential for physical and psychological dependence. (See Appendix A for a complete list of the various opiate analgesics.)

2. Natural alkaloids derived from opium (e.g., codeine, morphine), semisynthetic modifications of morphine (e.g., heroin [diacetylmorphine]), and the synthetic formulations that only slightly resemble the structure of morphine (e.g., meperidine, methadone) have traditionally been referred to pharmacologically as narcotic analgesics. This term reflects their major therapeutic use: pain relief or management. These drugs and substances of abuse also have been commonly called, simply, narcotics, a word derived from the Greek word *narke*, meaning numbness, or lack of feeling or sensation. Unfortunately, the term narcotic frequently causes confusion, because it has a completely different legal meaning (i.e., it legally includes all drugs and substances of abuse that are listed under the various "narcotic" acts and laws). For example, legally, cannabis, cocaine, heroin, and LSD are all classified as narcotics—even though, of these, only heroin would be pharmacologically classified as a narcotic. More recently, the term "opioid," which also includes the narcotic antagonists and the endogenous opioid peptides, has been suggested. However, the term "opiate analgesic," meaning a natural or synthetic substance that exerts morphine-like actions on the human CNS, seems to be the more appropriate term and is used in this text.

3. This poppy plant also is referred to as *Papaver paenoniflorum*, when grown for decorative purposes (e.g., flower arrangements), and "breadseed poppy," when grown for culinary purposes (e.g., poppyseed bread).

4. Afghanistan is the world's largest producer of opium (i.e., ~8,000 tons in 2008). This is the source of most of the heroin used in Europe and Eurasia.

5. Thebaine is a minor chemical derivative of opium and is chemically similar to codeine, but it generally produces psychostimulation rather than psychodepression. It is not therapeutically used and is almost never abused in its natural form. However, it is converted into a variety of opiate analgesics (e.g., buprenorphine, hydrocodone, nalbuphine, oxycodone, and oxymorphone) and opiate antagonists (e.g., naloxone, naltrexone). Thebaine is thus pharmacologically classified as an opiate (i.e., a natural derivative of the opium poppy) but not as a psychodepressant. Because of its potential to be chemically converted, both licitly and illicitly, into several different opiate analgesics, it has been designated a USDEA Schedule II drug (high potential for abuse).

6. The receptors also are found, and elicit their effects, in other body organ systems, including the blood (e.g., erythrocytes) and the GI system.

7. Opiate analgesics also may be used to manage the pain associated with labor and delivery. In addition, they are commonly used as antitussives for the management of nonproductive cough and are found in many cough and cold products, most of which are prescription products.

8. *Rapid* intravenous injection of the opiate analgesics is associated with a greater risk for hypotension and respiratory depression.

9. Opiate analgesic abuse occurs frequently among people whose chronic pain is being medically managed with opiate analgesic pharmacotherapy. People with chronic pain disorders whose pain is being managed with opiate analgesic pharmacotherapy appear to have a significantly higher risk for abusing these medications if they also are depressed and have somatization disorder. To avoid the well-known physical and psychological dependence that can occur with opiate analgesics, many health care providers have tended to undertreat pain disorders, particularly in patients who have an active or past history of drug and substance use disorders. This practice, while well-intentioned, is not recommended. Pain management should include pharmacologic and other pain management approaches, as needed, to promote optimal comfort and daily activities for people who live with pain disorders.

References

Amato, L., Davoli, M., Ferri, M., et al. (2002). Methadone at tapered doses for the management of opioid withdrawal. *Cochrane Database of Systematic Reviews*, (2), CD003409.

Cody, J.T., Valtier, S., & Kuhlman, J. (2001). Analysis of morphine and codeine in samples adulterated with Stealth. *Journal of Analytical Toxicology, 25*(7), 572-575.

Culberson, J.W., & Ziska, M. (2008). Prescription drug misuse/abuse in the elderly. *Geriatrics, 63*(9), 22-31.

Gilson, A.M., & Joranson, D.E. (2002). U.S. policies relevant to the prescribing of opioid analgesics for the treatment of pain in patients with addictive disease. *The Clinical Journal of Pain, 18*(4 Supplement), S91-S98.

Inturrisi, C.E. (2002). Clinical pharmacology of opioids for pain. *The Clinical Journal of Pain, 14*(4 Supplement), S3-S13.

Ives, T.J., Cheiminski, P.R., Hammett-Stabler, C.A., et al. (2006). Predictors of opioid misuse in patients with chronic pain: A prospective cohort study. *BMC Health Services Research, 6,* 46.

Johnson, K., Gerada, C., & Greenough, A. (2003). Treatment of neonatal abstinence syndrome. *Archives of Disease in Childhood. Fetal and Neonatal Edition, 88*(1), F2-F5.

Katz, N., Fernandez, K., Chang, A., et al. (2008). Internet-based survey of nonmedical prescription opioid use in the United States. *The Clinical Journal of Pain, 24*(6), 528-535.

Manchikanti, L., Giordano, J., Boswell, M.V., et al. (2007). Psychological factors as predictors of opioid abuse and illicit drug use in chronic pain patients. *Journal of Opioid Management, 3*(2), 89-100.

Merrill, J.O. (2002). Policy progress for physician treatment of opiate addiction. *Journal of General Internal Medicine, 17*(5), 361-368.

Osborn, D.A., Jeffery, H.E., & Cole, M.J. (2002). Sedatives for opiate withdrawal in newborn infants. *Cochrane Database of Systematic Reviews,* (3), CD002053.

Sharma, S.S. (2002). Sphincter of Oddi dysfunction in patients addicted to opium: An unrecognized entity. *Gastrointestinal Endoscopy, 55*(3), 427-430.

Zeiger, A.R., Patkar, A.A., Fitzgerald, R., et al. (2002). Changes in mu opioid receptors and rheological properties of erythrocytes among opioid abusers. *Addiction Biology, 7*(2), 207-217.

OPIUM (See Opiate analgesics)

OXAZEPAM

Names

BAN or INN Generic Synonyms: None

Brand/Trade: Alepam®; Serax®; Seresta®

Chemical: 7-Chloro-1,3-dihydro-3-hydroxy-5-phenyl-2H-1,4-benzodiazepin-2-one

Street: None

Pharmacologic Classification

Psychodepressant, sedative-hypnotic: benzodiazepine

Brief General Overview

Oxazepam is a "general use," intermediate-acting benzodiazepine. It is commonly used for the medical management of sleep disorders in elderly people and others who have diminished hepatic function, because of its limited hepatic metabolism. In addition, it has a shorter elimination half-life than other benzodiazepines and thus is not as commonly associated with hangover effects—another reason for use in the elderly.

Dosage Forms and Routes of Administration

Oxazepam is licitly produced by pharmaceutical manufacturers in North America. It is available in oral capsule and tablet formulations and is usually orally ingested. Most people who use oxazepam are elderly residents of extended-care facilities and nursing homes where oxazepam (or other benzodiazepines) is commonly used as a bedtime sedative-hypnotic.[1] Oxazepam also is used by people residing in other types of institutions, including prison inmates. "Double-doctoring" (i.e., obtaining the same prescription from more than one physician), prescription forgery, and diversion from extended-care facilities and nursing homes are methods that are commonly used by other oxazepam users to obtain their supplies.

Mechanism of CNS Action

The exact mechanism of action of oxazepam has not been determined. However, it appears to be mediated by, or work in concert with, the inhibitory neurotransmitter GABA (see Benzodiazepines monograph).

Pharmacodynamics/Pharmacokinetics

Oxazepam is completely absorbed (~95%) after oral ingestion. Peak blood concentrations are achieved in ~3 hours. Oxazepam is highly plasma protein bound (~98%) and has an apparent volume of distribution of 0.6 L/kg. Metabolism is primarily by glucuronidation, which does not significantly involve the hepatic microsomal enzyme system. The mean elimination half-life is ~8 hours (range, 6 to 11 hours), and the mean total body clearance is ~70 mL/minute.

Current Approved Indications for Medical Use

Anxiety disorders; behavioral management of elderly patients (see Note 1); insomnia, difficulty staying asleep

Desired Effect/Reason for Personal Use

Alcohol-like disinhibitory euphoria or "high"; anxiety or tension reduction; prevention/self-management of the oxazepam withdrawal syndrome

Toxicity

Acute: Ataxia; cognitive impairment; dizziness; drowsiness; headache; hepatic dysfunction; lethargy; memory impairment (transient amnesia); nausea; psychomotor impairment; rashes; syncope; vertigo; weakness

Chronic: Physical dependence; psychological dependence

Pregnancy & Lactation: FDA Pregnancy Category C (see Appendix B). Safety of oxazepam use by adolescent girls and women who are pregnant has not been established. The use of oxazepam by adolescent girls and women who are pregnant has been associated with cleft lip and palate in neonates. An increased risk for congenital malformations also has been associated with other benzodiazepines, including chlordiazepoxide (Librium®)

and diazepam (Valium®). In addition, use near term has resulted in the "floppy infant syndrome," characterized by neonatal hypotonia and poor sucking response. Regular long-term use of oxazepam during pregnancy also may result in the neonatal oxazepam withdrawal syndrome. Adolescent girls and women who are pregnant should not use oxazepam.

Safety of oxazepam use by adolescent girls and women who are breast-feeding has not been established. Oxazepam is excreted in breast milk in low concentrations. Although concentrations are low, elimination half-life is significantly prolonged in breast-fed neonates during the first week after birth because of their immature hepatic and renal function. Neonates and infants may display expected pharmacologic effects (e.g., drowsiness, lethargy) and may become physically dependent. Adolescent girls and women who are breast-feeding should not use oxazepam.

Abuse Potential

Physical dependence: Moderate (USDEA Schedule IV; low potential for abuse)
Psychological dependence: Moderate

Withdrawal Syndrome

Regular, long-term use of oxazepam is associated with physical and psychological dependence. Abrupt discontinuation of regular, long-term use (i.e., longer than 4 months) results in the oxazepam withdrawal syndrome (see Benzodiazepines monograph).

Overdosage

The signs and symptoms of oxazepam overdosage resemble those associated with other benzodiazepine overdosage (see Benzodiazepines monograph). Oxazepam overdosage requires emergency medical support of body systems, with attention to increasing oxazepam elimination. The benzodiazepine antagonist flumazenil (Anexate®, Romazicon®) may be required.[2]

Notes

1. Oxazepam is medically recommended only as short-term pharmacotherapy for the symptomatic management of anxiety or sleep disorders. However, it is commonly used on a long-term basis. Sometimes for economic reasons, extended-care facility staff members use oxazepam to help reduce their elderly patients' need for supervision and care by evening and night staff. These staff members are often few and have limited health care education or training. Oxazepam helps patients to fall asleep and to sleep through the night. Unfortunately, in addition to the risk for falls and other sequelae related to its psychodepressant actions and hangover effect, physical and psychological dependence inevitably occur.
2. Caution is required because flumazenil antagonism may precipitate the oxazepam withdrawal syndrome in people who are physically dependent on oxazepam.

Reference

Fraser, A.D., Zamecnik, J., Keravel, J., et al. (2001). Experience with urine drug testing by the Correctional Service of Canada. *Forensic Science International, 121*(1-2), 16-22.

OXYCODONE

Names

BAN or INN Generic Synonyms: Dihydrohydroxycodeinone

Brand/Trade: OxyContin®; Oxydose®; OxyFast®; OxyIR®; Roxicodone®; Supeudol®

Chemical: 4,5-Epoxy-14-hydroxy-3-methoxy-17-methyl-morphinan-6-one

Street: 40; 80; 40-Bar; Blue; Cotton; Hillbilly Heroin; Kicker; Killer; OC; Oceans; Os; O's; Ox; OX; Oxicotten; Oxies; Oxy; Oxy 80s; Oxycoffins; Oxycotton; Pain Killers; Poor Man's Heroin; Redneck Heroin; Percs; Rushbo

Pharmacologic Classification

Psychodepressant, opiate analgesic: pure agonist (semisynthetic)

Brief General Overview

Introduced into North America in 1963, oxycodone is a semisynthetic opiate analgesic derived from the opium alkaloid thebaine (see Opiate Analgesics monograph). It is a pure opiate analgesic agonist and produces typical opiate analgesic actions, including analgesia, constipation, cough suppression, mental clouding, miosis, mood change (both euphoria and dysphoria), nausea, sedation, respiratory depression, and vomiting. Oxycodone is well absorbed from the GI tract and does not undergo extensive first-pass hepatic metabolism. Thus, oxycodone is often a preferred oral opiate analgesic for long-term outpatient use, and prescribing of the drug increased significantly during the 1990s. Consequently, it is one of the most frequently prescribed opiate analgesics for the medical management of moderate to severe pain. Oxycodone is personally used for its psychodepressant actions. It also is used to prevent the opiate analgesic withdrawal syndrome among regular, long-term opiate analgesic users when they are unable to obtain their usual opiate analgesic (e.g., heroin).

Oxycodone is used orally and intravenously.[1,2] The rate of oxycodone use increased significantly during the 1990s, and intravenous use of oxycodone is now widespread across North America, particularly in large urban centers. The highest rate of use is observed among adolescents of European descent and men 20 to 40 years of age who have a previous history of drug and substance use. In rural areas, oxycodone use increases significantly, particularly among young, unmarried men of European descent, when other opiate analgesics (e.g., heroin) are difficult to obtain.

Dosage Forms and Routes of Administration

Oxycodone is available from licit pharmaceutical manufacturers in a variety of oral dosage forms (i.e., caplets, capsules, solutions, and tablets—in both standard and controlled-release formulations). It also is available as a rectal suppository.[3] Virtually all illicit oxycodone use involves legitimately produced pharmaceutical products—in most cases, OxyContin®.[4] These products are routinely diverted for personal use by employee pilferage, thefts from pharmacies, "double-doctoring", and sale for profit of legitimate prescriptions by elderly patients and others with chronic, painful medical conditions who desire the extra income.[5] Increasingly, users are obtaining their supplies of oxycodone over the Internet from on-line pharmacists and physicians.

People who are legitimately receiving oxycodone for pain relief may occasionally become physically dependent. However, the vast majority of current users of oxycodone use it for the euphoric effect or to prevent the opiate analgesic withdrawal syndrome when their preferred opiate analgesic of use (e.g., heroin) is unavailable or they are otherwise unable to obtain it.

Mechanism of CNS Action

Oxycodone appears to elicit its analgesic and other psychodepressant actions primarily by binding to endorphin receptors in the CNS. However, the exact molecular mechanism of action has not been determined. (See the Opiate Analgesics monograph.)

Pharmacodynamics/Pharmacokinetics

Approximately 60% to 90% of oxycodone is absorbed after oral ingestion, with an apparent volume of distribution of ~2.6 L/kg. Oxcodone's plasma protein binding is low (~45%), and its duration of analgesic action generally is 4 to 5 hours. Although it does not undergo extensive first-pass hepatic metabolism, it is extensively metabolized by the hepatic cytochrome P450 microsomal enzyme system, primarily to inactive metabolites. However, low concentrations of an active metabolite, oxymorphone (see monograph), have been identified. Oxycodone and its metabolites are excreted primarily by the kidneys, with up to 20% eliminated in unchanged form in the urine. The total plasma clearance of oxycodone in adults is ~0.8 L/minute. The mean elimination half-life is ~4 hours.

Current Approved Indications for Medical Use

Pain, moderate to severe

Desired Action/Reason for Personal Use[6]

Euphoria; pain relief/self-management; prevention/self-management of the opiate analgesic withdrawal syndrome, particularly among regular, long-term users of heroin

Toxicity

Acute: Cognitive impairment; constipation; dizziness; drowsiness; dry mouth; dysphoria; flushing of the skin; headache; hypotension; increased intracranial pressure; miosis; nausea; pruritus; psychomotor impairment; respiratory depression; somnolence; sweating; vomiting

Chronic: Physical dependence; psychological dependence; renal impairment[7]

Pregnancy & Lactation: FDA Pregnancy Category B (see Appendix B). Oxycodone use during pregnancy has not been associated with teratogenic effects. However, regular use during the last trimester of pregnancy may result in the neonatal opiate analgesic withdrawal syndrome.

Safety of oxycodone use by adolescent girls and women who are breast-feeding has not been established. Oxycodone is excreted in low concentrations in breast milk. Additional valid and reliable data are needed.

Abuse Potential

Physical dependence: High (USDEA Schedule II; high potential for abuse)
Psychological dependence: High

Withdrawal Syndrome

Abrupt discontinuation of regular, long-term oxycodone use may result in the opiate analgesic withdrawal syndrome. Signs and symptoms of this syndrome include abdominal cramps, anorexia, anxiety, backache, chills, diarrhea, hypertension, hyperventilation, irritability, joint pain, lacrimation, myalgia, mydriasis, perspiration, restlessness, rhinorrhea, tachycardia, vomiting, weakness, and yawning. (See the Opiate Analgesics monograph.)

Overdosage

Signs and symptoms of oxycodone overdosage may include bradycardia, cold and clammy skin, coma, hypotension, miosis, respiratory depression, skeletal muscle flaccidity, and somnolence (extreme). Severe oxycodone overdosage may result in apnea, circulatory collapse, cardiac arrest, and death. Overdosage deaths have been reported with inhalational (smoking), intravenous, and oral oxycodone use. Risk of overdosage is significantly increased by concurrent use of other psychodepressants, particularly alcohol. Oxycodone overdosage requires emergency medical support of body systems, with attention to establishing and maintaining adequate respiratory function and increasing oxycodone elimination. The opiate antagonist naloxone (Narcan®) is usually needed to reverse the respiratory depression associated with oxycodone overdosage. Repeated doses of naloxone may be required.[8,9]

Notes

1. People who become physically and psychologically dependent on oxycodone often progress from oral use to either intranasal sniffing (i.e., snorting) or intravenous use. For intravenous use, solid oral dosage formulations are crushed, dissolved, filtered, and injected. Intravenous use is complicated by the presence of talc and other inert ingredients that contribute to making injections painful, and it has been associated with pulmonary emboli and other sequelae (e.g., infection at the injection site, thrombophlebitis). Intravenous injection of rectal suppository formulations also has been reported.
2. Some attempts are being made by pharmaceutical manufacturers to reformulate current oral formulations of oxycodone to contain naloxone (an opiate analgesic antagonist), thereby significantly reducing or eliminating intravenous use of these formulations—as when pentazocine (Talwin®) was reformulated, for similar reasons, to pentazocine and naloxone (Talwin Nx®) more than two decades ago (see Pentazocine monograph).
3. Oxycodone also is available in several combination pharmaceutical products, including Endocet®, Oxycocet®, Percocet®, Percocet-Demi®, Roxicet®, and Tylox®, which also contain acetaminophen (a nonopiate analgesic), and Endodan®, Oxycodan®, Percodan®, and Percodan-Demi®, which also contain aspirin (a nonsteroidal anti-inflammatory analgesic).
4. In rare cases, illicit chemists have produced oxycodone from opiate analgesic precursors (i.e., codeine or thebaine).

5. Profit is not the only motive for these diversions, nor are patients the only drug diverters. Frequently, dentists, nurses, pharmacists, and physicians divert oxycodone (and other such drugs) from their patients or their place of employment to supply loved ones (such as sons, daughters, boyfriends, or girlfriends) with oxycodone in order to "keep them off of the streets" and out of jail.

6. Continued regular use of oxycodone may result in physical dependence, including tolerance to many of its actions (i.e., analgesia, euphoria, nausea, respiratory depression, and sedation). The tolerance is often variable, occurring in different degrees according to the characteristics of the individual user. To compensate for this tolerance, users must increase the dosage (and risk overdosage) to achieve desired actions.

7. The renal impairment associated with regular, long-term oxycodone use may be related to intravenous use, during which impurities may be injected along with the oxycodone. The impurities may cause granulomatous glomerulonephritis and other related pathology.

8. Administration of naloxone to a person who is physically dependent on an opiate analgesic, such as oxycodone, immediately precipitates the opiate analgesic withdrawal syndrome. Careful individualized clinical assessment, judgment, and monitoring are required in these situations.

9. Oxycodone is frequently available in combination products (see Note 3). When treating oxycodone overdosage, attention to the specific toxicities of all of the ingredients in these combination products and their medical management also is required.

References

Adams, N.J., Plane, M.B., Fleming, M.F., et al. (2001). Opioids and the treatment of chronic pain in a primary care sample. *Journal of Pain and Symptom Management, 22,* 791-796.

Forrester, M.B. (2007). Oxycodone abuse in Texas, 1998-2004. *Journal of Toxicology and Environmental Health. Part A: Current Issues, 70*(6), 534-538.

Gammaitoni, A.R., & Davis, M.W. (2002). Comparison of the pharmacokinetics of oxycodone administered in three Percocet formulations. *Journal of Clinical Pharmacology, 42,* 192-197.

Hays, L.R. (2004). A profile of OxyContin addiction. *Journal of Addictive Diseases, 23*(4), 1-9.

Hill, P., Dwyer, K., Kay, T., et al. (2002). Severe chronic renal failure in association with oxycodone addiction: A new form of fibrillary glomerulopathy. *Human Pathology, 33*(8), 783-787.

Joranson, D.E., Ryan, K.M., Gilson, A.M., et al. (2000). Trends in medical use and abuse of opioid analgesics. *JAMA: The Journal of the American Medical Association, 283*(13), 1710-1714.

Levy, M.S. (2007). An exploratory study of OxyContin use among individuals with substance use disorders. *Journal of Psychoactive Drugs, 39*(3), 271-276.

Lugo, R.A., & Kern, S.E. (2004). The pharmacokinetics of oxycodone. *Journal of Pain & Palliative Care Pharmacotherapy, 18*(4), 17-30.

Rao, R., & Desai, N.S. (2002). OxyContin and neonatal abstinence syndrome. *Journal of Perinatology, 22,* 324-325.

Sees, K.L., Di Marino, M.E., & Ruediger, N.K., et al. (2005). Non-medical use of OxyContin tablets in the United States. *Journal of Pain & Palliative Care Pharmacotherapy, 19*(2), 13-23.

Wasserman, S. (2001). States respond to growing abuse of painkiller. *State Legislature, 27*(9), 33-34.

Wunsch, M.J., Cropsey, K.L., Campbell, E.D., et al. (2008). OxyContin use and misuse in three populations: Substance abuse patients, pain patients, and criminal justice participants. *Journal of Opioid Management, 4*(2), 73-79.

OXYMORPHONE

Names

BAN or INN Generic Synonyms: None

Brand/Trade: Numorphan®

Chemical: 14-Hydroxy-dihydromorphinone

Street: None

Pharmacologic Classification

Psychodepressant, opiate analgesic: pure agonist (semisynthetic)

Brief General Overview

Oxymorphone is derived from morphine (see monograph). Compared with morphine, it reportedly produces equal analgesia with less respiratory depression. When injected, 1 mg of oxymorphone is equivalent to 10 mg of morphine. Oxymorphone also is structurally similar to hydromorphone (see monograph).

Dosage Forms and Routes of Administration

Oxymorphone is produced by licit pharmaceutical manufacturers in North America.[1] It is available in formulations for injection (i.e., intramuscular, intravenous, subcutaneous), oral immediate-release (IR) and extended-release (ER) tablets, and rectal suppositories. Although users generally inject oxymorphone intravenously, some users now grind the IR tablets to a fine powder and intranasally sniff (snort) the powder through a small tube (e.g., a beverage straw or rolled paper currency).

Mechanism of CNS Action

Oxymorphone is a potent opiate analgesic that appears to elicit its analgesic action primarily by binding to mu endorphin receptors in the CNS. However, the exact mechanism of action has not been determined. (See the Opiate Analgesics monograph.)

Pharmacodynamics/Pharmacokinetics

After oral ingestion, oxymorphone undergoes significant first-pass hepatic metabolism, resulting in low bioavailability (i.e., ~10%). Co-ingestion of alcohol with the ER oral tablet formulation (i.e., Opana ER®) can result in dose-dumping (i.e., the premature and exaggerated release of drug from its delivery system). After rectal insertion of the suppository formulation, the onset of action is rapid and generally occurs within 5 to 10 minutes. Analgesia persists for 3 to 6 hours following absorption of oxymorphone by the various routes of administration. Oxymorphone is extensively metabolized to several metabolites, including 6-hydroxyoxymorphone, an active metabolite. Oxymorphone is conjugated with glucuronic acid in the liver, resulting in oxymorphone-3-glucuronide, which is excreted in the urine. Additional valid and reliable data are not available.

Current Approved Indications for Medical Use

Pain disorders: acute pain, moderate to severe; pain disorders: terminal cancer pain, moderate to severe

Desired Effect/Reason for Personal Use

Euphoria; pain relief; prevention/self-management of the opiate analgesic withdrawal syndrome

Toxicity

Acute: Cognitive impairment; drowsiness; dysphoria; headache; itching; lightheadedness; miosis; nausea; respiratory depression; sedation (relatively mild); vomiting

Chronic: Physical dependence; psychological dependence

Pregnancy & Lactation: FDA Pregnancy Category "not established." Safety of oxymorphone use by adolescent girls and women who are pregnant has not been established. Regular long-term use may result in the neonatal opiate analgesic withdrawal syndrome (see Opiate Analgesics monograph). Adolescent girls and women who are pregnant should not use oxymorphone.

Safety of oxymorphone use by adolescent girls and women who are breast-feeding has not been established (see Opiate Analgesics monograph). Additional valid and reliable data are needed.

Abuse Potential

Physical dependence: High (USDEA Schedule II; high potential for abuse)
Psychological dependence: High

Withdrawal Syndrome

Physical and psychological dependence are associated with regular, long-term oxymorphone use. Abrupt discontinuation after regular, long-term use may result in the opiate analgesic withdrawal syndrome (see Opiate Analgesics monograph).

Overdosage

The signs and symptoms of oxymorphone overdosage resemble those associated with other opiate analgesic overdosage (see Opiate Analgesics monograph). Severe oxymorphone overdosage may result in apnea, cardiac arrest, circulatory collapse, and death. Oxymorphone overdosage requires emergency medical support of body systems, with attention to increasing oxymorphone elimination and the establishment and maintenance of adequate respiratory function. The opiate antagonist naloxone (Narcan®) is usually required to reverse the respiratory depression associated with oxymorphone overdosage.[2] Repeated doses of naloxone may be required.

Notes

1. In rare cases, illicit chemists have produced oxymorphone from opiate precursors (i.e., codeine or thebaine).
2. Caution is indicated, because the use of naloxone may precipitate the opiate analgesic withdrawal syndrome in patients who are physically dependent on oxymorphone.

References

Guay, D.R. (2007). Use of oral oxymorphone in the elderly. *Consultant Pharmacist, 22*(5), 417-430.

Inturrisi, C.E. (2002). Clinical pharmacology of opioids for pain. *The Clinical Journal of Pain, 18*(4, Supplement), S3-S13.

Matsumoto, A.K. (2007). Oral extended-release oxymorphone: A new choice for chronic pain relief. *Expert Opinion on Pharmacotherapy, 8*(10), 1515-1527.

Oral oxymorphone (Opana). (2007). *The Medical Letter on Drugs and Therapeutics, 49*(1251), 3-4.

Prommer, E. (2006). Oxymorphone: A review. *Supportive Care in Cancer, 14*(2), 109-115.

Sloan, P.A., & Barkin, R.L. (2008). Oxymorphone and oxymorphone extended release: A pharmacotherapeutic review. *Journal of Opioid Management, 4*(3), 131-144.

PARALDEHYDE

Names

BAN or INN Generic Synonyms: Paracetaldehyde

Brand/Trade[1]: Paral®

Chemical: 2,4,6-Trimethyl-1,3,5-trioxane

Street: None

Pharmacologic Classification

Psychodepressant, sedative-hypnotic: miscellaneous (acetaldehyde)

Brief General Overview

For over a century, from the mid-1800s to the mid-1900s, paraldehyde was widely used in lieu of physical restraints to manage the behavior of mental patients in institutional care and was the mainstay for the in-hospital medical management of the alcohol withdrawal syndrome in people with chronic alcoholism. With the discovery and development of other drugs (e.g., antimanics, antipsychotics, benzodiazepine sedative-hypnotics) and therapeutic modalities (e.g., electroconvulsive therapy, counseling), paraldehyde is now rarely used in North America or Europe as an anticonvulsant or sedative. However, it continues to be commonly used in other parts of the world, such as Africa, for the medical management of disorders that are rarely seen in North America, including convulsions associated with severe malaria in children.

Dosage Forms and Routes of Administration

Paraldehyde is produced by licit pharmaceutical manufacturers in North America. It is available as a sterile solution for intravenous injection (Canada only) and as oral and rectal liquids. Paraldehyde is extremely irritating to body tissues, and intramuscular and subcutaneous injections are not recommended because of the risk for sterile abscesses, extreme pain, and tissue damage at the injection site. Intravenous injection[2] has been associated with thrombophlebitis, as well as circulatory collapse, hypotension, pulmonary edema, and respiratory distress.

Paraldehyde is rarely personally used in North America, and its use is not expected to increase in the foreseeable future. When used, it is almost always orally ingested—usually mixed in a glassful of milk or iced fruit juice to mask its odor, improve its taste, and decrease its irritant effects on the mucous membranes of the mouth, throat, and stomach. When exposed to light and air, paraldehyde solutions rapidly decompose to acetaldehyde and acetic acid (i.e., vinegar).

Mechanism of CNS Action

The exact mechanism of paraldehyde's psychodepressant action has not been determined. However, it is believed to be due to a general depressant action on several areas of the CNS, including the ascending reticular activating system.

Pharmacodynamics/Pharmacokinetics

Paraldehyde solution is absorbed rapidly and well from the GI tract after oral ingestion. Peak blood concentrations are achieved within 30 to 60 minutes. However, these concentrations may be delayed for up to 2 hours following rectal administration. Paraldehyde is widely distributed in the body and is extensively metabolized (~90%) in the liver. It is depolymerized to acetaldehyde, which is oxidized by acetaldehyde dehydrogenase to acetic acid and, subsequently, to carbon dioxide and water. Approximately 7% of an oral dose of paraldehyde is excreted in unchanged form through the lungs, imparting a characteristic odor to the breath. The elimination half-life ranges from 3.5 to 9.5 hours (mean, 7.5 hours).

Current Approved Indications for Medical Use

Delirium tremens, associated with the alcohol withdrawal syndrome that is refractory to conventional pharmacotherapy (see Alcohol monograph); seizure disorders refractory to conventional pharmacotherapy

Desired Effect/Reason for Personal Use

Alcohol-like disinhibitory euphoria or "high"; relaxation; tranquility

Toxicity

Acute: Cognitive impairment; contact dermatitis; coughing (with intravenous injection only); dizziness; drowsiness; erythematous rash; gastric irritation (including hemorrhagic gastritis); muscle cramps; skin rash; sweating; trembling

Chronic: Metabolic acidosis; nephrosis; physical dependence; psychological dependence; toxic hepatitis

Pregnancy & Lactation: FDA Pregnancy Category D (see Appendix B). Paraldehyde readily crosses the placenta and appears in the fetal circulation. Neonates of mothers who use paraldehyde during labor may exhibit significant respiratory depression. Adolescent girls and women who are pregnant should not use paraldehyde.

Safety of paraldehyde use by adolescent girls and women who are breast-feeding has not been established. Additional valid and reliable data are needed.

Abuse Potential

Physical dependence: Moderate (USDEA Schedule IV; low potential for abuse)
Psychological dependence: Moderate

Withdrawal Syndrome

A paraldehyde withdrawal syndrome has not been reported.

Overdosage

Signs and symptoms of paraldehyde overdosage include abdominal cramps (severe), bradycardia, cloudy urine, coma, confusion, lethargy, muscle tremors, pulmonary edema, respiratory depression, stupor, urinary retention, and weakness (severe). Metabolic acidosis also may occur. A strong, characteristic odor of paraldehyde on the breath facilitates diagnosis of overdosage. Paraldehyde overdosage requires emergency medical support, with attention to increasing paraldehyde elimination. Induction of emesis is not recommended because of the mildly corrosive property of paraldehyde. There is no known antidote.

Notes

1. Generally available by generic name.
2. Paraldehyde interacts with plastic. Thus, glass syringes (not the usual plastic syringes used for injectable pharmacotherapy) must be used to administer injectable paraldehyde, and glass cups and metal spoons (not plastic cups and spoons) should be used for preparing and administering oral dosages.

References

Ban, T.A. (2001). Pharmacotherapy of mental illness—a historical analysis. *Progress in Neuro-Psychopharmacology & Biological Psychiatry, 25*(4), 709-727.

Chin, R.F., Neville, B.G., Peckham, C., et al. (2008). Treatment of community-onset childhood convulsive status epilepticus: A prospective, population-based study. *The Lancet Neurology, 7*(8), 696-703.

Githiga, I.M., Muchohi, S.N., Ogutu, B.R., et al. (2004, June 15). Determination of paraldehyde by gas chromatography in whole blood from children. *Journal of Chromatography B, Analytical Technologies in the Biomedical and Life Sciences, 805*(2), 365-369.

Townend, W., & Mackway-Jones, K. (2002). Towards evidence based emergency medicine: Best BETs from the Manchester Royal Infirmary. Phenytoin or paraldehyde as the second drug for convulsions in children. *Emergency Medicine Journal, 19*(1), 50.

PARAMETHOXYAMPHETAMINE

Names

BAN or INN Generic Synonyms: 4-Methoxyamphetamine

Brand/Trade: None

Chemical: p-Methoxy-α-methlyphenethylamine

Street: Death; False Ecstasy; Mitsubishi; Mitsubishi Double Stack; PMA

Pharmacologic Classification

Psychodelic, amphetamine-like psychodelic: phenethylamine

Brief General Overview

Paramethoxyamphetamine (PMA) is sold and used for its psychodelic actions. However, because of its known toxicity (i.e., ability to cause death), it is usually misrepresented when sold.[1] For example, during the early 1970s it was often sold as methylenedioxyamphetamine (MDA, Adam; see monograph), and during the early 2000s it was often sold as methylenedioxymethamphetamine (MDMA, Ecstasy; see monograph), particularly at raves.

Dosage Forms and Routes of Administration

PMA is produced in illicit chemical laboratories, primarily in Canada (i.e., greater Toronto, Ontario, area). A limited amount of PMA is legally produced in the United States for specific commercial applications and approved research. It is available in a number of dosage formulations that can be orally ingested, intravenously injected, or intranasally sniffed (i.e., snorted). PMA is most often available as a compressed white tablet with a Mitsubishi® symbol stamped on one side. PMA also is frequently found as an adulterant in tablets sold "on the street" and over the Internet as MDMA. American users are generally men of European descent, 18 to 35 years of age, who attend dance clubs and raves. In addition to PMA, they often use other club drugs, particularly MDMA.

Mechanism of CNS Action

The exact mechanism of PMA's psychodelic action has not been determined.

Pharmacodynamics/Pharmacokinetics

PMA's major metabolite, 4-hydroxyamphetamine, is formed by O-desmethylation, a reaction catalyzed by the hepatic microsomal isoenzyme CYP2D6. CYP2D6 is genetically polymorphic. People who are slow metabolizers of PMA are expected to have higher blood concentrations than those who are fast metabolizers. Thus, slow metabolizers may be at increased risk for fatal PMA toxicity. Additional valid and reliable data are not available.

Current Approved Indications for Medical Use

None

Desired Action/Reason for Personal Use

Energy; euphoria (mild); hallucinations (primarily visual, minor); MDMA-like actions (see 3,4-Methylenedioxymethamphetamine monograph)

Toxicity

Acute: Agitation; dehydration; erratic eye movements; hallucinations; hypertension; hyperthermia; muscle contractions/spasms; mydriasis; nausea; restlessness; tachycardia

Chronic: Valid and reliable data are not available.[2]

Pregnancy & Lactation: Valid and reliable data are not available.

Abuse Potential

Physical dependence: Low (USDEA Schedule I; use is prohibited)
Psychological dependence: Low[3]

Withdrawal Syndrome

A PMA withdrawal syndrome has not been reported.

Overdosage

Death, which usually occurs rapidly, is common and appears to be related to excessive CNS stimulation. Signs and symptoms of PMA overdosage include agitation, bruxism (grinding of the teeth), cardiac dysrhythmias, coma, convulsions, hemorrhage, hyper-thermia (severe),[4] hypoglycemia, pulmonary congestion, and respiratory distress. Autopsies have revealed coagulopathy, multiple organ failure, renal tubular necrosis, and rhabdomyolysis. PMA overdosage requires emergency medical support and monitoring of body systems, with attention to PMA elimination. There is no known antidote.

Notes

1. A few cases have been reported in which PMA is sold as a drug capable of enhancing or intensifying the effects of MDMA.
2. Although valid and reliable data are not available on the potential toxicities associated with regular, long-term use of PMA, the structural and pharmacologic similarities of PMA to MDMA, and its apparent significantly greater stimulation of serotonergic neurotransmission, warrant serious concern about neurotoxicity with regular, long-term PMA use. (See the Methylenedioxymethamphetamine monograph.)
3. In part because of the recognized risk of death associated with intentional PMA use.
4. Hyperthermia (between 39°C and 42°C) has been reported in fatal PMA overdosages.

References

Becker, J., Neis, P., Röhrich, J., et al. (2003). A fatal paramethoxymethamphetamine intoxication. *Legal Medicine, 5* (Supplement 1), S138-S141.

Byard, R.W., Rodgers, N.G., James, R.A., et al. (2002). Death and paramethoxyamphetamine—an evolving problem. *The Medical Journal of Australia, 176*(10), 496.

Galloway, J.H., & Forrest, A.R.W. (2002). *Caveat Emptor*: Death involving the use of 4-methoxyamphetamine. *The Veterinary Journal, 164*(3), 298.

Jaehne, E.J., Salem, A., & Irvine, R.J. (2007). Pharmacological and behavioral determinants of cocaine, methamphetamine, 3,4-methylenedioxymethamphetamine, and para-methoxyamphetamine-induced hyperthermia. *Psychopharmacology, 194*(1), 47-52.

Johansen, S.S., Hansen, A.C., Müller, I.B., et al. (2003). Three fatal cases of PMA and PMMA poisoning in Denmark. *Journal of Analytical Toxicology, 27*(4), 253-256.

Kraner, J.C., McCoy, D.J., & Evans, M.A. (2001). Fatalities caused by the MDMA-related drug paramethoxyamphetamine (PMA). *Journal of Analytical Toxicology, 25*(7), 645-648.

Ling, L.H., Marchant, C., Buckley, N.A., et al. (2001). Poisoning with the recreational drug paramethoxyamphetamine ("death"). *The Medical Journal of Australia, 174*(9), 453-455.

Martin, T.L. (2001). Three cases of fatal paramethoxyamphetamine overdose. *Journal of Analytical Toxicology, 25*(7), 649-651.

Mortier, K.A., Dams, R., Lambert, W.E., et al. (2002). Determination of paramethoxyamphetamine and other amphetamine-related designer drugs by liquid chromatography/sonic spray ionization mass spectrometry. *Rapid Communications in Mass Spectrometry, 16*(9), 865-870.

Pritzker, D., Kanungo, A., Kilicarslan, T., et al. (2002). Designer drugs that are potent inhibitors of CYP2D6. *Journal of Clinical Psychopharmacology, 22*(3), 330-332.

Refstad, S. (2003). Paramethoxyamphetamine (PMA) poisoning: A "party drug" with lethal effects. *Acta Anaethesiologica Scandinavica, 47*(10), 1298-1299.

PEMOLINE

Names

BAN or INN Generic Synonyms: None

Brand/Trade: Cylert®

Chemical: 2-Amino-5-phenyl-2-oxazolin-4-one

Street: None

Pharmacologic Classification

Psychostimulant, miscellaneous: oxazolidine compound

Brief General Overview

Pemoline is structurally unrelated to the amphetamines and methylphenidate (Ritalin®). However, it shares their same general spectrum of psychostimulant and other actions, except that it has minimal sympathomimetic effects (e.g., pemoline does not generally increase blood pressure or heart rate). Pemoline is personally used for its psychostimulant actions. However, it is not widely used, largely because of its limited availability. Users are most likely to be adolescent boys and girls who have a dual diagnosis of ADHD and a substance use disorder. Alcohol is often used in combination with pemoline by these adolescents.

Dosage Forms and Routes of Administration

Pemoline is produced by licit pharmaceutical manufacturers in North America. It is generally available as an oral capsule or tablet and is orally ingested.

Mechanism of CNS Action

The exact mechanism of pemoline's psychostimulant action has not been determined. However, available data suggest that it works through dopaminergic mechanisms.

Pharmacodynamics/Pharmacokinetics

Pemoline is rapidly absorbed after ingestion. Peak blood concentrations usually are achieved within 4 hours. Pemoline is weakly plasma protein bound (~50%). It achieves steady state in 2 to 3 days. Pemoline is metabolized primarily by the liver. Approximately 50% of pemoline is excreted in unchanged form in the urine. The mean elimination half-life is ~12 hours (range, 9 to 14 hours).

Current Approved Indications for Medical Use

Attention-deficit/hyperactivity disorder[1]

Desired Effect/Reason for Personal Use

Alertness, vigilance, or wakefulness; appetite/hunger suppression; decrease fatigue; euphoria; work productivity

Toxicity

Acute: Agitation; anorexia; choreoathetosis (rare); diarrhea; dizziness; dyskinesia; excitement; hallucinations; headache; insomnia (common); irritability; nausea; nystagmus; precipitation of motor and phonic tics (i.e., Tourette's syndrome); restlessness; seizures

Chronic: Exacerbation of psychosis; hepatic dysfunction/failure[2]; physical dependence; psychological dependence; weight loss (generally transient)

Pregnancy & Lactation: FDA Pregnancy Category B (see Appendix B). Safety of pemoline use by adolescent girls and women who are pregnant has not been established. Additional valid and reliable data are needed.

Safety of pemoline use by adolescent girls and women who are breast-feeding has not been established. Additional valid and reliable data are needed.

Abuse Potential

Physical dependence: Low (USDEA Schedule IV; low potential for abuse)
Psychological dependence: Low

Withdrawal Syndrome

A pemoline withdrawal syndrome has not been reported.

Overdosage

Signs and symptoms of acute pemoline overdosage include agitation, confusion, delirium, dyskinetic movements, euphoria, flushing, hallucinations, headache, hyperpyrexia, hyperreflexia, hypertension, muscle twitching, mydriasis, restlessness, seizures (may be followed by coma), sweating, tachycardia, tremors, and vomiting. Pemoline overdosage requires emergency medical support, with attention to increasing pemoline elimination. There is no known antidote.

Notes

1. Pemoline pharmacotherapy for symptomatic management of ADHD has been associated with fatal hepatic toxicity. Thus, use is generally reserved for patients who have failed to adequately respond to other available pharmacotherapy (e.g., methylphenidate [Ritalin®] or the mixed amphetamines [Adderall®]).
2. The hepatotoxicity is thought to be associated with a delayed hypersensitivity reaction.

References

Bonnet, U., & Davids, E. (2006). A rare case of dependence on pemoline. *Progress in Neuro-Psychopharmacology and Biological Psychiatry, 30*(7), 1340-1341.

Martin Morgado, B., Vaz Leal, F.J., Bolivar Perálvarez, M., et al. (2007). Efficacy of bupropion in the treatment of pemoline dependence. *Actas Españōlas de Psiguiatria, 35*(4), 277-278.

Novak, S.P., Kroutil, L.A., Williams, R.L., et al. (2007). The nonmedical use of prescription ADHD medications: Results from a national internet panel. *Substance Abuse Treatment, Prevention, and Policy, 2*, 32.

Riggs, P.D., Hall, S.K., Mikulich-Gilbertson, S.K., et al. (2004). A randomized controlled trial of pemoline for attention-deficit/hyperactivity disorder in substance-abusing adolescents. *Journal of the American Academy of Child & Adolescent Psychiatry, 43*(4), 420-429.

PENTAZOCINE

Names

BAN or INN Generic Synonyms: None

Brand/Trade: Talwin®; Talwin Nx®

Chemical: (2R*, 6R*, 11R*)-1,2,3,4,5,6-Hexahydro-6,11-dimethyl-3-(3-methyl-2-butenyl)-2,6-methano-3-benzazocin-8-ol

Street: Big T; Poor Man's Heroin; Tea; Tees; Ts

Pharmacologic Classification

Psychodepressant, opiate analgesic: mixed agonist/antagonist (synthetic)

Brief General Overview

Pentazocine was introduced into clinical use in North America in the 1960s as an effective analgesic that reputedly was not associated with physical or psychological dependence. This claim, which was later shown to be incorrect, was largely based on the drug's mixed opiate analgesic agonist and antagonist properties. By the early 1970s, two distinct groups of users were identified. The first group consisted of health care professionals, primarily physicians, who used pentazocine, usually by intravenous injection, to self-medicate their pain disorders (e.g., migraine headache), manage anxiety and stress (e.g., job-related stress), or other related mental disorders. They believed pentazocine would provide needed relief without producing physical dependence (i.e., addiction), as their medical references reported at that time. The second group of pentazocine users originally consisted of Native Americans and Aboriginal Canadians. Later users comprised people from every ethnic group who resided in socioeconomically disadvantaged inner city neighborhoods, particularly in southern Canada and the northwestern United States.[1] A decade into the new millennium, levels of pentazocine use in North America are low. However, it is still available and widely personally used for its psychodepressant actions in other countries worldwide (e.g., India).

Dosage Forms and Routes of Administration

Pentazocine is produced by licit pharmaceutical manufacturers in North America. It is available as oral tablets with and without naloxone (Talwin Nx® and Talwin®, respectively) and as an injectable for intramuscular and intravenous use. Users generally prefer to inject pentazocine intravenously, either by first crushing and dissolving the Talwin® tablets and then injecting the solution or by using the injectable product.

Mechanism of CNS Action

Pentazocine elicits its analgesic, psychodepressant, and respiratory depressant actions primarily by binding to endorphin receptors in the CNS. It appears to function primarily as a kappa receptor agonist. However, its exact mechanism of action has not been determined. (See also the Opiate Analgesics monograph.)

Pentazocine antagonizes the analgesic action of morphine and meperidine and produces incomplete reversal of their cardiovascular, respiratory, and psychodepressant actions. Pentazocine has approximately one-fiftieth the antagonistic action of naloxone (Narcan®), a pure opiate analgesic antagonist. The respiratory depressant action of pentazocine is equal to or less than that observed after a single dose of other opiate analgesics. Pentazocine's respiratory depression appears to have a ceiling effect.

Pharmacodynamics/Pharmacokinetics

Pentazocine's analgesic action occurs within 3 minutes after intravenous injection and within 30 minutes after oral ingestion, intramuscular injection, or subcutaneous injection. However, only ~20% of the oral dose reaches the systemic circulation, because of extensive first-pass hepatic metabolism. Analgesia lasts for 3 to 4 hours. Pentazocine is about 60% bound to plasma proteins. The elimination half-life is ~2 to 3 hours, and the total body clearance is ~1.4 L/minute. The elimination half-life may be significantly prolonged in people with hepatic dysfunction.

Current Approved Indications for Medical Use[2]

Pain disorders: acute pain, moderate to severe; chronic cancer pain, moderate to severe

Desired Effect/Reason for Personal Use

Euphoria; pain relief; prevention/self-management of the opiate analgesic withdrawal syndrome; sleepy, dreamlike state ("nod")

Toxicity

Acute: Blurred vision; cognitive impairment; confusion; constipation; disorientation; dizziness; drowsiness; flushed skin; hallucinations (usually visual); lightheadedness; miosis; nausea; pruritus; sedation; somnolence; syncope; tachycardia; tinnitus; urinary retention; vertigo; vomiting; weakness

Chronic: Mental depression; physical dependence; psychological dependence; sclerosis of the skin, severe[3]

Pregnancy & Lactation: FDA Pregnancy Category C (see Appendix B). Safety of the use of pentazocine by adolescent girls and women who are pregnant has not been established. Pentazocine crosses the placenta. Blood concentrations in neonates at delivery are equal to approximately 65% of maternal blood concentrations. Neonates born to mothers who have regularly used pentazocine during pregnancy or near term may display expected pharmacologic actions (e.g., drowsiness, lethargy, respiratory depression). They also may display signs and symptoms of the opiate analgesic withdrawal syndrome (see Opiate Analgesics monograph). Adolescent girls and women who are pregnant should not use pentazocine.

Safety of pentazocine use by adolescent girls and women who are breast-feeding has not been established. However, pentazocine is excreted in breast milk. Thus, adolescent girls and women who are breast-feeding should not use pentazocine. (Also see the Opiate Analgesics monograph.)

Abuse Potential

Physical dependence: Moderate (USDEA Schedule IV; low potential for abuse)
Psychological dependence: Moderate

Withdrawal Syndrome

Regular, long-term use of pentazocine is associated with physical and psychological dependence. Pentazocine has mixed opiate analgesic agonist/antagonist actions. Thus, it also may cause signs and symptoms of the opiate analgesic withdrawal syndrome in people who are physically dependent on pure opiate analgesic agonists (e.g., morphine). The combination oral tablet formulation (Talwin Nx®) contains both pentazocine and naloxone to discourage illicit intravenous injection of pentazocine.

Abrupt discontinuation of pentazocine by users after regular, long-term oral use may result in a reportedly mild form of the opiate analgesic withdrawal syndrome, the signs and symptoms of which include abdominal cramps, anxiety, fever, restlessness, and rhinorrhea.

Overdosage

Signs and symptoms of pentazocine overdosage are similar to the signs and symptoms associated with other opiate analgesic overdosage (see Opiate Analgesics monograph). However, pentazocine does not appear to produce the severe respiratory depression usually associated with pure opiate agonist overdosage. Regardless, pentazocine overdosage requires emergency medical support of body systems, with attention to increasing pentazocine elimination. Naloxone (Narcan®) is the specific and effective antagonist for the respiratory depression associated with pentazocine overdosage.[4]

Notes

1. During the early 1970s, aboriginal people in central Alberta, Canada, discovered that Talwin® tablets ("Ts"), when crushed and mixed in various ratios (e.g., 2 to 5) with the contents of tripelennamine (Pyribenzamine®) capsules ("Blues") and injected intravenously, could produce heroin-like actions. This discovery was made at a time when heroin was not readily available in rural prairie communities (i.e., heroin was more commonly available along the eastern and western seaboards of North America). The combination soon became known "on the street" as "poor man's heroin." Use spread from Indian reserve to Indian reserve across Canada and across the border into Indian reservations in the United States. From the reserves and reservations, it then spread to the inner cities and soon became a common cause for emergency room admissions.

   Another popular combination at that time was Talwin® and the psychostimulant methylphenidate (Ritalin®). This combination became widely known as "Ritz and Ts," "Ts and Ritz," and "Ts and Rs." This combination produced effects that caused it to become known as a "synthetic speedball" (i.e., intravenous injection of the combination of cocaine and heroin was called a "speedball"), but it was much less expensive.

   To stem the growing number of emergency room admissions and related overdosage deaths in the mid-1970s, Talwin® tablets were cleverly reformulated by the U.S. manufacturer (Winthrop) in 1983 as Talwin Nx®, which contains the opiate antagonist naloxone (i.e., Narcan®). The oral bioavailability of naloxone is limited. Thus, when Talwin Nx® tablets are ingested, only the pentazocine is absorbed and the intended opiate analgesic actions are produced; however, if Talwin Nx® tablets are illicitly crushed and intravenously injected, the bioavailability of naloxone becomes, by definition, 100% ($F = 1$). The naloxone is then able to competitively bind to the opiate receptors and, in so doing, block the desired psychodepressant actions of pentazocine. More than 20 years later, even though the success of Talwin Nx® combination tablets in curtailing illicit use and associated harmful effects has been demonstrated in the United States, Talwin® tablets (without naloxone) are still the only formulation available in Canada.
2. Pentazocine pharmacotherapy for the medical management of pain disorders should be considered to be obsolete because of the availability of other equally efficacious and less toxic opiate analgesics.
3. The severe skin sclerosis and injection site ulcers are associated with multiple intramuscular injections or inadvertent subcutaneous injection.
4. Caution is indicated, because naloxone may precipitate the opiate analgesic withdrawal syndrome in people who are physically dependent on pentazocine.

References

Agarwal, S., & Trivedi, M. (2007). Cutaneous complications of pentazocine abuse. *Indian Journal of Dermatology, Venereology, and Leprology, 73*(4), 280.

Cohen, B.M., & Murphy, B. (2008). The effects of pentazocine, a kappa agonist, in patients with mania. *International Journal of Neuropsychopharmacology, 11*(2), 243-247.

De, D., Dogra, S., & Kanwar, A.J. (2007). Pentazocine-induced leg ulcers and fibrous papules. *Indian Journal of Dermatology, Venereology, and Leprology, 73*(2), 112-113.

Prasad, H.R., Khaitan, B.K., Ramam, M., et al. (2005). Diagnostic clinical features of pentazocine-induced ulcers. *International Journal of Dermatology, 44*(11), 910-915.

PENTOBARBITAL

Names

BAN or INN Generic Synonyms: None

Brand/Trade: Nembutal®; Novo-Pentobarb®

Chemical: 5-Ethyl-5-(1-methylbutyl)barbituric acid

Street: Abbots; Canaries; Jackets; Mexican Yellows; Nebs; Nembs; Nembies; Nemmies; Nems; Yellow Angels; Yellow Birds; Yellow Bullets; Yellow Dolls; Yellow Jackets; Yellows

Pharmacologic Classification

Psychodepressant, sedative-hypnotic: barbiturate

Brief General Overview

Pentobarbital is a short-acting barbiturate with sedative-hypnotic action. It was one of the two barbiturates most widely clinically used and illicitly used[1] during the 1950s, 1960s, and 1970s. However, both clinical use and personal use of pentobarbital decreased significantly during the last two decades of the 20th century as a result of the development and clinical use of the benzodiazepines (see Benzodiazepines monograph).

Dosage Forms and Routes of Administration

Pentobarbital is produced by licit pharmaceutical manufacturers in North America. It is commercially available in a number of dosage formulations, including injectables for intramuscular and intravenous use; oral capsules, elixirs, and tablets; and rectal suppositories. Users virtually always inject pentobarbital intravenously or ingest it orally.

Mechanism of CNS Action

The exact mechanism of pentobarbital's psychodepressant actions has not been determined. However, pentobarbital appears to act primarily at the level of the thalamus, where it interferes with impulse transmission to the cortex. (See also the Barbiturates monograph.)

Pharmacodynamics/Pharmacokinetics

Pentobarbital is rapidly and completely absorbed after oral or rectal administration and generally has its onset of action within 15 to 30 minutes. Pentobarbital is ~40% plasma protein bound. It is extensively metabolized in the liver, with less than 5% excreted in unchanged form in the urine. Changes in the urine volume or pH do not significantly affect the urinary excretion of pentobarbital. The elimination half-life ranges from 25 to 50 hours and appears to be dose dependent.

Current Approved Indications for Medical Use[2]

Anxiety disorders: acute anxiety; sleep disorders: insomnia (short-term management)

Desired Effect/Reason for Personal Use

Alcohol-like disinhibitory euphoria or "high"; anxiety/tension reduction; prevention/self-management of the barbiturate withdrawal syndrome; relaxation; tranquility

Toxicity

Acute: CNS depression (severe); cognitive impairment; cough; hypotension (particularly with rapid intravenous injection); laryngospasm; nausea; pain at the injection site; respiratory depression[3]; vomiting

Chronic: Physical dependence; psychological dependence; suppression of REM sleep

Pregnancy & Lactation: FDA Pregnancy Category D (see Appendix B). Pentobarbital use near term may result in respiratory depression in neonates, and regular, long-term use during pregnancy may result in signs and symptoms of the neonatal barbiturate withdrawal syndrome (see Barbiturates monograph). Adolescent girls and women who are pregnant should not use pentobarbital.

Pentobarbital is excreted in breast milk. Breast-fed neonates and infants may display expected pharmacologic actions (e.g., drowsiness). They also may develop physical dependence (see Barbiturates monograph). Adolescent girls and women who are breast-feeding should not use pentobarbital.

Abuse Potential

Physical dependence: High (USDEA Schedule II; high potential for abuse)
Psychological dependence: High

Withdrawal Syndrome

Regular, long-term pentobarbital use is associated with the development of physical and psychological dependence. Abrupt discontinuation of regular, long-term use may result in the barbiturate withdrawal syndrome, signs and symptoms of which include delirium and convulsions that may be fatal. The barbiturate withdrawal syndrome requires appropriate medical management. Regular, long-term users of pentobarbital should avoid abrupt discontinuation of use, particularly when they have used high dosages, and should, when possible, seek medical treatment before discontinuing use.

Overdosage

Signs and symptoms of pentobarbital overdosage include cardiac depression, coma, hypotension, hypothermia (early sign), fever (late sign), sluggish or absent reflexes, respiratory depression, gradual circulatory collapse, and pulmonary edema. Pentobarbital overdosage requires emergency medical support of body systems, with attention to increasing pentobarbital elimination (e.g., hemoperfusion). There is no known antidote.

Notes

1. The other barbiturate that was commonly used at that time was secobarbital (see monograph).
2. The use of pentobarbital for the pharmacotherapeutic management of anxiety and sleep disorders is not generally recommended because of the ready availability of other equally efficacious and less toxic drugs (e.g., benzodiazepines; see the Benzodiazepines monograph).
3. Respiratory depression is particularly associated with the use of higher dosages of pentobarbital or rapid intravenous injection.

References

Carter, L.P., Richards, B.D., Mintzer, M.Z., et al. (2006). Relative abuse liability of GHB in humans: A comparison of psychomotor, subjective, and cognitive effects of supratherapeutic doses of triazolam, pentobarbital, and GHB. *Neuropsychopharmacology, 31*(11), 2537-2551.

Koyama, K., Suzuki, R., Yoshida, T., et al. (2007). Usefulness of serum concentration measurement for acute pentobarbital intoxication in patients. *Chudoku Kenkyu (The Japanese Journal of Toxicology), 20*(1), 45-53.

Tobias, J.D. (2000). Tolerance, withdrawal, and physical dependency after long-term sedation and analgesia of children in the pediatric intensive care unit. *Critical Care Medicine, 28*(6), 2122-2132.

Yanay, O., Brogan, T.V., & Martin, L.D. (2004). Continuous pentobarbital infusion in children is associated with high rates of complications. *Journal of Critical Care, 19*(3), 174-178.

PETHIDINE (see Meperidine)

PEYOTE (see Mescaline)

PHENCYCLIDINE

Names

BAN or INN Generic Synonyms: None

Brand/Trade: None

Chemical: l-(l-Phenylcyclohexyl)-piperidine

Street: Amoeba; AMP; Anchorage; Angel; Angel Death; Angel Dust; Angel Hair; Angel Mist; Angel Poke; Animal Trank; Animal Tranq; Animal Tranquilizer; *Aurora Borealis*; Black Dust; Black Whack; Blue Madman; Boat; Buff Naked; Busy Bee; Butt Naked; Cannabinol; Cigaroid; Cigarrode; CJ; Cliffhanger; Cliqum; Columbo; Cozmo's; Crazy Coke; Crazy Eddie; Cristal; Crystal; Crystal Joint; Crystal T; Crystal THC; Cycline; *Cyclona*; Cyclones; Death Wish; Detroit Pink; Devil's Dust; Dipper; Dippie; Disembalming Fluid; DOA; Do It Jack; Dummy Dust; Dust; Dust of Angels; Dusted Parsley; Elephant Trank; Elephant Tranquilizer; Embalming Fluid; Energizer; Erth; Fake STP; Fake THC; Fake X; Flakes; Fresh; Fry; Fuck Me Harder; Goon; Goon Dust; Gorilla Biscuits; Gorilla Pills; Gorilla Tab; Green Leaves; Green Tea; Half Track; Happy Sticks; HCP; Heaven & Hell; Herms; Hinkley; Hog; Horse Tracks; Horse Tranquilizer; Ill; Illy Momo; Jo Mama; K; Kaps; K-Blast; Killer Joints; KJ; Kools; Krystal; Krystal Joint; Leaky Bolla; Leaky Leak; Lemon 714; Lenos; Lethal Weapon; Little Ones; Live Ones; Love Boat; Lovelies; Lovely; Mad Dog; Madman; Magic; Magic Dust; Mean Green; Mint Leaf; Mint Weed; Monkey Dust; Monkey Tranquilizer; More; New Acid; New Magic; *Niebla*; Ocean and Stigman; O.P.P.; Orange Crystal; Ozone; *Paz*; PCP; PCPA; PeaCe Pill; Peace Weed; Peep; Peter Pan; Pig Killer; Pig Tranquilizer; Pit; Pits; *Polvo de Angel*; *Polvo de Estrellas*; Powdered Milk; Puffy; Purple Rain; Rocket Fuel; Sam Williams; Scaffle; Scuffle; Sheets; Sherman Avenue; Sherman Hemsley; Shermans; Sherm Sticks; Star Dust; Super Grass; Synthetic Cocaine; Synthetic THC; TAC; Taking A Cruise; Tic Tac; Tick; Tish; Titch; Trank; Wack; Waters; Wets; Whack; White Horizon; Worm; Yellow Fever; Zombi Buzz; Zoom; Zoot

Pharmacologic Classification

Psychodelic, miscellaneous: cataleptic (dissociative) general anesthetic

Brief General Overview

Phencyclidine (PCP) was originally used during the 1950s as a dissociative anesthetic (under the brand/trade names Sernyl® and Sernylan®) in humans undergoing surgery, but its association with cardiovascular and respiratory depression as well as postoperative delirium and hallucinations resulted in discontinuation of its use. Subsequently, it was used for over a decade (from the mid-1960s to the late 1970s) as an animal tranquilizer, but steadily increasing problems with illegal diversion and abuse led to discontinuation of its veterinary use. Phencyclidine is no longer legally produced in North America. However, it is still personally used for its psychodelic actions.

In the United States, it is estimated that approximately 1 out of every 20 adults between 18 and 25 years of age has used PCP in his or her lifetime. Accurate data on actual use are difficult to obtain, and it is possible that PCP use is greatly underreported. Several reasons have been proposed for the difficulty of obtaining accurate data regarding personal use: (1) subjects who tend to use PCP usually cannot be reached in a survey of high school seniors (i.e., they are frequently high school dropouts); (2) use of PCP does not often result in emergency room visits; and (3) PCP is not always detected in blood or urine drug and substance abuse screening tests (i.e., often it is not even screened for). Over the past 5 years, the highest availability of PCP and incidence of PCP use have been reported for the Los Angeles area of southern California.

Dosage Forms and Routes of Administration

PCP is produced by illicit chemical laboratories[1] as a white crystalline powder,[2] available in a variety of oral dosage forms (i.e., capsules, powder, solution, tablets), that dissolves rapidly in either water or alcohol.[3] Although it is usually orally ingested, it may be intranasally sniffed (snorted) or intravenously injected. It also may be used by pulmonary inhalation (i.e., smoked) by sprinkling the powder form on tobacco or marijuana and rolling it up into a cigarette or joint, respectively, or dipping the tobacco cigarette or marijuana joint into liquid PCP and then smoking it.[4]

Mechanism of CNS Action

The exact mechanism of PCP's psychodelic actions has not been determined. However, noncompetitive antagonism of the N-methyl-D-aspartate (NMDA) receptor channel complexes located in the cortex and limbic regions of the brain has been postulated as a contributory mechanism. This antagonism is thought to block the action of the excitatory amino acids aspartate and glutamate. PCP also inhibits GABA and increases dopamine concentrations (by both increasing its synthesis and inhibiting its presynaptic reuptake).

Pharmacodynamics/Pharmacokinetics

PCP, a weak base, is relatively well absorbed (i.e., 50% to 90%) after oral ingestion, intranasal sniffing (i.e., snorting), or pulmonary inhalation (i.e., smoking). PCP also is absorbed percutaneously. The acute effects of PCP begin within 2 to 5 minutes after pulmonary inhalation and within 30 to 60 minutes after oral ingestion. Effects are dose-related and can generally last for up to 15 hours. Additional valid and reliable data are not available.

Current Approved Indications for Medical Use

None

Desired Effect/Reason for Personal Use

Braveness or toughness[5]; dissociation from the environment; euphoria; feelings of increased strength; peace and tranquility; power, invincibility, or invulnerability; hallucinations (primarily visual, but also auditory); illusions; sensory and perceptual changes (e.g., time distortion, LSD-like; see Lysergic Acid Diethylamide monograph)

Toxicity

Acute: Aggression; agitation; amnesia; anorexia; anxiety; ataxia; bizarre behavior (often violent); blank stare; blurred vision; cognitive impairment; coma; confusion; convulsions (with overdosage); difficulty concentrating; difficulty speaking or incoherent speech; diminished responsiveness to pain; disorganized thought; disorientation; dysarthria; erratic behavior (often aggressive); exaggerated gait; feelings of alienation, intense; fever; hostility; irrational behavior; irritability; lethargy; mental depression; miosis; motor incoordination; muscle rigidity; mutism; nausea (severe); numbness of the extremities; nystagmus (horizontal and vertical); obsessive–compulsive behavior; panic; paranoia; psychosis[6]; rapid, involuntary eye movements; rapid, shallow breathing; rhabdomyolysis; respiratory arrest (with overdosage); salivation (excessive); schizophrenia (exacerbation of signs and symptoms); slurred speech; stupor; tachycardia; terror; violent behavior

Chronic: Anxiety; depression; flashbacks; neurocognitive impairment (e.g., memory loss; speech impairment, such as inability to speak, slurred speech, and stuttering); psychological dependence; psychosis; social withdrawal and isolation; suicidal ideation; violent behavior[7]; weight loss

Pregnancy & Lactation: Safety of PCP use by adolescent girls and women who are pregnant has not been established. PCP does not appear to be a human teratogen. However, adolescent girls and women who are pregnant are advised not to use PCP.[8]

Safety of PCP use by adolescent girls and women who are breast-feeding has not been established. However, PCP is excreted in breast milk and has been associated with behavioral problems, coma, irritability, and lethargy in breast-fed infants whose mothers used PCP. Adolescent girls and women who are breast-feeding should not use PCP.

Abuse Potential

Physical dependence: None to low (USDEA Schedule I; use is prohibited)
Psychological dependence: Moderate

Withdrawal Syndrome

A PCP withdrawal syndrome has not been reported.

Overdosage

PCP overdosage may result in aggressive and violent behavior directed toward the user or others. Other prominent signs and symptoms include diaphoresis, dystonic reactions (generally localized), hypertension, hyperthermia, muscle rigidity, nystagmus, rapidly fluctuating behavior (e.g., quiet catatonia to agitated and violent behavior), and tachycardia. Severe overdosage can result in coma, convulsions, and death. Death is generally due to respiratory arrest. PCP overdosage requires emergency medical support of body systems, with attention to increasing PCP elimination when poisoning is by the oral route. There is no known antidote. PCP-induced delusional disorder may emerge up to a week after a PCP overdosage and is characterized by cognitive impairment, a disheveled or eccentric appearance, dysphoria, rambling and incoherent speech, and ritualistic stereotypic behavior.

Notes

1. These laboratories can be found across North America but are primarily located in the Los Angeles metropolitan area.
2. It is relatively easily synthesized from chemical precursors that are readily available and fairly inexpensive.
3. PCP is often illicitly represented and sold as synthetic mescaline (see monograph) or synthetic tetrahydrocannabinol (THC; see Cannabis monograph).
4. The combination of marijuana and PCP is commonly referred to as chips, clickums, crystal super-grass, crystal weed, donk, dust blunt, *frios,* illies, killer weed, lava leaf, leak, lovelies, macho weed, peace weed, super grass, super weed, woolies, *yerba mala,* zombie weed, or zoom. It also is sometimes represented as embalming-fluid-soaked marijuana (see Cannabis monograph).
5. PCP, because of its unpredictable actions and effects, is considered to be a "macho" drug by some youth, particularly those who are of Hispanic descent, mostly male gang members. Thus, although lifetime PCP use declined during the 1980s and early 1990s, it is beginning to increase again.
6. The mechanism of PCP's action suggests the reason for causing psychosis. In fact, antagonism of the NMDA receptor has been proposed as a model for studying psychosis, particularly that associated with catatonic or negative features.
7. One of the most troublesome psychological effects associated with PCP use is its tendency to bring out or aggravate aggressiveness, anger, hostility, and underlying or latent psychological conditions (e.g., fears, depression). A clear association between PCP use and violent behavior has been widely observed and frequently reported. These observations tend to suggest that regular, long-term use of PCP is directly associated with violent behavior or toxic organic brain disorders. The violent behavior is often bizarre, sudden, and unexpected. Primitive sadistic behaviors (e.g., brutal murders, self-mutilation) also have been documented. Usually, users "blank out" and report no conscious memory of the events that occurred during the violent episode.
8. Some published studies and reports have noted lower birth weight in neonates exposed to PCP in utero than in neonates who were not exposed in utero. However, these differences appear clinically insignificant. The PCP-using mothers concurrently used other drugs and substances of abuse, particularly alcohol, marijuana, or tobacco, all of which can affect birth weight. In addition, the neonates of PCP-using mothers were delivered approximately 1 week earlier than those of non-PCP-using mothers. Thus, early delivery may have contributed to the observed lower birth weight.
   A source of concern related to risk for teratogenic effects of PCP use during pregnancy is the drug's mechanism of action (i.e., antagonism of N-methyl-D-aspartate [NMDA]). This antagonism, particularly during the third trimester when synaptogenesis, or the brain growth spurt, occurs, may result in yet unrecognized long-term neurocognitive impairment. This impairment may not be recognized until offspring reach school age.

References

Breese, G.R., Knapp, D.J., & Moy, S.S. (2002). Integrative role for serotonergic and glutamatergic receptor mechanisms in the action of NMDA antagonists: Potential relationships to antipsychotic drug actions on NMDA antagonist responsiveness. *Neuroscience and Biobehavioral Reviews, 26*(4), 441-455.

Compton, W.M. 3rd, Cottler, L.B., Ben Abdallah, A., et al. (2000). Substance dependence and other psychiatric disorders among drug dependent subjects: Race and gender correlates. *The American Journal on Addictions, 9*(2), 113-125.

Gouzoulis-Mayfrank, E., Heekeren, K., Neukirch, A., et al. (2005). Psychological effects of (S)-ketamine and N,N-dimethyltryptamine (DMT): A double-blind, cross-over study in healthy volunteers. *Pharmacopsychiatry, 38*(6), 301-311.

Olney, J.W., Wozniak, D.F., Farber, N.B., et al. (2002). The enigma of fetal alcohol neurotoxicity. *Annals of Medicine, 34*(2), 109-119.

Sharp, F.R., Tomitaka, M., Bernaudin, M., et al. (2001). Psychosis: Pathological activation of limbic thalamocortical circuits by psychomimetics and schizophrenia? *Trends in Neurosciences, 24*(6), 330-334.

Singer, M., Mirhej, G., Shaw, S., et al. (2005). When the drug of choice is a drug of confusion: Embalming fluid use in inner city Hartford, CT. *Journal of Ethnicity in Substance Abuse, 4*(2), 73-96.

PHENDIMETRAZINE

Names

BAN or INN Generic Synonyms: None

Brand/Trade: Anorex-SR®; Bontril®; Melfiat®; Obezine®; Phendiet®; Plegine®; Prelu-2®

Chemical: (+)-(2S,3S)-3,4-Dimethyl-2-phenylmorpholine

Street: BI-64s; Diet Pills; Green and Yellows

Pharmacologic Classification

Psychostimulant, miscellaneous

Brief General Overview

Phendimetrazine, a sympathomimetic amine, is commonly used as an anorectic, or appetite suppressant. Efficacy for weight loss in the absence of calorie reduction (i.e., diet) or increased energy expenditure (i.e., exercise) is highly suspect. Tachyphylaxis, or tolerance, has been demonstrated, particularly when the duration of use exceeds a few weeks. Since its introduction into clinical practice, phendimetrazine has also been personally used for its psychostimulant actions, as has occurred with virtually all of the other prescription anorectics. It is widely available over the Internet.

Dosage Forms and Routes of Administration

Phendimetrazine is produced by licit pharmaceutical manufacturers in North America. It is available in oral capsule and tablet formulations and is usually orally ingested. Most users are women 25 to 65 years of age of European descent, who were initially prescribed phendimetrazine by their physicians for weight reduction. However, they continue to use it for its psychostimulant actions. Increasingly, new users are being introduced to phendimetrazine by friends or acquaintances and are purchasing it over the Internet from on-line pharmacy sites.

Mechanism of CNS Action

Phendimetrazine's actions include psychostimulation and increased blood pressure. The exact mechanism of its anorexiant action, including appetite suppression, has not been determined. However, it appears that, as an indirect-acting sympathomimetic, it may be associated with norepinephrine stimulation of the CNS.

Pharmacodynamics/Pharmacokinetics

Phendimetrazine is readily absorbed after oral ingestion. Peak blood concentrations are achieved within 1 to 3 hours. Phendimetrazine is extensively metabolized in the liver to several metabolites, including the active metabolite phenmetrazine (~30%). The metabolites are eliminated primarily in the urine. The mean elimination half-life is ~20 hours.

Current Approved Indications for Medical Use[1]

Eating disorders: exogenous obesity (short-term use with appropriate diet and exercise program)

Desired Effect/Reason for Personal Use

Appetite/hunger suppression (weight reduction or maintenance); energy; euphoria

Toxicity

Acute: Agitation; blurred vision; convulsions; dehydration; dizziness; dry mouth; dysuria; headache; hyperreflexia; hyperstimulation; hypertension; hypotension; impotence; insomnia; myopia (transient and associated with ciliochoroidal effusion); nervousness; palpitations; restlessness; tachycardia; tremor; urticaria

Chronic: Dilated cardiomyopathy (rare); physical dependence; primary pulmonary hypertension (relatively rare but potentially fatal); psychological dependence; rhabdomyolysis (rare)

Pregnancy & Lactation: FDA Pregnancy Category "not established." Safety of phendimetrazine use by adolescent girls and women who are pregnant has not been established. Additional valid and reliable data are needed.

Safety of phendimetrazine use by adolescent girls and women who are breast-feeding has not been established. Additional valid and reliable data are needed.

Abuse Potential

Physical dependence: Moderate (USDEA Schedule III; moderate potential for abuse)
Psychological dependence: Moderate

Withdrawal Syndrome

Regular, long-term use of phendimetrazine has been associated with physical and psychological dependence. Abrupt discontinuation has been associated with an amphetamine-like withdrawal syndrome, with signs and symptoms of extreme fatigue and mental depression. EEG changes also have been reported. Abrupt discontinuation of regular, long-term phendimetrazine use should be avoided.

Overdosage

Signs and symptoms of acute phendimetrazine overdosage include belligerence, combativeness, confusion, hallucinations, hyperreflexia, hyperventilation, panic, restlessness, and tremor. Depression and fatigue usually follow the CNS stimulation. Cardiovascular signs and symptoms include dysrhythmias, hypertension or hypotension, and circulatory collapse. GI signs and symptoms include abdominal cramps, diarrhea, nausea, and vomiting. Fatal overdosage usually terminates in convulsions and coma. Acute phendimetrazine overdosage requires emergency medical support of body systems, with attention to increasing phendimetrazine elimination. There is no known antidote.

Note

1. The therapeutic efficacy of phendimetrazine was brought into question, and it has now been withdrawn from the European market. Use is not generally recommended.

References

Bray, G.A. (2005). Drug insight: Appetite suppressants. *Nature Clinical Practice Gastroenterology & Hepatology, 2*(2) 89-95.

Kwiker, D., Godkar, D., Lokhandwala, N., et al. (2006). Rare case of rhabdomyolysis with therapeutic doses of phendimetrazine tartrate. *American Journal of Therapeutics, 13*(2), 175-176.

Landau, D., Jackson, J., & Gonzalez, G. (2008). A case of demand ischemia from phendimetrazine: A case report. *Cases Journal, 1*(1), 105.

Lee, W., Chang, J.H., Roh, K.H., et al. (2007). Anorexiant-induced transient myopia after myopic laser in situ keratomileusis. *Journal of Cataract Refractive Surgery, 33*(4), 746-749.

Ryan, D.H. (2000). Use of sibutramine and other noradrenergic and serotonergic drugs in the management of obesity. *Endocrine, 13*(2), 193-199.

PHENOBARBITAL

Names

BAN or INN Generic Synonyms: Phenobarbitone

Brand/Trade[1]: Luminal®; Solfoton®

Chemical: 5-Ethyl-5-phenylbarbituric acid

Street: Barbs; Beans; Block Busters; Downers; Golf Balls; Goofballs; Goofers; Idiot Pills; Phennies; Pheno; Phenobarb; Purple Hearts; Sleepers; Stoppers

Pharmacologic Classification

Psychodepressant, sedative-hypnotic: barbiturate

Brief General Overview

Phenobarbital is a long-acting barbiturate. Its personal use has been related to its inappropriate prescribing by physicians. It has never been widely used as a drug and substance of abuse because it produces less euphoria and other desired effects than the intermediate-acting barbiturates (e.g., pentobarbital and secobarbital; see monographs), which are preferentially used for their psychodepressant actions.

Dosage Forms and Routes of Administration

Phenobarbital is produced by licit pharmaceutical manufacturers in North America. It is available in a number of dosage formulations, including injectables for intramuscular or intravenous use; oral capsules, drops, elixirs, and tablets; and rectal suppositories. When personally used, it is usually orally ingested.

Mechanism of CNS Action

The exact mechanism of phenobarbital's psychodepressant actions has not been determined. Phenobarbital appears to act primarily at the level of the thalamus, where it interferes with impulse transmission to the cortex. (See also the Barbiturates monograph.)

Pharmacodynamics/Pharmacokinetics

Phenobarbital is slowly but well absorbed (90% to 100%) after oral ingestion. Peak blood concentrations are generally achieved within 6 to 12 hours. Onset of action depends on its method of use but is generally within 60 minutes. After intravenous injection, onset of action occurs within 5 minutes. Onset of action after intramuscular injection is slightly slower than after oral ingestion or rectal insertion.

The duration of action is 6 to 12 hours. Phenobarbital is ~50% plasma protein bound and has an apparent volume of distribution of 0.5 L/kg. Of the barbiturates, phenobarbital is the least soluble and has the lowest distribution. Phenobarbital is not as extensively metabolized as the other barbiturates because of its low lipid solubility. Almost 25% is excreted in unchanged form in the urine.[2] The elimination half-life is ~4 days (range, 80 to 120 hours). Total body clearance is 4 to 5 mL/minute.

Current Approved Indications for Medical Use[3]

Management of the barbiturate withdrawal syndrome; seizure disorders (partial and tonic–clonic)

Desired Effect/Reason for Personal Use

Alcohol-like disinhibitory euphoria or "high" (mild); prevention/self-management of the barbiturate withdrawal syndrome; relaxation; tranquility

Toxicity

Acute: Cognitive impairment; dizziness; drowsiness; excitement (particularly among children); headache; nausea; neuropsychological impairment; psychomotor impairment; respiratory depression; sedation; skin rash; vomiting

Chronic: Aplastic anemia; megaloblastic anemia; mental depression; osteomalacia[4]; physical dependence; psychological dependence; suppression of REM sleep

Pregnancy & Lactation: FDA Pregnancy Category D (see Appendix B). Numerous reports in the published literature have associated the use of phenobarbital with various fetal and congenital malformations, including cleft lip and palate, congenital dislocated hip, microcephaly, and wide fontanelle. In addition, the neonatal phenobarbital withdrawal syndrome, developmental delay, and psychomotor retardation have been noted in neonates and infants born to mothers who regularly used phenobarbital during pregnancy. Adolescent girls and women who are pregnant should not use phenobarbital.

Phenobarbital is excreted in breast milk in sufficient quantities to cause drowsiness and lethargy among breast-fed neonates and infants, who also may become physically dependent. Adolescent girls and women who are breast-feeding should not use phenobarbital.

Abuse Potential

Physical dependence: Low to moderate (USDEA Schedule IV; low potential for abuse)
Psychological dependence: Low

Withdrawal Syndrome

Regular, long-term use of phenobarbital has been associated with the development of physical and psychological dependence. Sudden discontinuation of regular, long-term use may result in the barbiturate withdrawal syndrome, which is considered a medical emergency that can be fatal if not appropriately treated. (Also see the Barbiturates monograph.)

Overdosage

See the Barbiturates monograph.

Notes

1. Generally available by generic name.
2. The urinary excretion of phenobarbital, a weak acid, is increased in alkaline urine.
3. Although phenobarbital was widely used throughout much of the 20th century to treat both anxiety and insomnia because of its sedative-hypnotic actions, these indications for phenobarbital are now considered obsolete because of the availability of the benzodiazepines. The benzodiazepines are at least as efficacious as phenobarbital for these indications, and they are significantly less toxic.
4. As a hepatic enzyme inducer, phenobarbital induces hepatic metabolism. The osteomalacia is related to the induction of the hepatic metabolism of vitamin D.

References

Focosi, D., Kast, R.E., Benedetti, E., et al. (2008). Phenobarbital-associated bone marrow aplasia: A case report and review of the literature. *Acta Haematologica, 119*(1), 18-21.

Kaaja, E., Kaaja, R., Matila, R., et al. (2002). Enzyme-inducing antiepileptic drugs in pregnancy and the risk of bleeding in the neonate. *Neurology, 58*(4), 549-553.

Tobias, J.D. (2000). Tolerance, withdrawal, and physical dependency after long-term sedation and analgesia of children in the pediatric intensive care unit. *Critical Care Medicine, 28*(6), 2122-2132.

PHENTERMINE

Names

BAN or INN Generic Synonyms: None

Brand/Trade: Adipex-P®; Banobese®; Fastin®; Ionamin®; Obenix®

Chemical: α,α-Dimethylphenethylamine

Street: None

Pharmacologic Classification

Psychostimulant, miscellaneous

Brief General Overview

Like other drugs that are clinically used for symptomatic management of exogenous obesity, phentermine is commonly referred to as an anorexiant, anorectic, or anorexigenic. Phentermine use is relatively infrequent compared with that of other psychostimulants. It is one of the many psychostimulants used by tractor-trailer drivers (i.e., truckers). However, the majority of users are women 20 to 65 years of age of European descent, who use phentermine for its anorexiant actions.

Dosage Forms and Routes of Administration

Phentermine is licitly produced by pharmaceutical manufacturers in North America. It is available in oral capsule and tablet formulations, which are usually orally ingested. Increasingly, users are purchasing phentermine over the Internet from on-line pharmacies.

Mechanism of CNS Action

Phentermine appears to elicit its psychostimulant and related anorexiant actions by means of activation of the noradrenergic pathway of the sympathetic nervous system. However, the exact mechanism of these actions, including appetite suppression, has not been determined.

Pharmacodynamics/Pharmacokinetics

Phentermine is well absorbed (approximately 100%) after oral ingestion. Phentermine and its metabolites are excreted in the urine. Additional valid and reliable data are not available.

Current Approved Indications for Medical Use[1]

Eating disorders: Exogenous obesity (short-term use)

Desired Effect/Reason for Personal Use

Alertness; appetite/hunger suppression (weight reduction or management); energy; euphoria

Toxicity

Acute: Constipation; diarrhea; dry mouth; headache; hypertension; insomnia; irritability; overstimulation; palpitations; psychosis; restlessness; tachycardia; tremor; unpleasant taste; vomiting

Chronic: Cardiac arrest (rare); physical dependence; primary pulmonary hypertension (relatively rare, but potentially fatal); psychological dependence; valvular disease (including aortic valve rupture)

Pregnancy & Lactation: FDA Pregnancy Category "not established." Safety of phentermine use by adolescent girls and women who are pregnant has not been established. Additional valid and reliable data are needed.

Safety of phentermine use by adolescent girls and women who are breast-feeding has not been established. Additional valid and reliable data are needed.

Abuse Potential

Physical dependence: Moderate (USDEA Schedule IV; low potential for abuse)
Psychological dependence: Moderate

Withdrawal Syndrome

Valid and reliable data are not available. However, because of phentermine's pharmacologic similarity to the amphetamines, caution is advised (see Amphetamines monograph; also see Phendimetrazine monograph).

Overdosage

Signs and symptoms of phentermine overdosage include abdominal cramps, belligerence, cardiac arrest, circulatory collapse, combativeness, confusion, diarrhea, dizziness, dysrhythmias, hallucinations, hypertension or hypotension, hyporeflexia, hyperventilation, nausea, panic, restlessness, tachycardia, tremor, and vomiting. Depression and fatigue usually follow the CNS stimulation. Fatal phentermine overdosage usually terminates in coma and convulsions. Acute phentermine overdosage requires emergency medical support of body systems, with attention to increasing phentermine elimination. There is no known antidote.

Note

1. Phentermine was approved for short-term management of obesity during the 1970s, as was fenfluramine (Pondimin®). Commonly referred to as "phen-fen," the combined use of these two anorexiants became popular during the mid-1990s. Unfortunately, the combination, which was not part of the approved labeling of the two drugs, became associated with serious adverse reactions in women, including valvular heart disease. In the summer of 1997, the FDA began to issue public health advisory statements about the combined use of phentermine and fenfluramine and the risk for valvular heart disease. In response to a request from the FDA and increasing reports of the occurrence of valvular heart disease in women treated for obesity with this combination of drugs, the manufacturer of fenfluramine voluntarily withdrew it from the U.S. market on September 15, 1997.

References

Bray, G.A. (2000). A concise review on the therapeutics of obesity. *Nutrition, 16*(10), 953-960.

Couper, F.J., Pemberton, M., Jarvis, A., et al. (2002). Prevalence of drug use in commercial tractor-trailer drivers. *Journal of Forensic Sciences, 47*(3), 562-567.

Makaryus, J.N., & Makaryus, A.N. (2008), Cardiac arrest in the setting of diet pill consumption. *The American Journal of Emergency Medicine, 26*(6), 732.

Said, S.I. (2006). Mediators and modulators of pulmonary arterial hypertension. *American Journal of Physiology—Lung Cellular and Molecular Physiology, 291*(4), L547-L558.

Seghatol, F.F., & Rigolin, V.H. (2002). Appetite suppressants and valvular disease. *Current Opinion in Cardiology, 17*(5), 486-492.

Yosefy, C., Berman, M., & Beeri, R. (2006). Cusp tear in bicuspid aortic valve possibly caused by phentermine. *International Journal of Cardiology, 106*(2), 262-263.

PIPERAZINE DERIVATIVES[1]

Names

BAN or INN Generic Synonyms: None

Brand/Trade: None

Chemical: See Note 1

Street: A2; BZP; Fly; Legal E; Legal X; Nemesis; TFMPP

Pharmacologic Classification

Psychodelic, miscellaneous: piperazine derivatives

Brief General Overview

Piperazine and several of its derivatives are sold widely around the world as anthelmintic drugs. They are generally well absorbed from the GI tract after oral ingestion and have a relatively high therapeutic index. These drugs are promoted and sold, primarily over the Internet, as "legal Ecstasy" because of their legal status and the sharing of several common pharmacologic actions (e.g., hallucinations, increased blood pressure). Illicit use of these drugs reportedly began in Switzerland and spread to the United States in 2000. The piperazine derivatives are now frequently encountered on high school and college campuses across North America. Increasingly, they are being represented and sold as 3,4-methylenedioxymethamphetamine (MDMA, Ecstasy; see monograph).

Dosage Forms and Routes of Administration

The piperazine derivatives are produced by illicit chemical laboratories[2] in tablet form and are usually orally ingested. They are sold primarily over the Internet and at raves as a legal alternative to MDMA. Adolescents and young adults of European descent are the primary users. There appear to be no gender differences in reported use patterns.

Mechanism of CNS Action

The exact mechanism of the psychodelic actions of the piperazine derivatives has not been determined. However, it appears to involve action on the serotonergic system.

Pharmacodynamics/Pharmacokinetics

Valid and reliable data are not available.

Current Approved Indications for Medical Use

Treatment for worm infestations[3]

Desired Effect/Reason for Personal Use

Hallucinations; MDMA-like effects (including feelings of energy and euphoria and a desire to socialize (see 3,4-Methylenedioxymethamphetamine monograph); sensation of "floating in space"; stimulant actions (mild)

Toxicity

Acute: Hypertension; hyperthermia; locomotor activity (increased); respiratory depression; seizures; tachycardia

Chronic: Valid and reliable data are not available.

Pregnancy & Lactation: Safety of the use of piperazine derivatives by adolescent girls and women who are pregnant has not been established. However, no teratogenic effects have been noted when piperazine derivatives have been used by adolescent girls or women during pregnancy. They appear to be safe for both the mother and the fetus.

Safety of the use of piperazine derivatives by adolescent girls and women who are breast-feeding has not been established. Additional valid and reliable data are needed.

Abuse Potential

Physical dependence: None to low (USDEA: not a scheduled drug)
Psychological dependence: Low

Withdrawal Syndrome

A piperazine derivatives withdrawal syndrome has not been reported.

Overdosage

Piperazine derivatives have been rarely reported to be involved in fatal overdosages. However, there have been no reports of overdosage deaths involving the piperazine derivatives alone. Overdosages involving the piperazine derivatives have been associated with convulsions, hallucinations, and respiratory depression. Thus, overdosage involving the piperazine derivatives requires emergency medical support of body systems. There is no known antidote.

Notes

1. The piperazine derivatives most commonly produced for illicit sale and use in North America include benzylpiperazine (BZP) and trifluromethylphenylpiperazine (TFMPP).
2. BZP and TFMPP are licitly produced by pharmaceutical manufacturers in several countries, principally India. They are readily available over the Internet for direct sale in both individual and bulk quantities.
3. For over half a century, piperazine and some of its derivatives (e.g., diethylcarbamazine) have been used as anthelmintics for the treatment of parasitic infestations of the GI tract.

References

de Boer, D., Bosman, I.J., Hidvegi, E., et al. (2001). Piperazine-like compounds: A new group of designer drugs-of-abuse on the European market. *Forensic Science International, 121*(1-2), 47-56.

Maurer, H.H., Kraemer, T., Springer, D., et al. (2004). Chemistry, pharmacology, toxicology, and hepatic metabolism of designer drugs of the amphetamine (ecstasy), piperazine, and pyrrolidinophenone types: A synopsis. *Therapeutic Drug Monitoring, 26*(2), 127-131.

Staack, R.F., Fritschi, G., & Maurer, H.H. (2002). Studies on the metabolism and toxicological detection of the new designer drug N–benzylpiperazine in urine using gas chromatography-mass spectrometry. *Journal of Chromatography. B, Analytical Technology, Biomedical Life Sciences, 773*(1), 35-46.

Staack, R.F., & Maurer, H.H. (2005). Metabolism of designer drugs of abuse. *Current Drug Metabolism, 6*(3), 259-274.

Yoon, J., Yoo, E.A., Kim, J.Y., et al. (2008). Preparation of piperazine derivatives as 5-HT7 receptor antagonists. *Bioorganic & Medicinal Chemistry, 16*(10), 5405-5412.

PROPANE (see Volatile solvents & inhalants)

PROPOXYPHENE

Names

BAN or INN Generic Synonyms: Dextropropoxyphene

Brand/Trade: 642®; Darvon®; Darvon-N®; Dolene®; Novo-Propoxyn®

Chemical: [(2S,3R)-4-Dimethylamino-3-methyl-1,2-diphenyl-butan-2-yl]propanoate

Street: Footballs; Vons; Yellow Footballs; Yellows

Pharmacologic Classification

Psychodepressant, opiate analgesic: pure agonist (synthetic)

Brief General Overview

Propoxyphene is a relatively weak opiate analgesic that was first marketed in North America in 1957 under the Darvon® brand/trade name. Its analgesic potency is approximately equivalent to that of codeine. Propoxyphene was widely prescribed and personally used during the 1960s, 1970s, and 1980s. Since that time, both medical and personal use have significantly declined. However, it is still significantly used inappropriately in the medical management of the elderly in long-term care facilities.

Dosage Forms and Routes of Administration

Propoxyphene is produced by licit pharmaceutical manufacturers in North America. It is available for oral use as capsules, suspensions, and tablets. Propoxyphene is used by adolescent boys and girls, who usually orally ingest the dosage formulation that may be available to them. Adults, particularly those who are living "on the street," usually prefer to dissolve the capsules or tablets and intravenously inject the resultant propoxyphene solution for its "heroin-like rush." (See Heroin monograph.)

Mechanism of CNS Action

Propoxyphene elicits its analgesic, psychodepressant, and respiratory depressant actions by binding to endorphin receptors in the CNS, primarily the mu receptor. The exact mechanism of action has not been determined. (See also the Opiate Analgesics monograph.)

Pharmacodynamics/Pharmacokinetics

Propoxyphene is well absorbed after oral ingestion and has an onset of action within 15 to 60 minutes. Peak blood concentrations are achieved within 3 hours. Generally, the duration of action is 4 to 6 hours. Propoxyphene is extensively metabolized in the liver, mediated predominantly by cytochrome P4502D6 and 3A4. It is excreted almost entirely as metabolites in the urine. One metabolite, norpropoxyphene, is cardiotoxic. The elimination half-life of propoxyphene ranges from 6 to 12 hours (mean, 13 hours in young adults).

Current Approved Indications for Medical Use[1]

Pain disorders: acute pain, mild to moderate; chronic cancer pain, mild to moderate

Desired Effect/Reason for Personal Use

Euphoria; heroin-like "rush" (when injected intravenously); pain relief; prevention/self-management of the opiate analgesic withdrawal syndrome[2]

Toxicity

Acute: Cognitive impairment (particularly during the first few days of use); constipation; dizziness; drowsiness; dysphoria; headache; insomnia; lightheadedness; miosis; nausea; psychomotor impairment

Chronic: Physical dependence; psychological dependence; seizures[3]; toxic psychosis[3]

Pregnancy & Lactation: FDA Pregnancy Category C (see Appendix B). Safety of propoxyphene use by adolescent girls and women who are pregnant has not been established. Various physical malformations (e.g., beaked nose, congenital hip dislocation, micrognathia) and the signs and symptoms of the neonatal opiate analgesic withdrawal syndrome (e.g., irritability, seizures, tremors) have been reported. However, the data are inconclusive. As a precaution, adolescent girls and women who are pregnant should not use propoxyphene. (Also see the Opiate Analgesics monograph.)

Safety of propoxyphene use by adolescent girls and women who are breast-feeding has not been established. Low concentrations of propoxyphene are excreted in breast milk and appear to be unlikely to affect breast-fed neonates or infants. However, expected pharmacologic actions (e.g., sedation) have been noted in breast-fed neonates whose mothers used medically prescribed propoxyphene during the postpartum period. Adolescent girls and women who are breast-feeding should not use propoxyphene. (Also see the Opiate Analgesics monograph.)

Abuse Potential

Physical dependence: Low to moderate (USDEA Schedule IV; low potential for abuse)
Psychological dependence: Moderate

Withdrawal Syndrome

A propoxyphene withdrawal syndrome has not been reported.

Overdosage

Signs and symptoms of propoxyphene overdosage resemble those observed with other opiate analgesics and include respiratory depression (e.g., decrease in respiratory rate and tidal volume, Cheyne-Stokes respirations), extreme somnolence progressing to stupor or coma, initial constriction of the pupils (miosis) followed by dilation (mydriasis) as hypoxia increases, and circulatory collapse (also see Opiate Analgesics monograph). In addition, local and generalized seizures occur in most cases of severe propoxyphene overdosage. Propoxyphene overdosage, alone or in combination with alcohol or other psychodepressants, has been associated with a significant number of overdosage deaths. Fatalities within the first hour of overdosage are common. Thus, propoxyphene overdosage requires emergency medical support of body systems, with attention to increasing propoxyphene elimination. The opiate analgesic antagonist naloxone (Narcan®) is a specific antidote for the respiratory depression produced by propoxyphene.

Notes

1. The clinical use of propoxyphene for pain management is not generally recommended because of the availability of more efficacious and less toxic therapeutic alternatives.
2. Use of propoxyphene by people who are physically dependent on opiate analgesics is often not sufficient to fully suppress the opiate analgesic withdrawal syndrome.
3. Generally associated with regular, long-term, high-dosage propoxyphene use.

References

Barkin, R.L., Barkin, S.J., & Barkin, D.S. (2006). Propoxyphene (dextropropoxyphene): A critical review of a weak opioid analgesic that should remain in antiquity. *American Journal of Therapeutics, 13*(6), 534-542.

Desai, A.K., & Chibnall, J.T. (2004). Propoxyphene use in the elderly. *Journal of the American Geriatric Society, 52*(7), 1227.

Edwin, T., Nammalvar, N., & Ramanujam, V. (2001). Dextropropoxyphene dependence: A cautionary note. *The Journal of the Association of Physicians of India, 49*, 571-573.

Jonasson, B., Jonasson, U., & Saldeen, T. (2000). Among fatal poisonings dextropropoxyphene predominates in younger people, antidepressants in the middle aged and sedatives in the elderly. *Journal of Forensic Sciences, 45*(1), 7-10.

Jonasson, U., Jonasson, B., & Saldeen, T. (2000). Middle-aged men—a risk category regarding fatal poisoning due to dextropropoxyphene and alcohol in combination. *Preventive Medicine, 31*(2, Part 1), 103-106.

Kamal-Bahl, S.J., Doshi, J.A., Stuart, B.C., et al. (2003). Propoxyphene use by community-dwelling and institutionalized elderly Medicare beneficiaries. *Journal of the American Geriatric Society, 51*(8), 1099-1104.

O'Neill, W.M., Hanks, G.W., Simpson, P., et al. (2000). The cognitive and psychomotor effects of morphine in healthy subjects: A randomized controlled trial of repeated (four) oral doses of dextropropoxyphene, morphine, lorazepam and placebo. (2000). *Pain, 85*(1-2), 209-215.

Singh, S., Sleeper, R.B., & Seifert, C.F. (2007). Propoxyphene prescribing among populations older and younger than age 65 in a tertiary care hospital. *The Consultant Pharmacist, 22*(2), 141-148.

Wu, L.T., Pilowsky, D.J., & Patkar, A.A. (2008). Non-prescribed use of pain relievers among adolescents in the United States. *Drug and Alcohol Dependence, 94*(1-3), 1-11.

Zacny, J.P., & Goldman, R.E. (2004). Characterizing the subjective, psychomotor, and physiological effects of oral propoxyphene in non-drug-abusing volunteers. *Drug and Alcohol Dependence, 73*(2), 133-140.

PSILOCIN

Names

BAN or INN Generic Synonyms: Psilocine; Psilocyn; Psilotsin

Brand/Trade: None

Chemical: 4-Hydroxy-N,N-dimethyltryptamine

Street[1]: Fungus; God's Flesh; *Hombrecitos*; *Las Mujercitas*; *Los Ninos*; Magic Mushrooms; Mexican Mushrooms; Mushrooms; Musk; Philosopher's Stones; Pizza Toppings; Rooms; Sacred Mushrooms; Shrooms; Silly Putty; Simple Simon; Smurfhats; *Teonanácatl*; Toads; Truffles; Umbrellas; Wild Mushroom Tea

Pharmacologic Classification

Psychodelic, LSD-like psychodelic: indole/tryptamine

Brief General Overview

Psilocin, the principal psychodelic ingredient (together with psilocybin; see monograph) in "magic mushrooms," is found primarily in the *Psilocybe* and *Conocybe* mushrooms.[2] As such, it has been used for millennia by Native Americans, particularly in what is now Central America. Over a dozen species of psilocybe mushrooms (e.g., *Psilocybe baeocystis, Psilocybe cubensis [San Isidro], Psilocybe cyanescens* [Blue Halos], *Psilocybe mexicana, Psilocybe stuntzii, Psilocybe semilanceata* [Liberty Caps], *Psilocybe tampanensis*) exist. These and other psilocin-containing mushrooms (e.g., *Panaeolus cyanescens, Panaeolus subalteatus, Stropharia coronilla*) can be found in many parts of the world and have been used for their psychodelic actions and related effects (e.g., for traditional healing and magico-religious ceremonies) by many indigenous peoples, ostensibly "since the beginning of time."

Dosage Forms and Routes of Administration

Psilocin is obtained from psilocybe mushrooms that grow naturally in the wild, in meadows.[3] The mushrooms also may be cultivated from spores; as such, they can be purchased over the Internet for personal use. Although psilocin can be chemically synthesized, the process is costly and difficult. Thus, it is rarely synthesized. Psilocin is distributed in the form of dried mushrooms or as powder-filled capsules for oral use.[4] A solution, which is orally ingested, is sometimes made by soaking the dried mushrooms or dissolving the powder. Psilocin also can be injected intravenously, intranasally sniffed (i.e., snorted), or used by pulmonary inhalation (i.e., smoked).

Mechanism of CNS Action

The exact mechanism by which psilocin produces its psychodelic actions has not been determined. However, it appears to involve agonistic activity at the serotonin 2C receptor (i.e., 5-HT2C receptor). Tolerance can develop with repeated use, and users must discontinue psilocin use for several days to regain the original psychodelic effects. Cross-tolerance to the effects of related psychodelics (e.g., lysergic acid diethylamide [LSD] and mescaline; see monographs) also occurs.

Pharmacodynamics/Pharmacokinetics

Approximately 25% of psilocin is excreted in unchanged form in the urine after intravenous injection, intranasal sniffing, oral ingestion, or smoking. Additional valid and reliable data are not available.

Current Approved Indications for Medical Use

None

Desired Effect/Reason for Personal Use

Auditory and visual distortions (often vivid); ethnomedical healing among various aboriginal peoples of Mexico, Central America, and South America; perceptual distortion of space (feeling of "floating in space"); perceptual distortion of time (time-slowing); heightened sensory experiences; LSD-like effects (synesthesia: seeing sound or hearing color; see Lysergic Acid Diethylamide monograph); magico-religious and ceremonial use among various aboriginal peoples of Mexico, Central America, and South America

Toxicity

Acute: Confusion; disorientation; facial numbness; fear of disintegration of self; hypertension; hyperthermia; lightheadedness; mydriasis; nausea; panic; paranoia; poor concentration; preoccupation with trivial matters or thoughts; psychosis, paranoid schizophrenia (rare); sweating; tachycardia; tremor; vomiting

Chronic: Valid and reliable data are not available.

Pregnancy & Lactation: Valid and reliable data are not available.

Abuse Potential

Physical dependence: None (USDEA Schedule I; use is prohibited)
Psychological dependence: None to low

Withdrawal Syndrome

A psilocin withdrawal syndrome has not been reported.

Overdosage

Psilocin overdosage has not resulted in any reported fatalities. However, it is associated with severe psychological sequelae, including panic and psychosis. Psilocin overdosage requires emergency medical support of body systems, with attention to the management of any associated mental disorders. There is no known antidote.

Notes

1. Since the 1970s, what is generally sold illicitly as "magic mushrooms" is, actually, common edible mushrooms that have been adulterated (laced) with either lysergic acid diethylamide (LSD) or phencyclidine (PCP).
2. Other genera of mushrooms that contain psilocin include *Panaeolus* and *Stropheria (Stropharia)*.
3. Psilocin grows particularly well in cow pastures, where it can be found growing in the cow manure.
4. A rather unusual formulation of psilocin is composed of natural honey in glass jars topped with a 1 cm (about one-half inch) layer of *Psilocybe cubensis*. This formulation, which has been found to contain significant concentrations of psilocin, is commonly available for purchase in Europe, but its availability and use in North America have not been reported.

References

Hasler, F., Bourquin, D., Brenneisen, R., et al. (2002). Renal excretion profiles of psilocin following oral administration of psilocybin: A controlled study in man. *Journal of Pharmaceutical and Biomedical Analysis, 30*(2), 331-339.

Musshoff, F., Madea, B., & Beike, J. (2000). Hallucinogenic mushrooms on the German market—Simple instructions for examination and identification. *Forensic Science International, 113*(1-3), 389-395.

Sard, H., Kumaran, G., Morency, C., et al. (2005). SAR of psilocybin analogs: Discovery of a selective 5-HT 2C agonist. *Bioorganic Medicinal & Chemistry Letters, 15*(20), 4555-4559.

Stricht, G., & Käferstein, H. (2000). Detection of psilocin in body fluids. *Forensic Science International, 113*(1-3), 403-407.

PSILOCYBIN

Names

BAN or INN Generic Synonyms: Psilocybine

Brand/Trade: None

Chemical: O-Phosphoryl-4-hydroxy-N,N-ethyltryptamine

Street[1]: Fungus; God's Flesh; *Hombrecitos*; *Las Mujercitas*; *Los Ninos*; Magic Mushrooms; Mexican Mushrooms; Mushrooms; Musk; Philosopher's Stones; Pizza Toppings; Purple Passion; Sacred Mushrooms; Rooms; Shrooms; Silly Putty; Simple Simon; Smurfhats; *Teonanácatl*; Toads; Truffles; Umbrellas; Wild Mushroom Tea

Pharmacologic Classification

Psychodelic, LSD-like psychodelic: indole/tryptamine

Brief General Overview

Psilocybin, the principal psychodelic ingredient (together with psilocin; see monograph) in "magic mushrooms," is found primarily in the *Psilocybe* and *Conocybe* mushrooms.[2] As such, it has been used for millennia by Native Americans, particularly in what is now Central America. Over a dozen species of psilocybe mushrooms (e.g., *Psilocybe baeocystis*, *Psilocybe cubensis [San Isidro], Psilocybe cyanescens* [Blue Halos], *Psilocybe mexicana, Psilocybe stuntzii, Psilocybe semilanceata* [Liberty Caps], *Psilocybe tampanensis*) exist. These and other psilocybin-containing mushrooms (e.g., *Panaeolus cyanescens, Panaeolus subalteatus, Stropharia coronilla*) can be found in many parts of the world and have been used by many indigenous peoples for their psychodelic and related effects (e.g., for traditional healing and magico-religious ceremonies), ostensibly "since the beginning of time."

Dosage Forms and Routes of Administration

Psilocybin is obtained from psilocybe mushrooms that grow naturally in the wild, in meadows.[3] They also may be cultivated from spores; as such, they can be purchased over the Internet for illicit personal use. Although psilocybin can be chemically synthesized, the process is costly and difficult; thus, it is rarely synthesized.

Psilocybin is distributed in the form of dried mushrooms or powder-filled capsules. A solution is sometimes made by soaking the dried mushrooms or dissolving the powder. The solution is usually orally ingested. However, psilocybin also can be intravenously injected or intranasally sniffed (snorted). It also can be used by pulmonary inhalation (i.e., smoked). In the United States, users tend to be older adolescent boys and young men in their 20s, often in college or university, and they are usually of European descent.

Mechanism of CNS Action

The exact mechanism of action by which psilocybin produces its psychodelic actions has not been determined. However, it appears to involve NMDA antagonism and serotonin (i.e., 5-HT1A, 5-HT2A, and 5-HT2C) agonism. Tolerance can develop with repeated use, and users must discontinue psilocybin use for several days in order to regain the original desired psychodelic effects. Cross-tolerance to the effects of related psychodelics (e.g., lysergic diethylamide [LSD] and mescaline; see monographs) also occurs.

Pharmacodynamics/Pharmacokinetics

Following intravenous injection, intranasal sniffing, oral ingestion, or smoking, psilocybin is converted to psilocin in the body. Approximately 25% of psilocin is excreted in unchanged form in the urine. Additional valid and reliable data are not available.

Current Approved Indications for Medical Use

None

Desired Effect/Reason for Personal Use

Auditory and visual distortions (often vivid); ethnomedical healing among various aboriginal peoples of Mexico, Central America, and South America; perceptual distortion of space (feeling of "floating in space"); perceptual distortion of time (time-slowing); heightened sensory experiences; LSD-like effects (synesthesia: seeing sound or hearing color; see Lysergic Acid Diethylamide monograph); magico-religious and ceremonial use among various aboriginal peoples of Mexico, Central America, and South America

Toxicity

Acute: Anxiety; confusion; disorientation; facial numbness; fear of disintegration of self; flashbacks (rare); hypertension; hyperthermia; lightheadedness; mydriasis; nausea; nervousness; panic; paranoia; poor concentration; preoccupation with trivial matters or thoughts; psychosis, paranoid schizophrenia (rare); reaction time, prolonged; subjective experience of time, altered; sweating; tachycardia; tremor; vomiting

Chronic: Valid and reliable data are not available.

Pregnancy & Lactation: Valid and reliable data are not available.

Abuse Potential

Physical dependence: None (USDEA Schedule I; use is prohibited)
Psychological dependence: None to low

Withdrawal Syndrome

A psilocybin withdrawal syndrome has not been reported.

Overdosage

Psilocybin overdosage has not been fatal. However, it has been associated with severe psychological sequelae, including panic and psychosis. Psilocybin overdosage requires emergency medical support of body systems, with attention to the management of any associated mental disorders. There is no known antidote.

Notes

1. In many cases since the 1970s, what is sold "on the street" as magic mushrooms is actually common edible mushrooms that have been adulterated (laced) with either lysergic acid diethylamide (LSD) or phencyclidine (PCP).
2. Other genera of mushrooms that contain psilocybin include *Panaeolus* and *Stropheria* (*Stropharia*).
3. Psilocybin grows particularly well in cow pastures, where it can be found growing in the cow manure.

References

Carter, O.L., Burr, D.C., Pettigrew, J.D., et al. (2005). Using psilocybin to investigate the relationship between attention, working memory, and the serotonin 1A and 2A receptors. *The Journal of Cognitive Neuroscience, 17*(10), 1497-1508.

Carter, O.L., Pettigrew, J.D., Burr, D.C., et al. (2004). Psilocybin impairs high-level but not low-level motion perception. *Neuroreport, 15*(12), 1947-1951.

Espiard, M.L., Lecardeur, L., Abadie, P., et al. (2005). Hallucinogen persisting perception disorder after psilocybin consumption: A case study. *European Psychiatry, 20*(5-6), 458-460.

Gouzoulis-Mayfrank, E., Thelen, B., Maier, S., et al. (2002). Effects of the hallucinogen psilocybin on covert orienting of visual attention in humans. *Neuropsychobiology, 45*(4), 205-212.

Griffiths, R.R., Richards, W.A., McCann, U., et al. (2006). Psilocybin can occasion mystical-type experiences having substantial and sustained personal meaning and spiritual significance. *Psychopharmacology, 187*(3), 268-283.

Hasler, F., Grimberg, U., Benz, M.A., et al. (2004). Acute psychological and physiological effects of psilocybin in healthy humans: A double-blind, placebo-controlled dose-effect study. *Psychopharmacology, 172*(2), 145-156.

Riley, S.C., & Blackman, G. (2008). Between prohibitions: Patterns and meanings of magic mushroom use in the UK. *Substance Use & Misuse, 43*(1), 55-71.

Rimsza, M.E., & Moses, K.S. (2005). Substance abuse on the college campus. *Pediatric Clinics of North America, 52*(1), 307-319.

Wackermann, J., Wittmann, M., Hasler, F., et al. (2008). Effects of varied doses of psilocybin on time interval reproduction in human subjects. *Neuroscience Letters, 435*(1), 51-55.

Wittmann, M., Carter, O., Hasler, F., et al. (2007). Effects of psilocybin on time perception and temporal control of behaviour in humans. *Journal of Psychopharmacology, 21*(1), 50-64.

PSYCHODELIC MUSHROOMS (See *Amanita muscaria; Psilocin;* and *Psilocybin*)

SALVIA DIVINORUM

Names

BAN or INN Generic Synonyms: Divinorin A; Salvinorin A

Brand/Trade: None

Chemical: See "Mechanism of Action"

Street: Big Sal; Diviner's Mint; Diviner's Sage; *Hierba Maria; Hojas de la Pastora; Hojas de Maria;* Leaves of the Shepherdess; Magic Mint; *Maria Pastora;* Mexican Mint; Mystic Mint; *Pipiltzintzintli;* Sage of the Seers; Sally-D; *Salvia; Ska Maria; Ska Maria Pastora; Ska Pastora; Yerba de Maria*

Pharmacologic Classification

Psychodelic, miscellaneous: terpenoid

Brief General Overview

Salvia divinorum is a perennial herb of the *Lamiaceae* family. It is indigenous to the Sierra Mazateca region of Oaxaca, Mexico, where its magico-religious and shamanistic use in traditional healing ceremonies by indigenous peoples has been documented for well over 400 years. *Salvia divinorum* was "rediscovered" in the 1960s and reintroduced during the mid-1990s to the then current "drug scene," where its use gained popularity, particularly in Britain. *Salvia divinorum* is grown domestically and is personally used for its psychodelic actions. It also is imported into the United States and Canada from Mexico, Central America, and South America. The use of *Salvia divinorum* has been increasing over the past 5 years because it is both legal and relatively easy to obtain, being primarily available to users through Internet sales. North American users are likely to be adolescent boys and young men, particularly of European descent, who are often in college or university.

Dosage Forms and Routes of Administration

Traditionally, the fresh leaves of *Salvia divinorum* are chewed as a "quid" (i.e., a bundle of fresh leaves). The chewed leaves and juices are held in the cheek for maximal buccal absorption of the major psychodelic chemical (i.e., probably salvinorin A), in a manner somewhat similar to the chewing of coca leaves (see Cocaine monograph). The fresh leaves of *Salvia divinorum* also can be made into an oral infusion by finely grinding the leaves and extracting the juice, which is then drunk. However, North American users almost always smoke the dried leaves—in much the same way as cannabis or tobacco is smoked—so that the desired effects can be achieved more quickly by pulmonary inhalation.

Mechanism of CNS Action

The exact mechanism of *Salvia divinorum*'s psychodelic actions has not been determined. However, available data suggest that it involves salvinorin A (a neoclerodane diterpene found primarily in the leaves of *Salvia divinorum*), which acts as a potent agonist with the kappa endorphin receptor site. Salvinorin A appears to be the only one of the several salvinorins that has significant affinity for any of the endorphin receptors.

Pharmacodynamics/Pharmacokinetics

The principal active chemical in *Salvia divinorum*, salvinorin A, appears to be absorbed buccally when the fresh leaves are chewed. The onset of action after chewing a quid or bundle of leaves for 15 minutes is usually between 5 to 15 minutes. Associated effects generally persist for ~1 hour. When the leaves are made into an infusion and orally ingested, the psychodelic action of *Salvia divinorum* appears to be related to the degree of buccal absorption achieved before the oral infusion is actually swallowed. The onset of action after smoking the dried leaves is generally immediate (i.e., within 30 seconds), and actions persist for up to 30 minutes. Salvinorin A undergoes high first-pass hepatic metabolism ($F < 0.1$) and extensive hydrolysis by plasma esterases. Its mean elimination half-life is ~1 hour.

Current Approved Indications for Medical Use

None

Desired Effect/Reason for Personal Use

Ethnomedical or traditional healing among various aboriginal peoples of Mexico, Central America, and South America; hallucinations (primarily visual and similar to those associated with mescaline and psilocybin use; see monographs); magico-religious and cermonial use for the purposes of "divination" and healing[1] among various aboriginal peoples of Mexico, Central America, and South America; modified perception of external reality; psychospiritual awakening or rejuvenation

Toxicity

Acute: Dizziness; dysphoria; fear of disintegration of self; hallucinations (primarily visual); hyperthermia; intense feeling of derealization; laughter (uncontrolled); nausea; psychomotor impairment

Chronic: Regular, long-term use increases risk for suicide. Additional valid and reliable data are not available.

Pregnancy & Lactation: Valid and reliable data are not available.

Abuse Potential

Physical dependence: None to low (USDEA: not a scheduled drug)
Psychological dependence: Low

Withdrawal Syndrome

A *Salvia divinorum* withdrawal syndrome has not been reported.

Overdosage

Valid and reliable data are not available. However, on the basis of the observed toxicities and the relatively short duration of action, it is expected that minimal medical intervention would be required. Naloxone (Narcan®) has been theoretically suggested as a possible antidote. (See the Opiate Analgesics monograph.)

Note

1. Indigenous peoples in Mexico use *Salvia divinorum* for "divination" (i.e., to facilitate contacting the spirits of the dead). As such, use is generally reserved exclusively for healers (i.e., *curanderas* or *curanderos*) or shamans.

References

Chavkin, C., Sud, S., Jin, W., et al. (2004). Salvinorin A, an active component of the hallucinogenic sage salvia divinorum is a highly efficacious kappa-opioid receptor agonist: Structural and functional considerations. *The Journal of Pharmacology & Experimental Therapeutics, 308*(3), 1197-1203.

Dalgarno, P. (2007). Subjective effects of Salvia divinorum. *Journal of Psychoactive Drugs, 39*(2), 143-149.

Giroud, C., Felber, F., Augsburger, M., et al. (2000). Salvia divinorum: An hallucinogenic mint which might become a new recreational drug in Switzerland. *Forensic Science International, 112*(2-3), 143-150.

González, D., Riba, J., Bouso, J.C., et al. (2006). Pattern of use of subjective effects of Salvia divinorum among recreational users. *Drug and Alcohol Dependence, 85*(2), 157-162.

Grundmann, O., Phipp, S.M., Zadezensky, I., et al. (2007). Salvia divinorum and salvinorin A: An update on pharmacology and analytical methodology. *Planta Medica, 73*(10), 1039-1046.

Hanes, K.R. (2001). Antidepressant effects of the herb Salvia Divinorum: A case report. *Journal of Clinical Psychopharmacology, 21*, 634-635.

Hoover, V., Marlowe, D.B., Patapis, N.S., et al. (2008). Internet access to Salvia divinorum: Implications for policy, prevention, and treatment. *Journal of Substance Abuse Treatment, 35*(1), 22-27.

Lange, J.E., Reed, M.B., Croff, J.M., et al. (2008). College student use of Salvia divinorum. *Drug and Alcohol Dependence, 94*(1-3), 263-266.

Munro, T.A., Rizzacasa, M.A., Roth, B.L., et al. (2005). Studies toward the pharmacophore of salvinorin A, a potent kappa opioid receptor agonist. *Journal of Medicinal Chemistry, 48*(2), 345-348.

Prisinzano, T.E. (2005). Psychopharmacology of the hallucinogenic sage Salvia divinorum. *Life Sciences, 78*(5), 527-531.

Roth, B.L., Baner, K., Westkaemper, R., et al. (2002). Salvinorin A: A potent naturally occurring nonnitrogenous kappa opioid selective agonist. *Proceedings of the National Academy of Sciences of the United States of America, 99*(18), 11934-11939.

Singh, S. (2007). Adolescent salvia substance abuse. *Addiction, 102*(5), 823-824.

Vortherms, T.A., & Roth, B.L. (2006). Salvinorin A: From natural product to human therapeutics. *Molecular Interventions, 6*(5), 257-265.

SALVINORIN A (See *Salvia divinorum*)

SECOBARBITAL

Names

BAN or INN Generic Synonyms: Quinalbarbitone

Brand/Trade: Barbasec®; Novosecobarb®; Seconal®

Chemical: 5-Allyl-5-(1-methylbutyl)barbituric acid

Street: 40s; Border; Bullet; Canadian Bouncer; Cardinals; Devil; *Diablo Rojas*; Downs; F-40s; Forties; Ju-Ju; Lillys; Loads; M&Ms; Marshmallow Reds; Mexican Red; Pink Ladies; Pinks; Red Birds; Red Bullets; Red Devils; Red Dolls; Red Jackets; Red Jelly Beans; Red Lillies; Reds; *Rojas*; Sec; Seccy; Secs; Seggy; Sex; Strawberries

Pharmacologic Classification

Psychodepressant, sedative-hypnotic: barbiturate

Brief General Overview

Secobarbital is a short-acting barbiturate with sedative-hypnotic action. It was one of the two barbiturates most widely medically prescribed and personally used[1] during the 1950s, 1960s, and 1970s. However, its clinical and personal use decreased significantly during the last two decades of the 20th century as a result of the development and availability of the benzodiazepines (see Benzodiazepines monograph).

Dosage Forms and Routes of Administration

Secobarbital is produced by licit pharmaceutical manufacturers in North America. It is available in a variety of dosage formulations, including injectables for intramuscular and intravenous injection, oral capsules and tablets, and rectal suppositories. "Prescription addicts" tend to ingest the capsules and tablets. "Street addicts" tend to inject secobarbital intravenously.

Mechanism of CNS Action

The exact mechanism of secobarbital's psychodepressant actions has not been determined. However, secobarbital appears to act primarily at the level of the thalamus, where it interferes with impulse transmission to the cortex. (See also the Barbiturates monograph.)

Pharmacodynamics/Pharmacokinetics

Absorption of secobarbital after oral ingestion is generally rapid and complete (~90%). Once absorbed, distribution is rapid. Of the barbiturates, secobarbital has the highest degree of lipid solubility and, thus, the fastest distribution. Approximately 45% of secobarbital is bound to plasma proteins. The onset of action depends on the method of use but generally is within 10 to 15 minutes. The onset of action following rectal insertion is similar to that after oral ingestion. The onset of action following intramuscular injection is slightly faster than that following either oral ingestion or rectal insertion. The duration of action is 3 to 4 hours. Secobarbital is almost completely metabolized, with <5% excreted in unchanged form in the urine. The mean elimination half-life for adults is ~30 hours (range, 15 to 40 hours).

Current Approved Indications for Medical Use[2]

Sleep disorders: insomnia (short-term management)

Desired Effect/Reason for Personal Use

Alcohol-like disinhibitory euphoria or "high"; anxiety/stress reduction; prevention/self-management of the barbiturate withdrawal syndrome; relaxation; tranquility

Toxicity

Acute: Bradycardia; cognitive impairment; confusion; headache; hypotension; lethargy; psychomotor impairment; respiratory depression; skin rash

Chronic: Osteomalacia (rare); physical dependence; psychological dependence; suppression of REM sleep

Pregnancy & Lactation: FDA Pregnancy Category D (see Appendix B). Secobarbital use during pregnancy appears unlikely to result in congenital malformations. However, use near term or during labor may result in respiratory depression and the barbiturate withdrawal syndrome in neonates, which can be delayed in onset for up to 14 days. Adolescent girls and women who are pregnant should not use secobarbital.

Safety of secobarbital use by adolescent girls and women who are breast-feeding has not been established. Secobarbital is generally excreted in low concentrations in breast milk. Breast-fed neonates and infants may display expected pharmacologic actions (e.g., drowsiness, lethargy). They also may become physically dependent (see also Barbiturates monograph). Adolescent girls and women who are breast-feeding should not use secobarbital.

Abuse Potential

Physical dependence: High (USDEA Schedule II; high potential for abuse)
Psychological dependence: Moderate to high

Withdrawal Syndrome

Sudden discontinuation of regular long-term use of secobarbital may result in the barbiturate withdrawal syndrome. The barbiturate withdrawal syndrome is considered a medical emergency that can result in death if not managed appropriately. (See the Barbiturates monograph.)

Overdosage

See the Barbiturates monograph.

Notes

1. Pentobarbital was the other barbiturate that was commonly medically prescribed and illicitly abused during the 1950s, 1960s, and 1970s (see Pentobarbital monograph).
2. The use of secobarbital for the pharmacologic management of sleep disorders is not generally recommended because of the ready availability of other equally efficacious and less toxic drugs (e.g., benzodiazepines—see monograph).

Reference

Pagliaro, L.A., & Pagliaro, A.M. (2004). *Pagliaros' comprehensive guide to drugs and substances of abuse.* Washington, DC: American Pharmacists Association.

SODIUM OXYBATE (See Gamma-hydroxybutyrate)

SOLVENTS (See Volatile solvents & inhalants)

TEMAZEPAM

Names

BAN or INN Generic Synonyms: None

Brand/Trade: Restoril®

Chemical: 7-Chloro-1,3-dihydro-3-hydroxy-1-methyl-5-phenyl-2H-1,4-benzodiazepin-2-one

Street: Beans, Big T; Blackout; Brainwash; Drunk Pills; Eggs; Green Devils; Green Eggs; Hardball; Jellies; Jellys; King Kong Pills; Knockout Pills; Knockouts; Mazzies; Mind Erasers; Mommy's Big Helper; Mother's Big Helper; No-Gos; Norries; Oranges; Red and Blue; Rugby Balls; Ruggers; Tams; Temazies; Temmies; Terminators; Terms; Tramazi; Vitamin T; Wobbly Eggs

Pharmacologic Classification

Psychodepressant, sedative-hypnotic: benzodiazepine

Brief General Overview

Temazepam is an intermediate-acting benzodiazepine with hypnotic action. It was introduced into clinical practice in 1969 and has been widely used across North America, Europe, and Australia, as well as other parts of the world.

Dosage Forms and Routes of Administration

Temazepam is available in oral capsule form from licit pharmaceutical manufacturers. It also is readily available for purchase over the Internet from a number of on-line pharmacies and other sales sites. Most North American users are adults of European descent who obtain their temazepam by medical prescription. These users usually orally ingest their temazepam dose, sometimes with an alcoholic beverage. Other temazepam users may display more serious patterns of use. These users typically obtain their temazepam by buying it on-line over the Internet, "double-doctoring," forging prescriptions, or stealing it—primarily from nursing homes and pharmacies. These users usually intravenously inject their temazepam after dissolving the capsules.[1] While not yet a major problem in North America, the intravenous use of temazepam has been a significant problem in other countries, including Australia and the United Kingdom.

Mechanism of CNS Action

The exact mechanism of temazepam's hypnotic action has not yet been fully determined. However, it appears to be mediated by, or work in concert with, the inhibitory neurotransmitter GABA. Temazepam appears to produce hypnosis by binding to benzodiazepine receptors within the GABA receptor site complex. (See the Benzodiazepines monograph.)

Pharmacodynamics/Pharmacokinetics

Temazepam is rapidly and well absorbed after oral ingestion and has a mean bioavailability of ~90%. Therapeutic blood concentrations are achieved within 30 minutes, with peak blood concentrations occurring in 2 to 3 hours. Temazepam displays minimal first-pass hepatic metabolism (~8%) and has no active metabolites. Temazepam is moderately (approximately 96%) bound to plasma proteins. The mean apparent volume of distribution is 1 L/kg. Temazepam blood concentration levels decline biphasically, with a mean half-life of elimination of 10 hours (range, 3.5 to 18 hours). The mean total body clearance is 4.2 L/hour. Approximately 1% is excreted in unchanged form in the urine.

Current Approved Indications for Medical Use[2]

Sleep disorders: insomnia (short-term symptomatic management)

Desired Effect/Reason for Personal Use

Alcohol-like disinhibition euphoria or "high"; anxiety/stress reduction; also, purposely administered to others without their knowledge in the context of a drug-facilitated crime (e.g., robbery; sexual assault, including date rape)

Toxicity

Acute: Cognitive impairment; confusion; depression; dizziness; drowsiness; fatigue; hangover effect; headache; lethargy; nausea; memory impairment (anterograde amnesia); vomiting

Chronic: Physical dependence; psychological dependence

Pregnancy & Lactation: FDA Pregnancy Category X (see Appendix B). Safety of temazepam use by adolescent girls and women who are pregnant has not been determined. However, temazepam has caused teratogenic effects in several animal species. The similarity of these effects to those caused in humans by other benzodiazepines (see Benzodiazepines monograph) has resulted in a decision by FDA to contraindicate the use of temazepam during pregnancy. Adolescent girls and women who are pregnant should not use temazepam.

Temazepam is excreted in breast milk in quantities sufficient for breast-fed infants to display expected pharmacologic actions (e.g., drowsiness, lethargy, poor sucking). Adolescent girls and women who are breast-feeding should not use temazepam.

Abuse Potential

Physical dependence: Low to moderate (USDEA Schedule IV; low potential for abuse)
Psychological dependence: Moderate

Withdrawal Syndrome

A temazepam withdrawal syndrome, similar to the withdrawal syndromes associated with alcohol and with other benzodiazepines, has been observed upon abrupt discontinuation of regular, long-term use of temazepam. This syndrome is characterized by abdominal cramps, irritability, memory impairment, nervousness, rebound insomnia, and vomiting. Regular, long-term use should be gradually discontinued in order to avoid this syndrome. (See also the Benzodiazepines monograph.)

Overdosage

Temazepam overdosage may be fatal. Signs and symptoms of acute temazepam overdosage are related to its CNS depressant action and include confusion, dizziness, fainting, and somnolence. Overdosage involving large amounts of temazepam may result in respiratory depression, hypotension, and coma with reduced or absent reflexes. Temazepam overdosage requires emergency medical support of body systems, with attention to increasing temazepam elimination. The benzodiazepine antagonist flumazenil (Anexate®, Romazicon®) is a specific antidote for known or suspected benzodiazepine overdosage.[3]

Notes

1. Intravenous injection of temazepam is associated with greater morbidity (e.g., infections and ulcers at injection sites) and mortality than other methods of use. In addition, sometimes a specific characteristic of the drug formulation is particularly problematic (see, for example, the discussion of talc graulomas in the Pentazocine monograph). In the case of temazepam, intravenous injection of the dissolved capsules tends to result in thromboses in the injected arteries with resultant gangrene of the distal extremity, in some cases leading to amputation.
2. Also used by the U.S. military as a "no-go pill" to help pilots sleep after a mission.
3. Caution is required, because flumazenil antagonism may precipitate the temazepam withdrawal syndrome in people who are physically dependent on temazepam.

References

Bechtel, L.K., & Holstege, C.P. (2007). Criminal poisoning: Drug-facilitated sexual assault. *Emergency Medical Clinics of North America, 25*(2), 499-525.

Beynon, C.M., McVeigh, C., McVeigh, J., et al. (2008). The involvement of drugs and alcohol in drug-facilitated sexual assault: A systematic review of the evidence. *Trauma, Violence, & Abuse, 9*(3), 178-188.

Breen, C.L., Degenhardt, L.J., Bruno, R.B., et al. (2004). The effects of restricting publicly subsidised temazepam capsules on benzodiazepine use among injecting drug users in Australia. *The Medical Journal of Australia, 181*(6), 300-304.

Butler, J.M., & Begg, E.J. (2008). Free drug metabolic clearance in elderly people. *Clinical Pharmacokinetics, 47*(5), 297-321.

Degenhardt, L.J., Roxburgh, A., van Beek, I., et al. (2008). The effects of the market withdrawal of temazepam gel capsules on benzodiazepine injecting in Sydney, Australia. *Drug and Alcohol Review, 27*(2), 145-151.

Dobbin, M., Martyres, R.F., Clode, D., et al. (2003). Association of benzodiazepine injection with the prescription of temazepam capsules. *Drug and Alcohol Review, 22*(2), 153-157.

Elliott, S.P., & Burgess, V. (2005). Clinical urinalysis of drugs and alcohol in instances of suspected surreptitious administration ("spiked drinks"). *Science and Justice, 45*(3), 129-134.

Erman, M.K., Loewy, D.B., & Scharf, M.B. (2005). Effects of temazepam 7.5 mg and temazepam 15 mg on sleep maintenance and sleep architecture in a model of transient insomnia. *Current Medical Research and Opinion, 21*(2), 223-230.

Glass, J.R., Sproule, B.A., Herrmann, N., et al. (2003). Acute pharmacological effects of temazepam, diphenhydramine, and valerian in healthy elderly subjects. *Journal of Clinical Psychopharmacology, 23*(3), 260-268.

Glass, J.R., Sproule, B.A., Herrmann, N., et al. (2008). Effects of 2-week treatment with temazepam and diphenhydramine in elderly insomniacs: A randomized, placebo-controlled trial. *Journal of Clinical Psychopharmacology, 28*(2), 182-188.

Jaffe, J.H., Bloor, R., Crome, I., et al. (2004). A postmarketing study of relative abuse liability of hypnotic sedative drugs. *Addiction, 99(2), 165-173.*

Morgan, K., Dixon, S., Mathers, N., et al. (2004). Psychological treatment for insomnia in the regulation of long-term hypnotic drug use. *Health Techology Assessment, 8*(8), 1-68.

Nickol, A.H., Leverment, J., Richards, P., et al. (2006). Temazepam at high altitude reduces periodic breathing without impairing next-day performance: A randomized cross-over double-blind study. *Journal of Sleep Research, 15*(4), 445-454.

Paul, M.A., Gray, G., MacLellan, M., et al. (2004). Sleep-inducing pharmaceuticals: A comparison of melatonin, zaleplon, zopiclone, and temazepam. *Aviation, Space, and Environmental Medicine, 75*(6), 512-519.

Simons, R., Koerhuis, C.L., Valk, P.J., et al. (2006). Usefulness of temazepam and zaleplon to induce afternoon sleep. *Military Medicine, 171*(10), 998-1001.

Tiplady, B.., Bowness, E., Stien, L., et al. (2005). Selective effects of clonidine and temazepam on attention and memory. *Journal of Psychopharmacology, 19*(3), 259-265.

Voshaar, R.C., van Balkom, A.J., & Zitman, F.G. (2004). Zolpidem is not superior to temazepam with respect to rebound insomnia: A controlled study. *European Neuropsychopharmacology, 14*(4), 301-306.

TETRAHYDROCANNABINOL (See Cannabis)

THIOPENTAL (See Barbiturates)

TOBACCO (See Nicotine)

TOLUENE (See Glue)

TRAMADOL

Names

BAN or INN Generic Synonyms: None

Brand/Trade: Ralivia®; Tridural®; Ultram®; Ultram ER®; Zytram XL®

Chemical: (±)cis-2-[(Dimethylamino)methyl]-1-(3-methoxyphenyl)cyclohexanol

Street: None

Pharmacologic Classification

Psychodepressant, opiate analgesic congener[1]: mixed agonist/antagonist (synthetic)

Brief General Overview

Tramadol, a synthetic analogue of codeine, is a centrally acting analgesic with a potency estimated to be about one-tenth that of morphine. It was introduced into clinical practice in North America in 1995. Because preclinical data suggested a very low potential for abuse, it was not a "scheduled" drug under the U.S. Federal Controlled Substances Act. However, since its introduction, a number of confirmed cases of physical dependence (with tolerance), psychological dependence, and overdosage involving tramadol have been reported in the literature. Tramadol is personally used for its psychodepressant, analgesic, and other actions.

Dosage Forms and Routes of Administration

Tramadol is produced by licit pharmaceutical manufacturers in North America. It is available in oral tablet and oral extended-release capsule formulations. It is usually orally ingested. However, users are increasingly (1) chewing the oral extended-release formulations to obtain the entire dose at once, (2) crushing the oral dosage forms and intranasally sniffing (i.e., snorting) the resultant powder, and (3) dissolving the oral dosage forms and injecting the resultant solution intravenously. Over the past decade, tramadol has been increasingly purchased from pharmacies over the Internet—a practice greatly facilitated by its "nonscheduled" status. It is most commonly used by people who have chronic pain, including health care professionals, and people who are physically and psychologically dependent on the opiate analgesics.

Mechanism of CNS Action

The exact mechanism of tramadol's analgesic action has not been determined. However, both tramadol and its active metabolite, O-desmethyltramadol (M1), selectively bind to mu opiate receptors, which would account for the observed analgesic action.[2] In addition, tramadol inhibits the reuptake of selective monoamines (i.e., norepinephrine, serotonin), which also may contribute to tramadol's analgesic action, as well as to potential drug interactions.

Pharmacodynamics/Pharmacokinetics

Tramadol is well absorbed from the GI tract after oral ingestion ($F = 0.75$). The ingestion of food does not affect the rate nor the extent of tramadol absorption. Peak blood concentrations are achieved by ~2 hours. Analgesia generally occurs within 1 hour after ingestion, peaks within 2 to 3 hours, and lasts for 3 to 6 hours. Tramadol is only weakly bound to plasma proteins (approximately 20%) and has an apparent volume of distribution of ~3 L/kg. Tramadol is extensively metabolized, primarily by the polymorphic hepatic microsomal enzyme cytochrome P4502D6, to several metabolites, including an active metabolite, M1. Thus, people with different genotypes for CYP2D6 activity will display different pharmacokinetics and pharmacodynamics, as well as toxicity. Total body clearance is ~19 L/hour. The mean elimination half-life is about 6 hours. However, significant hepatic impairment (e.g., advanced cirrhosis; hepatic cancer) can reduce metabolic clearance by up to 50% and double the half-life of elimination. Approximately 30% of tramadol is excreted in unchanged form in the urine. Renal impairment significantly reduces the total body clearance of both tramadol and M1.

Current Approved Indications for Medical Use

Pain disorders: acute and chronic pain (moderate to severe)

Desired Effect/Reason for Personal Use

Euphoria; pain relief

Toxicity[3]

Acute: Agitation; anorexia; asthenia; blurred vision; cognitive impairment; constipation; dizziness; drowsiness; dry mouth; dysphoria; flushing; headache; hypotension (orthostatic); nausea; nervousness; pruritus; respiratory depression (significantly less than that noted with morphine); seizures[4]; sneezing; somnolence; sweating; tremors; vomiting

Chronic: Physical dependence; psychological dependence

Pregnancy & Lactation: FDA Pregnancy Category C (see Appendix B). Safety of tramadol use by adolescent girls and women who are pregnant has not been established. However, tramadol crosses the placental barrier, and use during labor has resulted in fetal death and stillbirth, neonatal seizures, and a neonatal tramadol withdrawal syndrome. Adolescent girls and women who are pregnant should not use tramadol.

Safety of tramadol use by adolescent girls and women who are breast-feeding has not been established. A small amount (about 0.1%) of the maternal dose of tramadol is excreted in breast milk. However, this small amount should not normally be harmful to breast-fed neonates or infants. Additional valid and reliable data are needed.

Abuse Potential

Physical dependence: High (USDEA: not a scheduled drug)
Psychological dependence: Moderate to high

Withdrawal Syndrome

Abrupt discontinuation of regular, long-term tramadol use, particularly high-dosage use, may result in an acute tramadol withdrawal syndrome. The signs and symptoms of this syndrome include anxiety, diarrhea, insomnia, nausea, pain, piloerection, rigors, sweating, tremors, and upper respiratory tract signs and symptoms. In addition, atypical signs and symptoms may occur in ~10% of cases of tramadol withdrawal, including anxiety (extreme), confusion, hallucinations (rare), panic attacks, paranoia, and paresthesias. Regular, long-term use of tramadol should be gradually discontinued in order to avoid the occurrence of this withdrawal syndrome.

Overdosage

Signs and symptoms of tramadol overdosage include bradycardia, coma, hypotension, miosis, myocardial infarction, respiratory depression, and seizures. Tramadol overdosage can be fatal and should be treated as a medical emergency requiring support of body systems, with attention to maintaining adequate ventilation and increasing tramadol elimination. There is no known antidote. The opiate antagonist naloxone (Narcan®) does not consistently counteract the lethality of tramadol overdosage.[5] It only reverses some of the signs and symptoms of overdosage and may actually increase the risk for seizures. The seizures may require management with diazepam (see monograph) pharmacotherapy.

Notes

1. Although acting at the opiate receptor (see "Mechanism of CNS Action"), tramadol is neither a natural nor a synthetic derivative of opium. Therefore, it is not considered a true or classic opiate analgesic and, consequently, is not subject to control under the U.S. Federal Controlled Substances Act.
2. However, tramadol-induced analgesia is only partially antagonized by naloxone (Narcan®).
3. A high percentage of people of northern African or southern European descent are ultra-rapid metabolizers of tramadol to its active metabolite, M1. These carriers of the CYP2D6 gene duplication have a significantly higher incidence of related adverse drug reactions.
4. Seizure risk is increased among users who (1) have a preexisting seizure disorder, (2) concomitantly use other epileptogenic drugs (e.g., amphetamines, tricyclic antidepressants), or (3) use high dosages of tramadol.
5. Caution is required, because naloxone may precipitate the tramadol withdrawal syndrome in people who are physically dependent on tramadol.

References

Brinker, A., Bonnel, R.A., & Beitz, J. (2002). Abuse, dependence, or withdrawal associated with tramadol. *The American Journal of Psychiatry, 159*(5), 881.

Freye, E., & Levy, J. (2000). Acute abstinence syndrome following abrupt cessation of long-term use of tramadol (Ultram): A case study. *European Journal of Pain, 4*(3), 307-311.

Gan, S.H., Ismail, R., Wan Adnan, W.A., et al. (2007). Impact of CYP2D6 genetic polymorphism on tramadol pharmacokinetics and pharmacodynamics. *Molecular Diagnosis & Therapy, 11*(3), 171-181.

Garcia-Quetglas, E., Azanza, J.R., Sádaba, B., et al. (2007). Pharmacokinetics of tramadol enantiomers and their respective phase I metabolites in relation to CYP2D6 phenotype. *Pharmacological Research, 55*(2), 122-130.

Kirchheiner, J., Keulen, J.T., Bauer, S., et al. (2008). Effects of the CYP2D6 gene duplication on the pharmacokinetics and pharmacodynamics of tramadol. *Journal of Clinical Psychopharmacology, 28*(1), 78-83.

Kotb, H.I., Fouad, I.A., Fares, K.M., et al. (2008). Pharmacokinetics of oral tramadol in patients with liver cancer. *Journal of Opioid Management, 4*(2), 99-104.

Leo, R.J., Narendran, R., & DeGuiseppe, B. (2000). Methadone detoxification of tramadol dependence. *Journal of Substance Abuse Treatment, 19*(3), 297-299.

Murthy, B.V., Pandya, K.S., Booker, P.D., et al. (2000). Pharmacokinetics of tramadol in children after i.v. or caudal epidural administration. *British Journal of Anaesthesia, 84*(3), 346-349.

Payne, K.A., Roelofse, J.A., & Shipton, E.A. (2002). Pharmacokinetics of oral tramadol drops for postoperative pain relief in children aged 4 to 7 years—A pilot study. *Anesthesia Progress, 49*(4), 109-112.

Pollice, R., Casacchia, M., Bianchini, V., et al. (2008). Severe tramadol addiction in a 61 year-old woman without a history of substance abuse. *International Journal of Immunopathology & Pharmacology, 21*(2), 475-476.

Reeves, R.R., & Liberto, V. (2001). Abuse of combinations of carisoprodol and tramadol. *Southern Medical Journal, 94*(5), 512-514.

Ripple, M.G., Pestaner, J.P., Levine, B.S., et al. (2000). Lethal combination of tramadol and multiple drugs affecting serotonin. *The American Journal of Forensic Medicine and Pathology, 21*(4), 370-374.

Senay, E.C., Adams, E.H., Geller, A., et al. (2003). Physical dependence on Ultram (tramadol hydrochloride): Both opioid-like and atypical withdrawal symptoms occur. *Drug and Alcohol Dependence, 69*(3), 233-241.

Stamer, U.M., Musshoff, F., Kobilay, M., et al. (2007). Concentrations of tramadol and O-desmethyltramadol enantiomers in different CYP2D6 genotypes. *Clinical Pharmacology & Therapeutics, 82*(1), 41-47.

Stamer, U.M., Stüber, F., Muders, T., et al. (2008). Respiratory depression with tramadol in a patient with renal impairment and CYP2D6 gene duplication. *Anesthesia and Analgesia, 107*(3), 926-929.

Withdrawal syndrome and dependence: Tramadol too. *Prescrire International, 12*(65), 99-100.

TRIAZOLAM

Names

BAN or INN Generic Synonyms: None

Brand/Trade: Alti-Triazolam®; Apo-Triazo®; Gen-Triazolam®; Halcion®; Novo-Triolam®; Nu-Triazo®

Chemical: 8-Chloro-6-(o-chlorophenyl)-1-methyl-4H-s-triazolo[4,3-α][1,4]benzodiazepine

Street: Halcyon; Halcyon Daze; Up Johns

Pharmacologic Classification

Psychodepressant, sedative-hypnotic: benzodiazepine

Brief General Overview

Triazolam is a short-acting benzodiazepine sedative-hypnotic. It was primarily developed as an aid to falling asleep. However, the therapeutic use of triazolam has undergone much controversy and debate. Approximately a decade ago, triazolam was removed from clinical use in England and several other European countries because of its association with fatal accidents, particularly among elderly people in whom it caused confusion and both memory and psychomotor impairment. It was suggested that these adverse effects contributed to their falls and other injuries. Although the safety of triazolam for clinical use has been questioned and its use is controversial, it remains available and is still in use in North America. Women are more likely than men to be prescribed triazolam and are also more likely to develop physical and psychological dependence. Triazolam is personally used for its psychodepressant actions.

Dosage Forms and Routes of Administration

Triazolam is produced by licit pharmaceutical manufacturers in North America. It is available in oral tablet form and is orally ingested. People who use triazolam are primarily patients who were prescribed triazolam for the long-term management of anxiety disorders and insomnia. Although most users orally ingest triazolam, some place whole or partial tablets under the tongue, where they are allowed to dissolve and the triazolam is absorbed sublingually. A large percentage of users are professional women (e.g., nurses, teachers) of European descent and patients in long-term care or residential treatment facilities.

Mechanism of CNS Action

Triazolam appears to increase stage 2 sleep and decrease REM sleep. The exact mechanism of its action has not been determined. However, it appears to be mediated by, or to work in concert with, the inhibitory neurotransmitter GABA. Thus, its action appears to be accomplished by binding to benzodiazepine receptors in the GABA complex. (See the Benzodiazepines monograph.)

Pharmacodynamics/Pharmacokinetics

Triazolam is rapidly but only moderately absorbed (mean bioavailability of 45%) after oral ingestion. Peak blood concentrations are achieved within 2 hours. Bioavailability is increased (mean, 55%) with sublingual administration. Triazolam is moderately plasma protein bound (~90%) and has an apparent volume of distribution of ~1 L/kg. It is metabolized extensively in the liver, primarily by CYP3A, to inactive metabolites, including α-hydroxytriazolam (the major metabolite) and 4-hydroxytriazolam. These metabolites are excreted in the urine as conjugated glucuronides (~2% in unchanged form). Triazolam has a short elimination half-life of ~3 hours (range, 1.5 to 5.5 hours). Mean total body clearance is ~25 L/hour. The pharmacokinetics of triazolam display significant age effects. Although peak blood concentrations and total bioavailability may be significantly higher and clearance significantly lower in elderly people, the time to peak blood concentration and differences in elimination half-life generally are insignificant.

Current Approved Indications for Medical Use

Sleep disorders: insomnia (short-term management)

Desired Effect/Reason for Personal Use

Alcohol-like disinhibitory euphoria or "high"; prevention/self-management of the benzo-diazepine withdrawal syndrome; self-management of anxiety and related mental disorders

Toxicity

Acute: Amnesia; ataxia; cognitive impairment; confusion; drowsiness; headache; lethargy; lightheadedness; memory impairment, including anterograde amnesia, particularly with large doses; mental depression; psychomotor impairment; slurred speech

Chronic: Physical dependence; psychological dependence

Pregnancy & Lactation: FDA Pregnancy Category X (see Appendix B). Safety of triazolam use by adolescent girls and women who are pregnant has not been established. On the basis of animal studies and the association of other benzodiazepines with congenital malformations, particularly when used during the first trimester of pregnancy, FDA contraindicated the use of triazolam during pregnancy. Maternal use of therapeutic dosages of benzodiazepines during the last weeks of pregnancy has resulted in neonatal CNS depression and the neonatal benzodiazepine withdrawal syndrome as a result of transplacental distribution (see Benzodiazepines monograph). Adolescent girls and women who are pregnant should not use triazolam.

Safety of triazolam use by adolescent girls and women who are breast-feeding has not been established. Triazolam is excreted in breast milk. Breast-fed neonates and infants may display expected pharmacologic actions (e.g., drowsiness, lethargy). They also may become physically dependent (see Benzodiazepines monograph). Adolescent girls and women who are breast-feeding should not use triazolam.

Abuse Potential

Physical dependence: Moderate (USDEA Schedule IV; low potential for abuse)
Psychological dependence: Moderate

Withdrawal Syndrome

Regular, long-term use of triazolam (and other benzodiazepines) is associated with the development of physical and psychological dependence. A withdrawal syndrome has been associated with abrupt discontinuation of regular, long-term benzodiazepine use. Signs and symptoms of withdrawal range from mild dysphoria and insomnia to more severe signs and symptoms such as abdominal and muscle cramps, convulsions, sweating, tremors, and vomiting. The severity and duration of the withdrawal syndrome appear to be related to the dosage used and the duration of regular, long-term use. (See the Benzodiazepines monograph.)

Overdosage

Signs and symptoms of triazolam overdosage generally are extensions of its pharmacologic actions and include confusion, excessive drowsiness, incoordination, slurred speech, and, ultimately, coma. Respiratory depression, apnea, and death have been associated with triazolam overdosage alone (usually associated with suicide attempt or completion) or in combination with the use of alcohol. In the latter cases, blood concentrations of triazolam and alcohol have been lower than those usually associated with overdosage death for each drug alone. Triazolam overdosage requires emergency medical support of body systems, with attention to increasing triazolam elimination. The benzodiazepine antagonist flumazenil (Anexate®, Romazicon®) is the specific antidote for benzodiazepine overdosage.[1]

Note

1. Caution is required, because flumazenil antagonism may precipitate the benzodiazepine withdrawal syndrome in people who are physically dependent on triazolam.

References

Abraham, J. (2002). Transnational industrial power, the medical profession and the regulatory state: Adverse drug reactions and the crisis over safety of Halcion in the Netherlands and the UK. *Social Science & Medicine, 55*(9), 1671-1690.

Fillmore, M.T., Rush, C.R., Kelly, T.H., et al. (2001). Triazolam impairs inhibitory control of behavior in humans. *Experimental and Clinical Psychopharmacology, 9*(4), 363-371.

Fraser, A.D. (1998). Use and abuse of the benzodiazepines. *Therapeutic Drug Monitoring, 20*(5), 481-489.

Gabe, J. (2001). Benzodiazepines as a social problem: The case of halcion. *Substance Abuse & Misuse, 36*(9-10), 1233-1259.

Greenblatt, D.J., Gan, L., Harmatz, J.S. (2005). Pharmacokinetics and pharmacodynamics of single-dose triazolam: Electroencephalography compared with the Digit-Symbol Substitution Test. *British Journal of Clinical Pharmacology, 60*(3), 244-248.

Greenblatt, D.J., Harmatz, J.S., von Moltke, L.L., et al. (2000). Comparative kinetics and response to the benzodiazepine agonists triazolam and zolpidem: Evaluation of sex-dependent differences. *The Journal of Pharmacology and Experimental Therapeutics, 293*(2), 435-443.

Levine, B., Grieshaber, A., Pestaner, J., et al. (2002). Distribution of triazolam and alpha-hydroxytriazolam in a fatal intoxication case. *Journal of Analytical Toxicology, 26*(1), 52-54.

Lin, D.L., Huang, T.Y., Liu, H.C., et al. (2005). Urinary excretion of alpha-hydroxytriazolam following a single dose of halcion. *Journal of Analytical Toxicology, 29*(2), 118-123.

Maubach, K.A., Martin, K., Choudhury, H.I., et al. (2004), Triazolam suppresses the induction of hippocampal long-term potentiation. *Neuroreport, 15*(7), 1145-1149.

Mintzer, M.Z., & Griffiths, R.R. (2002). Alcohol and triazolam: Differential effects on memory, psychomotor performance and subjective ratings of effects. *Behavioural Pharmacology, 13*(8), 653-658.

Mintzer, M.Z., Griffiths, R.R., Contoreggi, C., et al. (2001). Effects of triazolam on brain activity during episodic memory encoding: A PET study. *Neuropsychopharmacology, 25*(5), 744-756.

Moriya, F., & Hashimoto, Y. (2003). A case of fatal triazolam overdose. *Legal Medicine, 5*(Supplement 1), S91-S95.

Ohshima, T. (2005). Criminal injury case using vegetable juice intermixed with triazolam. *Journal of Clinical Forensic Medicine, 12*(4), 212-213.

Roehrs, T., Bonahoom, A., Pedrosi, B., et al. (2002). Nighttime versus daytime hypnotic self-administration. *Psychopharmacology (Berlin), 161*(2), 137-142.

Simpson, C.A., & Rush, C.R. (2002). Acute performance-impairing and subject-rated effects of triazolam and temazepam, alone and in combination with ethanol, in humans. *Journal of Psychopharmacology, 16*(1), 23-34.

Tanaka, R. (2002). Toxicological interactions between alcohol and benzodiazepines. *Journal of Toxicology. Clinical Toxicology, 40*(1), 69-75.

Tsujikawa, K., Kuwayama, K., Miyaguchi, H., et al. (2005). Urinary excretion profiles of two major triazolam metabolites, alpha-hydroxytriazolam and 4-hydroxytriazolam. *Journal of Analytical Toxicology, 29*(4), 240-243.

Tweedy, C.M., Milgrom, P., Kharasch, E.D., et al. (2001). Pharmacokinetics and clinical effects of sublingual triazolam in pediatric dental patients. *Journal of Clinical Psychopharmacology, 21*(3), 268-272.

Vansickel, A.R., Hays, L.R., & Rush, C.R. (2006). Discriminative-stimulus effects of triazolam in women and men. *The American Journal of Drug and Alcohol Abuse, 32*(3), 329-349.

Voderholzer, U., Riemann, D., Hornyak, M., et al. (2001). A double-blind, randomized and placebo-controlled study on the polysomnographic withdrawal effects of zopiclone, zolpidem and triazolam in healthy subjects. *European Archives of Psychiatry and Clinical Neuroscience, 251*(3), 117-123.

Yamadera, H., Suzuki, H., Kudo, Y., et al. (2002). The study of polysomnography and sleepiness the morning after administration of triazolam and brotizolam. *Psychiatry and Clinical Neurosciences, 56*(3), 297-298.

TRICHLOROETHANE (See Volatile solvents & inhalants)

3,4,5-TRIMETHOXYAMPHETAMINE

Names

BAN or INN Generic Synonyms: None

Brand/Trade: None

Chemical: (±)-3,4,5-Trimethoxy-α-methylphenethylamine

Street: Mescalamphetamine; TMA

Pharmacologic Classification

Psychodelic, amphetamine-like psychodelic: phenethylamine

Brief General Overview

3,4,5-Trimethoxyamphetamine (TMA) is an MDA-like compound that was first synthesized in 1933. It produces amphetamine-like effects (e.g., anorexia, mydriasis, tachycardia) at lower dosages and mescaline-like effects (e.g., hallucinations, synesthesia) at higher dosages. The toxicity that frequently accompanies the use of higher dosages has tended to limit its personal use.

Dosage Forms and Routes of Administration

TMA is produced by illicit chemists.[1]

Mechanism of CNS Action

Valid and reliable data are not available.

Pharmacodynamics/Pharmacokinetics

Valid and reliable data are not available.

Current Approved Indications for Medical Use

None

Desired Effect/Reason for Personal Use

Dissociation from environment; euphoria; hallucinations (primarily visual); heightened emotions; pseudohallucinations; rapid flow of ideas; sense of well-being; synesthesia; tactile sensations (heightened)

Toxicity

Acute: Anorexia; blurred vision; bruxism (teeth grinding or clenching); confusion; headache (mild); hypertension; hyperventilation; insomnia; mydriasis; nausea; panic; sweating (excessive); tachycardia; tremor (slight)

Chronic: Valid and reliable data are not available.

Pregnancy & Lactation: Valid and reliable data are not available.

Abuse Potential

Physical dependence: Low (USDEA Schedule I; use is prohibited)
Psychological dependence: Low

Withdrawal Syndrome

A TMA withdrawal syndrome has not been reported.

Overdosage

Valid and reliable data are not available.

Note

1. Trimethoxyamphetamine has six possible aromatic positional isomers (i.e., 2,3,4-, 2,3,5-, 2,3,6-, 2,4,5-, 2,4,6-, and 3,4,5-trimethoxyamphetamine), which differ only in the respective positions of the three methoxy groups on the central benzene ring. At least three of these (e.g., 2,4,5-, 2,4,6-, and 3,4,5-trimethoxyamphetamine) possess psychodelic action.

References

Takahashi, M., Nagashima, M., Suzuki, J., et al. (2008). Analysis of phenethylamines and tryptamines in designer drugs using gas chromatography-mass spectrometry. *Journal of Health Science, 54*(1), 89-96.

Tsujikawa, K., Kanamori, T., Kuwayama, K., et al. (2006, January-December). Analytical profiles for 3,4,5-, 2,4,5-, and 2,4,6-trimethoxyamphetamine. *U.S. Drug Enforcement Administration Resources, Microgram Journal, 4*, 1-12.

Zaitsu, K., Katagi, M., Kamata, H., et al. (2008). Discrimination and identification of the six aromatic positional isomers of trimethoxyamphetamine (TMA) by gas chromatography-mass spectrometry (GC-MS). *Journal of Mass Spectrometry, 43*(4), 528-534.

VOLATILE SOLVENTS & INHALANTS

Names

BAN or INN Generic Synonyms: None

Brand/Trade: See individual monographs: Acetone, Butane, Freon, Gasoline, Glue, and Nitrous Oxide

Chemical: See individual monographs: Acetone, Butane, Freon, Gasoline, Glue, and Nitrous Oxide

Street: See individual monographs: Acetone, Butane, Freon, Gasoline, Glue, and Nitrous Oxide

Pharmacologic Classification

Psychodepressants, volatile solvents & inhalants

Brief General Overview

The volatile *solvents* are a diverse group of chemical compounds that are liquid at room temperature and evaporate readily when exposed to air. The volatile *inhalants* are primarily anesthetic gases (e.g., nitrous oxide) but also include some other gases such as propane, all of which are inhaled in much the same way as volatile solvents. These psychodepressants are generally easy to obtain and use, and the large surface area of the lungs ensures their rapid absorption and onset of action. Virtually any marketed product that contains a volatile organic solvent is capable of being used for its major psychodepressant actions.

The major volatile solvents include chlorinated hydrocarbons (e.g., toluene, which may be found in airplane glues, correction fluids, lacquer thinners, plastic cements, and spray paints); acetone (see monograph), which may be found in nail polish remover, model (e.g., airplane, car) glue, and rubber cements; benzene, which may be found in cleaning fluids, rubber cements, and tire tube repair kits; butane (see monograph), which may be found in cigarette lighters, hair spray, and spray paint; trichloroethylene and trichloroethane, which may be found in contact cement, degreasers, dry cleaner formulations, refrigerants, Liquid Paper® or Wite-Out® correction fluid, and PVC cement; fluorinated hydrocarbons (e.g., freons; see monograph), which may be found in aerosols, air conditioning units, refrigerants, and propellants #11 and #12; gasoline (see monograph); paint thinner; and xylene, which is used in chemical production and manufacturing. The volatile gases include anesthetic gases, particularly nitrous oxide (see monograph), and propane, which is commonly used as a motor vehicle fuel or as a fuel for cooking or heating in the home.

Among eighth-graders, reported lifetime prevalence of volatile solvent and inhalant use peaked during the mid-1990s and since then has remained relatively constant at about 20%. Boys who are of Hispanic descent or who are Native American, as well as those who live in small towns and rural areas, disproportionately report use of volatile solvents and inhalants.

Largely because of easy accessibility and relatively low cost, the number of new volatile solvent and inhalant users in North America appears to be increasing. The volatile solvents and inhalants, personally used for their psychodepressant actions, are now the fourth most commonly used drugs and substances of abuse (after alcohol, cannabis, and tobacco) among adolescents. Of the wide variety of volatile solvents and inhalants currently available in North America, the most frequently used products are air fresheners, computer "air dusters," gasoline, glue, lighter fluid, paint thinners, permanent marking pens (i.e., permanent markers), shoe polish, and spray paint. Some common signs and symptoms of volatile solvent and inhalant use are presented in Table 8.

TABLE 8
Common Signs and Symptoms Associated with Volatile Solvent and Inhalant Use[a]

Anorexia
Apathy
Cache of solvents or inhalants in unusual location (e.g., bedroom closet, school locker)
Dazed appearance
Disorientation
"Drunken" appearance
Empty solvent or spray paint containers in unusual location (e.g., bedroom, school locker)
Nausea
Nosebleeds
Paint stains on clothes or face
Perioral pyodermas
Poor grooming and hygiene
Rapid mood change
Rash around the mouth or nose
Red nose
Rhinitis
Runny eyes
Slurred speech
Sores around the mouth or nose
Spray paint speckles around the mouth or nose
Strong chemical odor to the breath
Strong chemical odor from clothing
Sudden decrease in academic performance
Sudden decrease in school attendance
Volatile solvent-soaked clothes or rags
Weight loss

[a]These signs and symptoms may be indicative of volatile solvent or inhalant use when they are uncharacteristic of an individual's usual behavior or circumstance and are not explained by other causes.
Source: Pagliaro, L.A., & Pagliaro, A.M. (2004). *Pagliaros' comprehensive guide to drugs and substances of abuse.* Washington, DC: American Pharmacists Association.

Dosage Forms and Routes of Administration[1]

The personal use of volatile solvents and inhalants is variously referred to by users as "airblasting," "bagging," "gasing," "huffing," "oiling," "painting," "penny cleaning," "sacking," "sniffing," "spraying," or "Texas shoe-shining." The volatile solvents usually are poured onto or into a rag, balloon, or plastic bag and their vapor inhaled through the mouth or sniffed through the nostrils. Other methods of use include spraying an aerosol product directly into the mouth or nose, placing a solvent-soaked rag in the mouth and inhaling, and removing the lid of a solvent container and inhaling the fumes directly. These methods of use are commonly referred to as "bagging" or "huffing." Users often warm the container by holding it in their hands or over an external heat source, such as a stove or the radiator of a car. Warming the container significantly increases the volatility of the solvents, thus providing a larger dose when inhaled and intensifying the resultant "high."

Mechanism of CNS Action

The volatile solvents and inhalants depress the CNS through a variety of mechanisms that have not been fully elucidated. The result of use is a rapid, short-lived, disinhibition euphoria—very similar to acute alcohol intoxication. The volatile solvents have no generally approved medical use, and little is known about their actual human pharmacology because they were never intended for human personal use involving inhalation. The inhalant gases were developed for use during surgical procedures as anesthetics; thus, there is more information about their therapeutic use and toxicities in humans (also see the Acetone, Butane, Freon, Gasoline, Glue, and Nitrous Oxide monographs).

Pharmacodynamics/Pharmacokinetics

When inhaled into the lungs, volatile solvents and inhalants are readily absorbed into the bloodstream and rapidly reach the brain. The effects of the volatile solvents and inhalants occur within minutes of inhalation, and their psychodepressant effects can last from 10 to 60 minutes depending on the solvent or inhalant used and its dose. Additional valid and reliable data are not available. (Also see the Acetone, Butane, Freon, Gasoline, Glue, and Nitrous Oxide monographs.)

Current Approved Indications for Medical Use

None

Desired Effect/Reason for Personal Use

Alcohol-like disinhibitory euphoria or "high"

Toxicity[2,3]

Acute: The acute signs of toxicity observed in people who use volatile solvents include anorexia; body organ damage, including the heart, liver, kidneys, and lungs; cognitive impairment; fatigue; headache; memory impairment; nausea; psychomotor impairment; slowed, unclear thinking; slurred speech; and thirst. The extent of these acute toxic effects depends on the solvent used, the amount used, and the duration of use. If the user is otherwise healthy, the toxicities associated with the acute use of volatile solvents are usually temporary and reversible. Halogenated hydrocarbons (e.g., bromochlorodifluoromethane, trichloroethane, trichloroethylene) are volatile solvents commonly found in Wite-Out® correction fluid and fire extinguishers. The toxicity of these products is predominantly myocardial and similar to that of the volatile anesthetic gas halothane. These compounds are negative inotropes and thus can cause significant direct myocardial depression and resultant decreased cardiac output through their sensitization of the myocardium to catecholamines, resulting in increased generation of ectopic foci of electrical activity in the heart. These effects may result in ventricular fibrillation and death, a phenomenon that is commonly referred to as "sudden sniffing death" (see following discussion).[4]

Asphyxiation: Asphyxiation has been associated directly with the method of volatile solvent use. Usually a plastic bag is placed over the nose and mouth or the head. This method of use creates the risk of death due to fainting or losing consciousness and subsequent suffocation because the plastic bag remains in place over the nose and mouth. Death in these cases also is associated with the amount of the volatile solvent used. The use of any of these substances in sufficient quantities can depress the CNS enough to cause respiratory arrest.

Death by Accidental Injury: Death by accidental injury typically results from falls and other events that may be associated with the poor judgment and impulsive behavior of the user while intoxicated with a volatile solvent. Death by accidental injury also may be due to fires associated with the use of these flammable substances or to head injuries sustained when users lose consciousness (i.e., "pass out").

Sudden Sniffing Death: Sudden sniffing death has resulted from heart failure or severe respiratory depression. The use of halogenated (e.g., fluorinated) hydrocarbons (e.g., freon), in particular, has been associated with fatal cardiac dysrhythmias. However, any volatile solvent can cause paralysis of the respiratory centers if a large enough dose is absorbed. In most cases, acute sudden sniffing death occurs when users have been engaged in some type of strenuous activity (e.g., running) or have experienced some sudden unexpected stress (e.g., being discovered by a parent or teacher) immediately after heavy use. Both strenuous activity and unexpected stress cause the sudden release of epinephrine in the body. It is believed that volatile solvents increase the heart's sensitivity to the stimulant action of epinephrine and thus contribute to the "heart attack" in the user.

Chronic: Chronic gasoline inhalation can result in a gradually progressive poly-neuropathy. However, it is frequently difficult to ascertain the specific compound responsible for the observed toxicities because the volatile solvents are most often available and used as a complex mixture of compounds. Toluene is one of the most common compounds in volatile solvents, and its use causes a central neuropathy characterized by encephalopathy resulting in behavioral changes (e.g., self-mutilation), hallucinations, ataxia, and convulsions. Chronic use results in CNS deterioration characterized by neuropsychiatric disorders and persistent cerebellar ataxia and peripheral neurotoxicity. Although reflexes are normal, muscle weakness and rhabdomyolysis have been reported. Renal toxicity with severe electrolyte disturbances also has been reported in adults, as have renal calculi. These toxic effects are suspected to be due to increased renal excretion of hippurate, a metabolite of toluene. The profound weakness that may be observed has been related to electrolyte imbalance. Other effects, including abdominal pain, hematemesis, nausea, and vomiting, have been reported to be associated with gastric irritation caused by another toluene metabolite.

Body Organ Damage: Chronic use of volatile solvents may cause damage to several body organs, including the bone marrow, the kidneys, and the liver. In addition, it has been found that volatile solvent-induced alterations in the cell membrane of nervous tissue may be responsible for magnetic resonance imaging (MRI) signal abnormalities observed in the brain white matter of regular, long-term or chronic solvent users. Chlorinated hydrocarbons are particularly toxic to the human body.

Physical and Psychological Dependence: The use of some volatile solvents and inhalants, such as toluene, has been associated with physical and psychological dependence. For most volatile solvents and inhalants, however, the abuse potential and physical dependence liability are still not well understood.

Pregnancy & Lactation: Valid and reliable data are not available.

Abuse Potential

Physical dependence: Moderate (USDEA: not a scheduled drug)
Psychological dependence: Moderate

Withdrawal Syndrome

A volatile solvent and inhalant withdrawal syndrome has not been substantiated. Tolerance to the actions of the volatile solvents can occur with regular long-term use. It is not clear whether physiological withdrawal occurs when regular use is discontinued. Several signs and symptoms (e.g., anxiety, depression, dizziness, insomnia, irritability, tremors) are commonly observed in users when volatile solvent use is discontinued. However, it has not been established whether these signs and symptoms are physical or psychological in origin.

Overdosage

Signs and symptoms of volatile solvent and inhalant overdosage primarily involve impairment of consciousness. Volatile solvent and inhalant overdosage requires emergency medical support, with attention to minimizing continuing exposure to the volatile solvent or inhalant (e.g., removing the user from the site of exposure; removing the source of exposure, including the user's clothing if contaminated by the volatile solvent or inhalant). There is no known antidote.

Notes

1. During the mid-19th century several volatile inhalants, including chloroform, ether, and the newly discovered nitrous oxide (laughing gas), were used by partygoers for fun. More recently, the recreational inhalation of anesthetic gases has been confined mostly to hospital personnel, including operating room and emergency room technicians, nurses, anesthetists, surgeons, and anesthesiologists, presumably because of the lack of awareness by the general public of the existence of these substances and their relative inaccessibility. Nonetheless, in a review of 32 cases of nitrous oxide use, nonmedical users included commercial suppliers of the gas and industrial users. Nitrous oxide is commonly used as the propellant in canned whipped cream (e.g., whippets), which has become a readily available and legal source of supply. In addition, nitrous oxide can be diverted from the automobile industry, where it is used to boost performance of racing cars. Also, the use of anesthetics (e.g., nitrous oxide, halothane, methoxyflurane, enflurane, and isoflurane) stolen from hospitals and medical suppliers for their recreational use has been reported. Although the rate of chronic use appears to be low in comparison with similar drugs and substances of abuse, surveys of

medical and dental students indicate that 10% to 20% have used anesthetic gases.

2. The CNS and peripheral nervous system are the primary organ systems adversely affected by volatile solvents. Most volatile solvents seem to cause a rapid disinhibition mediated by depression of the CNS with resultant euphoria. Occurring concomitantly are drowsiness and gross and fine motor incoordination, with impaired ambulation and slurred speech. Hallucinations have been reported occasionally, and amnesia also can occur.

3. Volatile solvents are usually not available to the public as pure single chemicals but as mixtures containing two or more ingredients in a commercial product. A variety of additives are used to improve performance, stability, or production of these products. Often a second minor ingredient, which does not cause the "high," is more dangerous to the health of the user than the major "high"-producing ingredient. In addition, the various ingredients can sometimes work together to cause serious toxicity or death, even though toxicity would not result if they were used individually.

    In addition, manufacturers frequently change the ingredients or their concentrations in volatile solvent products (e.g., labels that read "new," "improved," "reformulated," "extra strength") so that a product that was previously safe and nontoxic may cause serious toxicity or death. For example, during the early 1970s, seven young men used a popular lacquer thinner that they had safely used many times before. However, the product had been reformulated to decrease production costs during an oil embargo. The result was death from respiratory failure for one of the men, permanent respiratory paralysis for two of the men, and severe muscle and nerve damage for four of the men, who subsequently required the use of wheelchairs. From this tragic example, it is apparent that the potential for serious toxicity accompanies the use of all volatile solvents.

4. The use of nonhalogenated hydrocarbons, including butane (see monograph), isobutane, and propane, also has been associated with fatal cardiac dysrhythmias.

References

Anderson, C.E., & Loomis, G.A. (2003). Recognition and prevention of inhalant abuse. *American Family Physician, 68*(5), 869-874.

Freedenthal, S., Vaughn, M.G., Jenson, J.M., et al. (2007). Inhalant use and suicidality among incarcerated youth. *Drug and Alcohol Dependence, 90*(1), 81-88.

Howard, M.O., Balster, R.L., Cottler, L.B., et al. (2008). Inhalant use among incarcerated adolescents in the United States: Prevalence, characteristics, and correlates of use. *Drug and Alcohol Dependence, 93*(3), 197-209.

Jones, G.R., & Singer, P.P. (2008). An unusual trichloroethanol fatality attributed to sniffing trichloroethylene. *Journal of Analytical Toxicology, 32*(2), 183-186.

LoVecchio, F., & Fulton, S.E. (2001). Ventricular fibrillation following inhalation of Glade Air Freshener. *European Journal of Emergency Medicine, 8*(2), 153-154.

Spiller, H.A. (2004). Epidemiology of volatile substance abuse (VSA) cases reported to US poison centers. *The American Journal of Drug and Alcohol Abuse, 30*(1), 155-165.

ZALEPLON

Names

BAN or INN Generic Synonyms: None

Brand/Trade: Sonata®; Starnoc®

Chemical: N-3-(3-Cyanopyrazolo-[1,5-a]pyrimidin-7-yl)phenyl-N-ethylacetamide

Street: None

Pharmacologic Classification

Psychodepressant, sedative-hypnotic: miscellaneous (pyrazolopyrimidine)

Brief General Overview

Zaleplon is a hypnotic with a relatively rapid onset of action and minimal next-day residual effects (i.e., hangover effects) due to its short half-life of elimination (see "Pharmacodynamics/Pharmacokinetics"). It is personally used for its psychodepressant actions.

Dosage Forms and Routes of Administration

Zaleplon is legally produced as an oral capsule formulation by licit pharmaceutical manufacturers in North America.

Mechanism of CNS Action

Zaleplon is a pyrazolopyrimidine with hypnotic action. Its exact mechanism of action has not been determined. However, it appears to work in concert with the inhibitory neurotransmitter GABA. Zaleplon, although not a benzodiazepine, acts at the benzo-diazepine recognition site of $GABA_A$ receptors, particularly the omega-1 receptor situated on the alpha subunit of the $GABA_A$ receptor complex, and potentiates the GABA-evoked chloride current. It shares many mechanistic features with both triazolam (see monograph) and zolpidem (see monograph).

Pharmacodynamics/Pharmacokinetics

Zaleplon has a limited oral bioavailability ($F = 0.3$) because of extensive first-pass hepatic metabolism. However, it is rapidly absorbed following oral ingestion and achieves peak effects within 1 hour. Zaleplon is ~60% bound to plasma proteins and has a volume of distribution of 1.3 L/kg. Zaleplon is extensively metabolized to several inactive metabolites, primarily 5-oxo-zaleplon (by aldehyde oxidase) and desmethylzaleplon (by CYP3A4). Less than 1% of zaleplon is excreted in unchanged form in the urine. Zaleplon's mean elimination half-life is ~1 hour, and its mean total body clearance is 65 L/hr.

Current Approved Indications for Medical Use

Sleep disorders: insomnia (short-term symptomatic management)

Desired Effect/Reason for Personal Use

Alcohol-like disinhibitory euphoria or "high" (relatively mild); anxiety/stress reduction

Toxicity

Acute: Cognitive impairment; dizziness; dry mouth; headache; lethargy; lightheadedness; memory impairment; psychomotor impairment

Chronic: Mental depression; physical dependence; psychological dependence

Pregnancy & Lactation: FDA Pregnancy Category C (see Appendix B). Safety of zaleplon use by adolescent girls and women who are pregnant has not been established. Additional valid and reliable data are needed.

Safety of zaleplon use by adolescent girls and women who are breast-feeding has not been established. Zaleplon is excreted in breast milk (in small amounts). Additional valid and reliable data are needed.

Abuse Potential

Physical dependence: Low (USDEA Schedule IV; low potential for abuse)
Psychological dependence: Low to moderate

Withdrawal Syndrome

A zaleplon withdrawal syndrome is expected but has not been reported.

Overdosage

Zaleplon overdosage is rarely fatal. Signs of zaleplon overdosage include coma, confusion, psychomotor impairment, respiratory impairment, and somnolence. Zaleplon overdosage requires emergency medical support of body systems, with attention to maintaining respiratory function and increasing zaleplon elimination. There is no known antidote. However, because zaleplon shares many similarities with the benzodiazepines, the benzodiazepine antagonist flumazenil (Anexate®, Romazicon®) may be of some assistance.[1]

Note

1. Caution is indicated, because the use of flumazenil may precipitate a benzodiazepine withdrawal syndrome if the zaleplon user also is physically dependent upon a benzodiazepine.

References

Doghramji, P.P. (2001). Treatment of insomnia with zaleplon, a novel sleep medication. *International Journal of Clinical Practice, 55*(5), 329-334.

Dooley, M., & Plosker, G.L., (2000). Zaleplon: A review of its use in the treatment of insomnia. *Drugs, 60*(2), 413-445.

Israel, A.G., & Kramer, J.A. (2002). Safety of zaleplon in the treatment of insomnia. *The Annals of Pharmacotherapy, 36*(5), 852-859.

Mangano, R.M. (2001). Efficacy and safety of zaleplon at peak plasma levels. *International Journal of Clinical Practice, 1*(Supplement 116), 9-13.

Paul, M.A., Gray, G., Kenny, G., et al. (2003). Impact of melatonin, zaleplon, zopiclone, and temazepam on psychomotor performance. *Aviation, Space, and Environmental Medicine, 74*(12), 1263-1270.

Stillwell, M.E. (2003). Zaleplon and driving impairment. *Journal of Forensic Sciences, 48*(3), 677-679.

Stone, B.M., Turner, C., Mills, S.L., et al. (2002). Noise-induced sleep maintenance insomnia: Hypnotic and residual effects of zaleplon. *British Journal of Clinical Pharmacology, 53*(2), 196-202.

Troy, S.M., Lucki, I., Unruh, M.A., et al. (2000). Comparison of the effects of zaleplon, zolpidem, and triazolam on memory, learning, and psychomotor performance. *The Journal of Clinical Pharmacology, 20*(3), 328-337.

Vermeeren, A., Riedel, W.J., van Boxtel, M.P., et al. (2002). Differential residual effects of zaleplon and zopiclone on actual driving: A comparison with a low dose of alcohol. *Sleep, 25*(2), 224-231.

Verster, J.C., Volkerts, E.R., Schreuder, A.H., et al. (2002). Residual effects of middle-of-the-night administration of zaleplon and zolpidem on driving ability, memory functions, and psychomotor performance. *Journal of Clinical Psychopharmacology, 22*(6), 576-583.

Weitzel, K.W., Wickman, J.M., Augustin, S.G., et al. (2000). Zaleplon: A pyrazolopyrimidine sedative-hypnotic agent for the treatment of insomnia. *Clinical Therapeutics, 22*(11), 1254-1267.

ZIPEPROL

Names

BAN or INN Generic Synonyms: None

Brand/Trade[1]: None

Chemical: o-(α-Methoxybenzyl)-4-(β-methoxyphenethyl)-1-piperazineethanol

Street: None

Pharmacologic Classification

Psychodepressant, miscellaneous opiate analgesic[2]: antitussive (synthetic)

Brief General Overview

Zipeprol is personally used for its psychodepressant actions. Although its use is primarily limited to South Korea, North American adolescents who are dependents of military families stationed in South Korea have been reported to use zipeprol. In addition, isolated cases of zipeprol use have been reported across the United States, particularly along the Mexico–U.S. border. Use also has been reported in France and Italy.

Dosage Forms and Routes of Administration

Zipeprol is produced as an oral liquid by licit foreign pharmaceutical manufacturers for the treatment of cough. Adolescent boys who use zipeprol usually orally ingest it at several times its recommended antitussive dosage.[3]

Mechanism of CNS Action

The exact mechanism of action of zipeprol has not been determined. It does, however, possess high affinity for mu and kappa opiate receptor binding sites and displays weak agonist activity at higher dosages.

Pharmacodynamics/Pharmacokinetics

Zipeprol is absorbed buccally, as well as following oral ingestion. It is rapidly and extensively metabolized,[4] with less than 5% excreted in unchanged form in the urine. Additional valid and reliable data are not available.

Current Approved Indications for Medical Use

Cough suppression[1]

Desired Effect/Reason for Personal Use

Alcohol-like disinhibitory euphoria or "high"; hallucinations; self-management of the opiate analgesic withdrawal syndrome (at higher dosages, zipeprol suppresses some of the associated signs and symptoms)

Toxicity[5]

Acute: Amnesia; confusion; hallucinations; seizures

Chronic: Psychological dependence

Pregnancy & Lactation: Safety of zipeprol use by adolescent girls and women who are pregnant has not been established. A single case of zipeprol-associated fetotoxicity was reported in the clinical literature. This case involved the occurrence of a typical opiate analgesic withdrawal syndrome in the neonate of a mother who regularly used zipeprol during pregnancy. Additional valid and reliable data are needed.

Safety of zipeprol use by adolescent girls and women who are breast-feeding has not been established. It is not known if zipeprol is excreted in breast milk. Additional valid and reliable data are needed.

Abuse Potential

Physical dependence: Low (USDEA: not a scheduled drug)
Psychological dependence: Low to moderate

Withdrawal Syndrome

Limited available data suggest an opiate analgesic-like withdrawal syndrome of low to moderate intensity. It has been reported that the withdrawal syndrome can be precipitated in regular, long-term zipeprol users by the administration of the opiate analgesic antagonist naloxone (Narcan®).

Overdosage

Zipeprol overdosage can be fatal.[6] Severe, acute overdosage requires emergency medical support of body systems, with attention to maintaining respiratory function. Although available data are limited, the use of naloxone (Narcan®), a pure opiate analgesic antagonist, should be attempted as a possible antidote.[7]

Notes

1. Zipeprol is not currently used clinically in North America, but it is available in South Korea under the brand/trade name Zinolta®. Zipeprol also has been available in Europe under the brand/trade names Mirsol®, Respilene®, and Respirase®.
2. On the basis of its pharmacologic characteristics, zipeprol is most likely an opiate (similar to dextromethorphan; see monograph). However, sufficient valid and reliable data are not available to allow definitive classification.
3. This pattern of use is quite similar to that observed with dextromethorphan (see monograph) and, reportedly, dextromethorphan is often used in combination with zipeprol to obtain stronger hallucinogenic effects.
4. The metabolism of zipeprol is principally by N-dealkylation, hydroxylation, methylation, and oxidation.
5. Only limited valid and reliable data are available.
6. In South Korea, where the use of zipeprol is common among adolescents, zipeprol overdosage fatalities steadily increased during the 1990s.
7. Caution is indicated, because the use of naloxone may precipitate an opiate analgesic-like withdrawal syndrome in people who are physically dependent on zipeprol.

References

Pagliaro, L.A., & Pagliaro, A.M. (2004). *Pagliaros' comprehensive guide to drugs and substances of abuse.* Washington, DC: American Pharmacists Association.

ZOLPIDEM

Names

BAN or INN Generic Synonyms: None

Brand/Trade: Ambien®; Ambien CR®; Lunata®; Stella®; Stilnox®

Chemical: N,N,6-Trimethyl-2-p-tolylimidazo[1,2-α]pyridine-3-acetamide

Street: Nappien; Tic-Tacs

Pharmacologic Classification

Psychodepressant, sedative-hypnotic: miscellaneous (imidazopyridine)

Brief General Overview

Zolpidem is a short-acting hypnotic. Although chemically distinct from the benzo-diazepines, its pharmacologic actions are similar in many regards. Zolpidem was introduced into clinical practice in the United States in 1983 as a drug that had little risk for abuse, development of physical or psychological dependence, or occurrence of a withdrawal syndrome when regular, long-term use was abruptly discontinued. However, as with many other drugs and substances of abuse once thought to be free of physical and psychological dependence, these promises turned out to be false.

Dosage Forms and Routes of Administration

Zolpidem is produced by licit pharmaceutical manufacturers. It is available in an oral tablet formulation and is usually orally ingested, although it can be crushed and intranasally sniffed (snorted). More rarely, it is "cooked" (i.e., dissolved in warm liquid), cooled, and intravenously injected. In North America, most zolpidem users are women, 20 to 40 years of age and of European descent, who use zolpidem in larger dosages and for longer periods of time than were prescribed by their physicians. In addition, as with the benzodiazepines (see Benzodiazepines monograph), it has been widely misused by health care workers in extended-care and other facilities for the behavioral management of elderly patients, particularly during the night.

Mechanism of CNS Action

The exact mechanism of zolpidem's psychodepressant action has not been determined. It appears to be mediated or work in concert with the benzodiazepine receptors that are found predominantly in association with the $GABA_A$ receptor, preferentially binding to the α-1 subunit.

Pharmacodynamics/Pharmacokinetics

Zolpidem is rapidly and moderately well absorbed ($F = 0.7$) after oral ingestion. Peak blood concentrations generally are achieved within 1.5 hours. However, ingesting zolpidem with food delays and decreases its absorption. Zolpidem is ~92% bound to plasma proteins and has an apparent volume of distribution of 0.7 L/kg. It is metabolized extensively in the liver and its metabolites are primarily excreted in the urine. Less than 1% of zolpidem is excreted in unchanged form in the urine. Metabolism is dependent on mixed cytochrome P450 isoenzymes, particularly CYP3A4. The mean elimination half-life is 2.5 hours (range, 1.5 to 4.5 hours). The half-life of zolpidem may be prolonged in people with hepatic dysfunction, but is not significantly affected by renal dysfunction. Zolpidem clearance is significantly lower in women (i.e., 3.5 mL/minute/kg) than men (i.e., 6.7 mL/minute/kg).

Current Approved Indications for Medical Use[1]

Sleep disorders: insomnia (short-term symptomatic management)

Desired Effect/Reason for Personal Use

Alcohol-like disinhibitory euphoria or "high"; hallucinations and visual illusions; prevention/self-management of the zolpidem withdrawal syndrome; also, zolpidem is purposely given to others, without their knowledge, in the context of the perpetration of drug-facilitated crime (e.g., robbery; sexual assault, including date rape)

Toxicity

Acute: Ataxia; blurred vision; cognitive impairment; confusion; constipation; delirium[2]; dizziness; drowsiness; dry mouth; GI distress; hallucinations (visual, particularly at extremely high dosages); hangover effects; headaches; heartburn; impaired judgment; increased appetite; lightheadedness; memory impairment (anterograde amnesia); nausea; nightmares; postural sway; psychomotor impairment; red eyes; ringing in the ears (tinnitus); sleepwalking (somnambulism); tremors; weakness

Chronic: Hip fracture[3]; physical dependence[4]; psychological dependence

Pregnancy & Lactation: FDA Pregnancy Category B (see Appendix B). Safety of zolpidem use by adolescent girls and women who are pregnant has not been established. Zolpidem crosses the placenta. Additional valid and reliable data are needed.

Safety of zolpidem use by adolescent girls and women who are breast-feeding has not been established. Additional valid and reliable data are needed.

Abuse Potential

Physical dependence: Low to moderate (USDEA Schedule IV; low potential for abuse)[4]
Psychological dependence: Moderate

Withdrawal Syndrome

Although originally denied when zolpidem was first introduced into clinical practice, a zolpidem withdrawal syndrome has since been identified. It is similar to the benzodiazepine withdrawal syndrome (see Benzodiazepines monograph) and comprises a variety of signs and symptoms, including seizures and drug-induced psychosis, when regular, long-term use of high daily dosages is suddenly discontinued. The standard 7-day diazepam withdrawal program of tapering diazepam (Valium®) doses (see Diazepam monograph) has been used to successfully manage the zolpidem withdrawal syndrome. Signs and symptoms of withdrawal are minimal after short-term use of zolpidem at recommended dosages.

Overdosage

Signs and symptoms of zolpidem overdosage primarily involve impairment of consciousness, which can range from drowsiness to light coma; miosis; and respiratory depression. Zolpidem overdosage requires emergency medical support of body systems, with attention to maintaining adequate respiratory function and increasing zolpidem elimination. There is no known antidote. However, the benzodiazepine antagonist flumazenil (Anexate®, Romazicon®) reportedly has been found to be of some benefit in the management of zolpidem overdosage[5] (see "Mechanism of CNS Action").

Notes

1. The U.S. military uses zolpidem, as well as temazepam (see monograph), as "no-go pills" to help pilots sleep after a mission, particularly after they have been using "go pills."
2. The risk for delirium is particularly high in elderly women.
3. Regular, long-term use of zolpidem by elderly people reportedly doubles the risk for hip fracture as a result of associated accidents and falls (see "Acute Toxicity" for contributory mechanisms).

4. The risk for physical dependence appears to be significantly increased in people with a history of alcohol abuse.

5. Caution is indicated, because the use of flumazenil may precipitate a benzodiazepine-like withdrawal syndrome in people who are physically dependent on zolpidem.

References

Aragona, M. (2000). Abuse, dependence, and epileptic seizures after zolpidem withdrawal: Review and case report. *Clinical Neuropharmacology, 23*(5), 281-283.

Askew, J.P. (2007). Zolpidem addiction in a pregnant woman with a history of second-trimester bleeding. *Pharmacotherapy, 27*(2), 306-308.

Brodeur, M.R., & Stirling, A.L. (2001). Delirium associated with zolpidem. *The Annals of Pharmacotherapy, 35*(12), 1562-1564.

Correas Lauffer, J., Braquehais Conesa, D., Barbudo Del Cura, E., et al. (2002). Abuse, tolerance and dependence of zolpidem: Three case reports. *Actas Españolas Psiquiatria, 30*(4), 259-262.

Cubala, W.J., & Landowski, J. (2007). Seizure following sudden zolpidem withdrawal. *Progress in Neuro-Psychopharmacology and Biological Psychiatry, 31*(2), 539-540.

Cubala, W.J., Landowski, J., & Wichowicz, H.M. (2008). Zolpidem abuse, dependence and withdrawal syndrome: Sex as susceptibility factor for adverse effects. *British Journal of Clinical Pharmacology, 65*(3), 444-445.

Drover, D., Lemmens, H., Naidu, S., et al. (2000). Pharmacokinetics, pharmacodynamics, and relative pharmacokinetic/pharmacodynamic profiles of zaleplon and zolpidem. *Clinical Therapeutics, 22*(12), 1443-1461.

Greenblatt, D.J., Harmatz, J.S., von Moltke, L.L., et al. (2000). Comparative kinetics and response to the benzodiazepine agonists triazolam and zolpidem: Evaluation of sex-dependent differences. *The Journal of Pharmacology and Experimental Therapeutics, 293*(2), 435-443.

Hajak, G., Müller, W.E., Wittchen, H.U., et al. (2003). Abuse and dependence potential for the non-benzodiazepine hypnotics zolpidem and zopiclone: A review of case reports and epidemiological data. *Addiction, 98*(10), 1371-1378.

Holm, K.J., & Goa, K.L. (2000). Zolpidem: An update of its pharmacology, therapeutic efficacy and tolerability in the treatment of insomnia. *Drugs, 59*(4), 865-889.

Hypnotic dependence: Zolpidem and zopiclone too. (2001). *Prescrire International, 10*(51), 15.

Kao, C.L., Huang, S.C., Yang, Y.J., et al. (2004). A case of parenteral zolpidem dependence with opioid-like withdrawal symptoms. *Journal of Clinical Psychiatry, 65*(9), 1287.

Liappas, I.A., Malitas, P.N., Dimopoulos, N.P., et al. (2003). Zolpidem dependence case series: Possible neurobiological mechanisms and clinical management. *Journal of Psychopharmacology, 17*(1), 131-135.

Logan, B.K., & Couper, F.J. (2001). Zolpidem and driving impairment. *Journal of Forensic Sciences, 46*(1), 105-110.

Madrak, L.N., & Rosenberg, M. (2001). Zolpidem abuse. *The American Journal of Psychiatry, 158*, 1330-1331.

Nakamura, M., Ishii, M., Niwa, Y., et al. (2005). Temporal changes in postural sway caused by ultrashort-acting hypnotics: Triazolam and zolpidem. *Journal for Oto-Rhino-Laryngology, Head and Neck Surgery, 67*(2), 106-112.

Rappa, L.R., Larose-Pierre, M., Payne, D.R., et al. (2004). Detoxification from high-dose zolpidem using diazepam. *The Annals of Pharmacotherapy, 38*(4), 590-594.

Toner, L.C., Tsambiras, B.M., Catalano, G., et al. (2000). Central nervous system side effects associated with zolpidem treatment. *Clinical Neuropharmacology, 23*(1), 54-58.

Troy, S.M., Lucki, I., Unruh, M.A., et al. (2000). Comparison of the effects of zaleplon, zolpidem, and triazolam on memory, learning, and psychomotor performance. *Journal of Clinical Psychopharmacology, 20*(3), 328-337.

Vartzopoulos, D., Bozikas, V., Phocas, C., et al. (2000). Dependence on zolpidem in high dose. *International Clinical Psychopharmacology, 15*(3), 181-182.

Verster, J.C., Volkerts, E.R., Olivier, B., et al. (2007). Zolpidem and traffic safety—The importance of treatment compliance. *Current Drug Safety, 2*(3), 220-226.

Victorri-Vigneau, C., Dailly, E., Veyrac, G., et al. (2007). Evidence of zolpidem abuse and dependence: Results of the French Centre for Evaluation and Information on Pharmacodependence (CEIP) network survey. *British Journal of Clinical Pharmacology, 64*(2), 198-209.

Voderholzer, U., Riemann, D., Hornyak, M., et al. (2001). A double-blind, randomized and placebo-controlled study on the polysomnographic withdrawal effects of zopiclone, zolpidem and triazolam in healthy subjects. *European Archives of Psychiatry and Clinical Neuroscience, 251*(3), 117-123.

Wang, P.S., Bohn, R.L., Glynn, R.J., et al. (2001). Zolpidem use and hip fractures in older people. *Journal of the American Geriatrics Society, 49*(12), 1685-1690.

ZOPICLONE

Names

BAN or INN Generic Synonyms: Racemic (R,S)zopiclone; (±)-zopiclone

Brand/Trade: Amovane®; Imovane®; Rhovane®; Zimovane®

Chemical[1]: 4-Methyl-1-piperazinecarboxylic acid 6-(5-chloro-2-pyridinyl)-6,7-dihydro-7-oxo-5H-pyrrolo[3,4-b]pyrazin-5-yl ester

Street: Vane; Z-Drug; Zimy; Zim Zims; Zoppies

Pharmacologic Classification

Psychodepressant, sedative-hypnotic: miscellaneous (cyclopyrrolone)

Brief General Overview

Zopiclone is a short-acting pyrrolopyrazine-derivative hypnotic. Although its chemical structure is unrelated to the benzodiazepines, it shares a virtually identical spectrum of pharmacologic action. It became commercially available in Europe in 1986 and in the United States in 2005. It is one of the most widely used hypnotics in the world.

Dosage Forms and Routes of Administration

Zopiclone is produced in North America by licit pharmaceutical manufacturers and is available in an oral tablet formulation. The primary users of zopiclone are men and women, including elderly men and women. They generally orally ingest the tablets, often with an alcoholic beverage in order to reportedly increase zopiclone's associated "euphoria." Most of these users obtain zopiclone by prescription. However, a significant number obtain it from illicit sources—"on the street" or over the Internet. Some people who are enrolled in treatment programs for their problematic patterns of drug and substance use use zopiclone during treatment because it is not generally screened for in the urine drug tests that are often required by these programs.

Mechanism of CNS Action

The exact mechanism of zopiclone's psychodepressant action has not been determined. However, it appears to work in concert with the inhibitory neurotransmitter $GABA_A$

in a manner very similar to, if not identical with, that of the benzodiazepines (see Benzodiazepines monograph). It has been demonstrated that zopiclone binds to the $GABA_A$ receptor, resulting in nonspecific activation of all α subtypes in a manner similar to that of the classic benzodiazepines (e.g., diazepam; see monograph).

Pharmacodynamics/Pharmacokinetics

Zopiclone is rapidly and well absorbed following oral ingestion ($F > 0.75$). Peak blood concentrations are reached in <2 hours. However, the ingestion of high-fat meals may delay the onset of peak blood concentrations and psychodepressant actions. Zopiclone is weakly bound to plasma proteins (i.e., ~50%) and has an apparent volume of distribution of ~120 L. It is extensively metabolized in the liver, principally by the hepatic isoenzymes CYP3A4 and CYP2E1, to a number of metabolites, particularly zopiclone-N-oxide (inactive) and N-desmethylzopiclone (active). Only 5% of zopiclone is excreted in unchanged form in the urine. Zopiclone has a mean elimination half-life of ~5 hours (range, 4 to 7 hours).

Current Approved Indications for Medical Use

Sleep disorders: insomnia (short-term, symptomatic management)

Desired Action/Reason for Personal Use

Alcohol-like disinhibitory euphoria or "high"; also, purposely administered to intended victims without their knowledge in the context of drug-facilitated crime (e.g., robbery; sexual assault, including date rape)[2]

Toxicity

Acute: Anxiety; asthenia; bitter, metallic taste; cognitive impairment; confusion; constipation; daytime fatigue; dizziness; drowsiness; dry mouth; dyspepsia; headache; memory impairment (anterograde amnesia); psychomotor impairment

Chronic: Mental depression; physical dependence; psychological dependence

Pregnancy & Lactation: FDA Pregnancy Category C (see Appendix B). Safety of zopiclone use by adolescent girls and women who are pregnant has not been established. Caution is warranted because of its pharmacologic similarity to the benzodiazepines (see Benzodiazepines monograpch). Additional valid and reliable data are needed.

Safety of zopiclone use by adolescent girls and women who are breast-feeding has not been established. However, zopiclone is excreted in significant concentrations in breast milk (i.e., 50% of maternal plasma concentrations). Adolescent girls and women who are breast-feeding should not use zopiclone.

Abuse Potential

Physical dependence: Low (USDEA Schedule IV; low potential for abuse)
Psychological dependence: Low to moderate

Withdrawal Syndrome

A zopiclone withdrawal syndrome similar to the withdrawal syndromes associated with regular, long-term alcohol and benzodiazepine use has been observed upon abrupt discontinuation of regular, long-term zopiclone pharmacotherapy or personal use. This syndrome is characterized by agitation, anxiety, confusion, delirium, hallucinations, headache, irritability, nightmares, palpitations, rebound insomnia, seizures (rare), tachycardia, and tremor. Regular, long-term use of zopiclone should be gradually discontinued in order to avoid the occurrence of this syndrome.

Overdosage

Zopiclone overdosage is generally not life-threatening when the overdosage solely involves zopiclone. Signs and symptoms of overdosage include ataxia, coma, confusion, hypotension, hypoxia, lethargy, respiratory depression, and somnolence. Zopiclone overdosage requires emergency medical support of body systems, with attention to maintaining cardiac and respiratory function. The benzodiazepine antagonist flumazenil (Anexate®; Romazicon®) may be of assistance.[3]

Notes

1. A single-isomer formulation of zopiclone (i.e., Eszopiclone, see monograph) also is available.
2. Zopiclone's relatively short half-life of elimination and its pattern of prescription use for elderly men and women receiving nursing and other personal care services in their own homes, extended care facilities, or other institutional care, contribute to this risk.
3. Caution is indicated, because the use of flumazenil may precipitate a benzodiazepine-like withdrawal syndrome in people who are physically dependent on zopiclone.

References

Bannan, N., Rooney, S., & O'Connor, J. (2007). Zopiclone misuse: An update from Dublin. *Drug and Alcohol Review, 26*(1), 83-85.

Cienki, J.J., Burkhart, K.K., Donovan, J.W. (2005). Zopiclone overdose responsive to flumazenil. *Clinical Toxicology, 43*(5), 385-386.

Cimolai, N. (2007). Zopiclone: Is it a pharmacologic agent for abuse? *Canadian Family Physician, 53*(12), 2124-2129.

Dolder, C., Nelson, M., & McKinsey, J. (2007). Use of non-benzodiazepine hypnotics in the elderly: Are all agents the same? *CNS Drugs, 21*(5), 389-405.

Drug Enforcement Administration, Department of Justice. (2005). Schedules of controlled substances: Placement of Zopiclone into schedule IV. Final rule. *Federal Register, 70*(63), 16935-16937.

Flynn, A., & Cox, D. (2006). Dependence on zopiclone. *Addiction, 101*(6), 898.

Fung, H.T., Lai, C.H., Wong, O.F., et al. (2008). Two cases of methemoglobinemia following zopiclone ingestion. *Clinical Toxicology, 46*(2), 167-170.

Hajak, G., Müller, W.E., Wittchen, H.U., et al. (2003). Abuse and dependence potential for the non-benzodiazepine hypnotics zolpidem and zopiclone: A review of case reports and epidemiological data. *Addiction, 98*(10), 1371-1378.

Kassam, A., Carter, B., & Patten, S.B. (2006). Sedative hypnotic use in Alberta. *The Canadian Journal of Psychiatry, 51*(5), 287-294.

Kintz, P., Villain, M., & Cirimele, V. (2008). Chemical abuse in the elderly: Evidence from hair analysis. *Therapeutic Drug Monitoring, 30*(2), 207-211.

Kuntze, M.F., Bullinger, A.H., & Mueller-Spahn, F. (2002). Excessive use of zopiclone: A case report. *Swiss Medical Weekly, 132*(35-36), 523.

Leonhart, M.M. (2005). Rules—2005. *Federal Register, 70*(29), 7449-7451.

Mahomed, R., Paton, C., & Lee, E. (2002). Prescribing hypnotics in a mental health trust: What consultant psychiatrists say and what they do. *The Pharmaceutical Journal, 268*, 657-659.

Mistri, H.N., Jangid, A.G., Pudage, A., et al. (2008). HPLC-ESI-MS/MS validated method for simultaneous quantification of zopiclone and its metabolites, N-desmethyl zopiclone and zopiclone-N-oxide in human plasma. *Journal of Chromatography B Analytical Technologies in the Biomedical and Life Sciences, 864*(1-2), 137-148.

Sivertsen, B., Omvik, S., Pallesen, S., et al. (2006). Cognitive behavioral therapy vs zopiclone for treatment of chronic primary insomnia in older adults: A randomized controlled trial. *JAMA, The Journal of the American Medical Association, 295*(24), 2851-2858.

Villain, M., Chèze, M., Tracqui, A., et al. (2004). Testing for zopiclone in hair application to drug-facilitated crimes. *Forensic Science International, 145*(2-3), 117-121.

Wong, C.P., Chiu, P.K., & Chu, L.W. (2005). Zopiclone withdrawal: An unusual cause of delirium in the elderly. *Age and Ageing, 34*(5), 526-527.

Appendix A

Classification of the Drugs and Substances of Abuse[1]— The Psychodepressants, Psychostimulants, and Psychodelics[2]

Psychodepressants

Opiate analgesics

Pure agonists, natural
    Codeine
    Morphine
Pure agonists, synthetic or semisynthetic
    Alfentanil
    Fentanyl
    Heroin
    Hydrocodone
    Hydromorphone
    Meperidine
    Methadone
    Oxycodone
    Oxymorphone
    Propoxyphene
Mixed agonists/antagonists, synthetic
    Buprenorphine
    Butorphanol
    Nalbuphine
    Pentazocine
Miscellaneous opiate analgesics
    Dextromethorphan[3]
    Kratom[4]
    Tramadol[5]
    Zipeprol[6]

Sedative-hypnotics

Barbiturates
    Amobarbital
    Butabarbital
    Pentobarbital
    Phenobarbital
    Secobarbital
Benzodiazepines
    Alprazolam
    Bromazepam
    Chlordiazepoxide
    Clonazepam
    Clorazepate
    Diazepam
    Estazolam
    Flunitrazepam
    Flurazepam
    Lorazepam
    Nitrazepam
    Oxazepam
    Temazepam
    Triazolam
Miscellaneous sedative-hypnotics
    Alcohol
    Carisoprodol
    Chloral hydrate
    Dimenhydrinate
    Diphenhydramine
    Eszopiclone
    Ethchlorvynol
    Gamma-hydroxybutyrate
    Kava
    Meprobamate
    Methaqualone
    Paraldehyde
    Zaleplon
    Zolpidem
    Zopiclone

Volatile solvents & inhalants

Volatile solvents
    Acetone
    Butane
    Gasoline
    Glue
Inhalant gases
    Freon
    Nitrous oxide

Psychostimulants

Amphetamines
    Amphetamine
    Dextroamphetamine
    Methamphetamine
    Mixed amphetamines
Miscellaneous psychostimulants
    Armodafinil
    Atomoxetine
    Betel cutch
    Caffeine

Catha edulis
Cocaine
Diethylpropion
Ephedrine
Ibogaine[7]
Kratom[4]
Mazindol
Methcathinone
Methylphenidate
Modafinil
Nicotine
Pemoline
Phendimetrazine
Phentermine

Psychodelics

Amphetamine-like psychodelics— phenethylamines

4-Bromo-2,5-dimethoxyphenethylamine
2,5-Dimethoxy-4-methylamphetamine
Mescaline
3,4-Methylenedioxyamphetamine
3,4-Methylenedioxyethylamphetamine
3,4-Methylenedioxymethamphetamine
N–Methyl-1-(3,4-methylenedioxyphenyl)-
  2-butanamine
4-Methylthioamphetamine
Nutmeg
Paramethoxyamphetamine
3,4,5-Trimethoxyamphetamine

LSD & LSD-like psychodelics

Indoles
  Amanita muscaria
  Harmala alkaloids
  Lysergic acid amide
  Lysergic acid diethylamide
Tryptamines[8,9]
  Alpha-ethyltryptamine[10]
  N,N-Diethyltryptamine
  N,N-Dipropyltryptamine[10]
  5-Hydroxy-N,N-dimethyltryptamine[11]
  5-Methoxy-N,N-dimethyltryptamine[10]
Indoles/Tryptamines
  Alpha-methyltryptamine
  N,N-Dimethyltryptamine
  5-Methoxy-N,N-diisopropyltryptamine
  Psilocin
  Psilocybin

Miscellaneous psychodelics

Cannabis
Ibogaine[7]
Ketamine
Phencyclidine
Piperazine derivatives
Salvia divinorum

Notes

1. Listed by generic name. Also see individual monographs for a comprehensive listing of brand/trade, chemical, and "street" names.
2. The term "psychedelic" (i.e., mind manifesting) was actually first used for this group of drugs and substances of abuse in 1957 by Humphry Osmond (1917–2004). The term has continued to be used by others to differentiate the psychedelics—drugs and substances that induce variable states of self-transcendence and mystical unity—from the hallucinogens— drugs and substances that produce a temporary madness. Various other terms reflect the specific professional stance of the person proposing the term or the identified action of this class of drugs and substances of abuse. These terms include "psychotogens" (inducers of psychosis), "psychotomimetics" (mimickers of psychosis), "schizophrenomimetics" (mimickers of schizophrenia), "mysticomimetics" (mimickers of mystic states), and "psychotomystics" (mimickers of psychosis and mystic states). "Phantasticants" and other terms reflect the vivid sensory experiences associated with the use of many of these drugs and substances of abuse.
   In addition, with the synthesis of 3,4-methylenedioxymethamphetamine (MDMA, Ecstasy) and related drugs and substances of abuse, the terms "empathogens" and "entactogens" ("hug" drugs) have been used to reflect their actions in regard to promoting "feelings of closeness and love" or their ability to increase "feelings of belonging." A probably more precise, but less commonly used, term is "illusinogens," which reflects the visual phenomena (i.e., illusions or misperceptions) often associated with use of the psychodelics. In keeping with the terms used for the other two major groups of drugs and substances of abuse (psychodepressants and psychostimulants), the term psychodelics is used throughout this text, as was done in the first edition.

3. Dextromethorphan is an opiate derived, synthetic antitussive.

4. At higher dosages, *kratom* works as a psychodepressant, primarily at the endorphin mu and kappa opiate analgesic receptors. At lower dosages, it acts as a psychostimulant (see monograph).

5. Tramadol is an opiate analgesic congener.

6. Zipeprol, an antitussive, shares many properties with dextromethorphan (see monograph).

7. At lower dosages, ibogaine works as a psychostimulant, primarily affecting the NMDA receptors. At higher dosages, it acts as a psychodelic, primarily involving the serotonin receptors.

8. Virtually all of the tryptamines are classified as "LSD-like" psychodelics because of their observed psychotropic actions. However, they also are classified as "tryptamines" in this taxonomy because each has the amino acid tryptamine as its core chemical structure.

9. Psilocybin (i.e., O-phosphoryl-4-hydroxy-N,N-ethyltryptamine) and psilocin (i.e., 4-hydroxy-N,N-dimethyltryptamine) also can be added to this taxonomy.

10. Not currently widely used. Available data are extremely limited. Therefore, individual monographs are not included in this text.

11. Also known as bufotenine. There is some question as to its psychodelic action, but the lack of psychodelic activity in human subjects may be simply due to its poor ability to cross the blood–brain barrier.

Appendix B

FDA Pregnancy Categories

A: Controlled Studies Show No Risk. Adequate, well-controlled studies in pregnant women have failed to demonstrate a risk to the fetus in any trimester of pregnancy.

B: No Evidence of Risk in Humans. Adequate, well-controlled studies in pregnant women have not shown increased risk of fetal abnormalities despite adverse findings in animals, or, in the absence of adequate human studies, animal studies show no fetal risk. The chance of human fetal harm is remote but remains a possibility.

C: Risk Cannot Be Ruled Out. Adequate, well-controlled human studies are lacking, and animal studies have shown a risk to the fetus or are lacking as well. There is a chance of human fetal harm if the drug is administered during pregnancy, but the potential benefits may outweigh the potential risk.

D: Positive Evidence of Risk. Studies in humans, or investigational or postmarketing reports, have demonstrated fetal risk. Nevertheless, potential benefits from use of the drug may outweigh the potential risk. For example, the drug may be acceptable if needed in a life-threatening situation or with serious disease for which safer drugs cannot be used or are ineffective.

X: Contraindicated in Pregnancy. Studies in animals or humans, or investigational or postmarketing reports, have demonstrated positive evidence of fetal abnormalities or risk that clearly outweighs any possible benefit to the patient. Use is unacceptable.

Appendix C

Abbreviations

A

A1, A2A	adenosine receptors, types 1 and 2A
ADHD	attention-deficit/hyperactivity disorder
AET	alpha-ethyltryptamine
AIDS	acquired immunodeficiency syndrome
AMF	alphamethylfentanyl
AMT	alpha-methyltryptamine

B

| BAN | British Approved Name |
| BZD-1, BZD-2 | benzodiazepine receptors, types 1 and 2 |

C

2 C-B	4-bromo-2,5-dimethoxyphenethylamine
CB_1, CB_2	cannabinoid receptors, types 1 and 2
CNS	central nervous system
COPD	chronic obstructive pulmonary disease
CTZ	chemoreceptor trigger zone
CYP	cytochrome P450 microsomal enzyme system

D

DAT	dopamine transporter
D1, D2	dopamine receptors, types 1 and 2
DM	dextromethorphan
DMT	N,N-dimethyltryptamine
DOM	2,5-dimethoxy-4-methylamphetamine
DSM-IV-TR	*Diagnostic and Statistical Manual of Mental Disorders, Fourth Edition, Text Revision*
DTs	delirium tremens

E

ECG	electrocardiogram
EEG	electroencephalogram
ER	extended-release

F

F	fraction of drug absorbed (total systemic bioavailability)
FAS	fetal alcohol syndrome
FDA	U.S. Food and Drug Administration

G

GABA   gamma-aminobutyric acid
GC-MS   gas chromatography with mass spectometry
GHB   gamma-hydroxybutyrate
GI   gastrointestinal
gram%   gram percent (grams per 100 mL)

H

H1, H2   histamine receptors, types 1 and 2
HIV   human immunodeficiency virus
hr   hour(s)
5-HT   5-hydroxytryptamine (serotonin)
5-HT1A,   Serotonin receptors, types 1A, 1C, 2, 2A, and 2C
  5-HT1C, 5HT2,
  5-HT2A, 5HT2C

I

INN   International Nonproprietary Name
IQ   intelligence quotient
IR   immediate-release

K

kg   kilogram(s)
km   Michaelis-Menten constant

L

L   liter(s)
LD_{50} The dose that, if administered, would result in the death of 50% of a specific
                  population of subjects (i.e., the median lethal dose)
LSA   lysergic acid amide
LSD   lysergic acid diethylamide

M

MAO-B   monoamine oxidase B
MBDB   N-methyl-1-(3,4-methylenedioxyphenyl)-2-butanamine
mcg   microgram(s)
MDA   3,4-methylenedioxyamphetamine
MDE   3,4-methylenedioxyethamphetamine
MDEA   3,4-methylenedioxyethylamphetamine
MDMA   3,4-methylenedioxymethamphetamine
5-MeO-DIPT   5-methoxy-N,N-diisopropyltryptamine
mg   milligram(s)
mL   milliliter(s)
4-MTA   4-methylthioamphetamine

N

nACh	nicotinic acetylcholine
nAChR	nicotinic acetylcholine receptor
NMDA	N-methyl-D-aspartate
NPF	nonpharmaceutical fentanyl

O

11-OH-THC	11-hydroxy-delta-9-tetrahydrocannabinol

P

PCP	phencyclidine
pH	potential of hydrogen (hydrogen ion concentration)
PMA	paramethoxyamphetamine
ppm	parts per million

R

REM	rapid eye movement

S

SERT	serotonin transporter
SIDS	sudden infant death syndrome

T

THC	tetrahydrocannabinol (delta-9-tetrahydrocannabinol)
THCCOOH	11-nor-9-carboxy-delta-9-tetrahydrocannabinol
TMA	3,4,5-trimethoxyamphetamine
T_{max}	time to reach maximal blood concentration

U

USDEA	U.S. Drug Enforcement Administration
U.S.	United States

W

WW II	World War II

Subject Index

This index contains the major subject entries for all drugs and substances of abuse presented in this text. Monograph titles are listed in boldface according to their USAN generic names. Notes are designated by (n), figures by (f), and tables by (t).

A

Absorption
    See individual monographs (pharmacodynamics/ pharmacokinetics)
Abuse
    See prescription drug abuse
    See also individual monographs (abuse potential)
Acetone, 1–3
    abuse potential, 2
    medical use, 2, 3(n3)
    memory impairment, 2
    methods of use, 1, 3(n2)
    pharmacologic classification, 1
    reasons for personal use, 2
    toxicity, 2, 3(n4)
    users, 1
Addiction, xvi–xvii(n6)
    See individual monographs (abuse potential)
Adolescents
    alcohol, 4, 9(n7)
    alprazolam, 16
    betel cutch, 44
    bidis, 263–264(n3)
    4-bromo-2,5-dimethoxy- phenethylamine, 50
    butane, 55
    butorphanol, 58
    caffeine, 62, 65(n 12)
    cannabis, 69
    cigarillos, 259, 264(n9)
    dextromethorphan, 109
    dimenhydrinate, 121
    diphenhydramine, 121

ephedrine, 125
flunitrazepam, 139, 140, 141(n5)
freon, 145, 147(n5)
gamma-hydroxybutyrate, 148
gasoline, 153
glue, 156
lysergic acid diethylamide, 192
mescaline, 204
methamphetamine, 212
methylphenidate, 237
mixed amphetamines, 243–244
nicotine, 258–259
nitrous oxide, 269, 271(n2)
oxycodone, 286
pemoline, 297–298
piperazine derivatives, 317
propoxyphene, 319
psilocybin, 325
Salvia divinorum, 328
tobacco, 258–259
volatile solvents & inhalants, 346
zipeprol, 354
Adulteration, xv
    barbiturates, 37–38(n3)
    cocaine, 97(n2), 98(n11)
    glue, 157(n1)
    heroin, 165(n2), 166(n5)
    3,4-methylenedioxy- methamphetamine, 229, 317
    mushrooms, 20(n5), 324(n1), 326(n1)
    opiate analgesics, 278
    paramethoxyamphetamine, 295
    phencyclidine, 309(n3)
    psilocin, 324(n1)
    psilocybin, 326(n1)
    volatile solvents & inhalants, 351(n3)
    See also combination drug and substance use
Adverse effects
    See toxicity
Aerosols
    See propellant gases
AET
    See alpha-ethyltryptamine
Afghanistan
    hashish, 72
    opium, 275–276, 282(n4)
Africa

cannabis, 70(t), 72
Catha edulis, 82(n1, 9)
cola nuts, 65(n1)
hashish, 72
ibogaine, 174, 176(n3, 4)
methaqualone, 217
paraldehyde, 292
African Americans
    See North Americans of African descent
Aggressive behavior
    See violent behavior
Agranulocytosis
    definition, 98(n11)
Alcohol, 3–11
    abuse potential, 6
    adverse effects, 5, 8–9(t)
    binge drinking, 4
    blood alcohol concentration, 5
    breast cancer, 5, 8(t), 9(n8)
    breast-feeding, 6
    cardiotoxicity, 8, 10(n9)
    chemical name, 3
    Chinese cooking wine, 4
    "Cisco," 76(n12)
    classification, 3
    cocaine and, 98(n9)
    combination use, 4, 39, 85(n1), 98(n9), 104(n1), 110(n1), 112, 113(n1), 123(n3), 139, 150, 150(n4), 165, 172, 186(n6), 220, 226, 231, 298
    congenital effects, 6, 10(n16)
    crime and, 5
    date rape, 5, 9(n6)
    deaths, 7, 9
    delirium tremens, 7
    dosage forms, 4
    driving impairment, 4, 5, 9(n7)
    energy drinks and, 4
    fetal alcohol spectrum disorder, 6
    fetal alcohol syndrome, 6, 7(f)
    generic synonyms, 3
    hepatic metabolism, 5
    liver impairment, 6
    Lysol® Spray, 4
    mechanism of action, 4
    medical use, 5, 9(n4)
    memory impairment, 5, 8(t)
    mental depression, 6, 8(t)

Drug Name Index

All drugs and substances of abuse discussed in this text are listed here by generic name (USAN; indicated in boldface), brand/trade names (designated by ®), BAN or INN generic synonyms, and current available street names. Generally, only the first or primary page number is provided for each drug name entry. Multiple page numbers for a street name entry usually indicate that it has been used to denote more than one drug or substance of abuse. Monograph notes are identified by (n) and monograph tables by (t).

"13," 67
"151," 93
"2000," 161
"2s", 49
222®, 101
"24-7," 93
"25," 191
"256," 93
"30s", 67
"3750s", 76(n12)
"40", 286
"40s", 330
"420," 67
"542s", 139
642®, 319
"714s", 217
"747," 161
"80," 286

A

A, 21, 191
A1, 93
A2, 317
A2CBs/A2C-Bs, 49
Abbots, 33, 303
A-Bomb, 161
Abu-Sufian, 67

Abyssinia Salad, 79
Abyssinian Tea, 79
Acapulco Gold, 67
Acapulco Red, 67
Accelerant, 21, 211
AC/DC, 101
Ace, 21, 67
Acelerante, 211
Acetone, 1
Acid, 191
Acid-25, 191
Actiq®, 135
Adam, 224, 228
Adderall®/AdderallXR®,107(n1),243
Addies, 243
Adipex-P®, 314
Adolph, 207
AET, 14
Affe, 21
Affies, 21
Afgani Indica, 67
Afi, 67
African, 67
African Black, 67
African Bush, 67
African Salad, 79
Aftershave, 4
Aimies, 21
AIP, 161
Air Ketum, 184
Airplane, 67
Ajmalicine, 186(n9)
AK-47, 67
Albert Hoffman, 195(n4)
Al Capone, 161
Alcohol, 3
Ale, 3
Alepam®, 283
Alertec®, 248
Alfalfa, 258
Alfenta®, 11
Alfentanil, 11
Al Green, 67
Alice, 191
Alice in Wonderland, 195(n4)
All American Drug, 93
Allerdryl®, 121
Allernix®, 121
Alphabet, 191
Alpha-ethyltryptamine, 14
Alphamethylfentanyl, 13(n1)
Alphamethylphenethylamine, 27(n1), 105
Alpha-methyltryptamine, 14
Alprazolam, 16

Alprazolam Intensol®, 16
Alquitran, 161
Al Sharpton, 67
Alti-Triazolam®, 340
Amanita muscaria, 18
Amaska, 44
Amber Brew, 3
Ambien®, 356
Ambien CR®, 356
Amelia, 161
AMF, 13(n1)
Amf, 21
Amfepramone, 114
Amfetamines, 21
Amidone, 207
3-(2-Aminopropyl) indole, 14
Amobarbital, 21
Amoeba, 306
Amovane®, 360
AMP, 21
Amp/Amps, 21, 211
Amphetamine, 21
Amphetamines, 21
Amphets, 21
Amsterdam, 67
AMT, 14
Amy, 21
Anandamide, 72
Anadenanthera peregrina, 160(n2)
Anastasia, 228
Anchorage, 306
Anexate®, 42
Angel, 93, 306
Angel Death, 306
Angel Dust, 306
Angel Hair, 306
Angel Mist, 306
Angel Poke, 306
Angel's Food, 3
Angie, 93
Angola, 67
Animal, 191
Animal Trank/Tranq/Tranquilizer, 306
Anorex-SR®, 310
Antifreeze, 161
Apache, 135
Aperitif, 3
A-Plus, 21
Apo-Alpraz®, 16
Apo-Triazo®, 340
Aquachloral®, 83
Aquachloral Supprettes®, 83
Arathi, 67
Arathi Highlands, 67

403

G

G, 147, 211
Gage, 67
Gagers/Gaggers, 219
Gak, 211
Galloping Horse, 161
Gallup, 161
Gamma 10, 147
Gamma-butyrolactone, 148, 151(n12)
Gamma-hydroxybutyrate, 147
Gamma Hydroxybutyric Acid, 147
Gamma-OH, 147
Gamot, 161
Ganesh, 195(n4)
Gange, 67
Ganja, 67
Gary Abletts, 228
Garys, 228
Gas (amphetamines), 21
Gas (butane), 55
Gas (freon), 145
Gas (gasoline), 153
Gas (methcathinone), 219
Gas (nitrous oxide), 269
Gash, 67
Gasoline, 153
Gato, 161
Gauge, 67
Gauge Butt, 67
GBH, 147
GBL, 151(n12)
GBs, 21
Gea, 177
Geek, 211
Geep, 211
Gen-Triazolam®, 340
George, 161
George Smack, 161
Georgia Home Boy, 147
German Boy, 207
Ggob, 219
Ghana, 67
GHB, 147
GH Buddy, 147
Ghost, 161, 192
Gi, 177
Gift of the Sun, 93
Gift-of-the-Sun-God, 93
Giggle Smoke, 67
Giggle Weed, 67
Girl, 93, 161
Girlfriend, 93
Glacines, 161
Glade® Air Freshener, 56
Glad Stuff, 93, 251
Glass, 211
Glories, 192
Glue, 155
Gluey, 155
Go, 21, 211
Goblet of Jam, 67
God's Drug, 251
God's Flesh, 322, 324
Go-ee, 21
Goey, 219
Go Fast, 211, 219

Gold, 67
Gold Bars, 16
Gold Dust, 93
Gold Star, 67
Golden, 67
Golden Eagle, 241
Golden Girl, 161
Golden Leaf, 67
Golf Balls, 312
Golpe, 161
G.O.M., 251
Goma, 161
Gone Time, 38, 86
Gong/Gonj, 67
Gonzolez, 211
Goob, 219
Good and Plenty, 161
Good Butt, 67
Goodfella, 135
Good Giggles, 67
Good Goods, 67
Good H, 161
Good Horse, 161
Good Ole M, 251
Goody-Goody, 67
Goofballs, 33, 312
Goof Butt, 67
Goofers, 38, 86, 312
Goofy's, 192
Googs, 228
Gook, 147
Goon, 306
Goon Dust, 306
Goop, 147
Goose Egg, 211
Go pills, 211
Gorilla Biscuits, 217, 306
Gorilla Pills, 33, 306
Gorilla Tab, 306
Graba, 79, 80
Grandpa's Cough Syrup, 3
Grant, 258
Granulated Orange, 211
Grapefruit Hydro, 67
Grape Parfait, 192
Grass, 67
Grass Brownies, 67
Grasshopper, 67
Grata, 67
Gra-Tom, 184
Grave Bodily Harm, 147
Gravel, 93
Gravol®, 121
Great Bear, 135
Great Hormones at Bedtime, 147
Green, 67, 180
Green and Yellows, 310
Green Bars, 16
Green Buds, 67
Green Devils, 333
Green Double Domes, 192
Green Eggs, 333
Green Frogs, 83
Green Goddess, 67
Greenies, 21, 105, 228
Green Leaves, 306

Green Single Dome, 192
Green Tea, 306
Green Wedge, 192
Green Whiskey, 204
Greeter, 67
Gremmies, 67
Greta, 67
Grey Shields, 192
Griefo, 67
Griefs, 67
Grievous Bodily Harm, 147
Grifa, 67
Griff/Griffa/Griffo, 67
G-Riffic/G-Riffick, 147
Grim Creeper, 67
Grits, 93
Grog, 3, 177
Grolid, 67
Guarana, 65(n4)
Gum, 228
Gumption, 211
Gunga/Gunge/*Gunja*, 67
Gungeon/Gungun, 67
Gutkha, 44
GWM, 228
Gyve, 67

H

H, 161
H & C, 98(n6)
H Caps, 161
Habitrol®, 258
Hache, 161
Hagigat®, 80
Hail, 93
Haircut, 67
Hair Spray, 346
Hairy, 161
Hairy Ogre, 67
Halcion®, 340
Halcyon, 340
Halcyon Daze, 340
Half Moon, 204
Half Track, 306
Hamburger, 93
Handlebars, 16
Hang Liu, 67
Hanhich, 67
Hanyak, 211
Happy Cigarette, 67-68
Happy Drug, 228
Happy Dust, 93
Happy Pill, 228
Happy Powder, 93
Happy Smoke, 68
Happy Sticks, 76(n12), 306
Happy Trails, 93
Hardball, 93, 333
Hard Candy, 161
Hardcore, 251
Hard Crystal, 211
Hard Stuff, 3
Harmala alkaloids, 158
Harmaline, 158
Harmine, 158